# Healthcare Goes Digital: Mobile Health and Electronic Health Technology in the 21st Century

# Healthcare Goes Digital: Mobile Health and Electronic Health Technology in the 21st Century

Guest Editor

**Daniele Giansanti**

MDPI

Basel • Beijing • Wuhan • Barcelona • Belgrade • Novi Sad • Cluj • Manchester

*Guest Editor*
Daniele Giansanti
Centre Tisp
Istituto Superiore di Sanità
Rome
Italy

*Editorial Office*
MDPI AG
Grosspeteranlage 5
4052 Basel, Switzerland

This is a reprint of the Special Issue, published open access by the journal *Healthcare* (ISSN 2227-9032), freely accessible at: https://www.mdpi.com/journal/healthcare/special_issues/0P14J89UOQ.

For citation purposes, cite each article independently as indicated on the article page online and as indicated below:

| |
|---|
| Lastname, A.A.; Lastname, B.B. Article Title. *Journal Name* **Year**, *Volume Number*, Page Range. |

**ISBN 978-3-7258-5079-2 (Hbk)**
**ISBN 978-3-7258-5080-8 (PDF)**
**https://doi.org/10.3390/books978-3-7258-5080-8**

# Contents

# About the Editor

**Daniele Giansanti**

Giansanti Daniele is a Research Director at the Istituto Superiore di Sanità.

More importantly, he also conducts varied research at ISS (the Italian NIH) (2000–today) in the following fields:

Biomedical engineering and medical physics with the development of wearable and portable devices (three national patents).

Telemedicine and e-Health, with technology assessment and the integration of new systems in the field of telerehabilitation, domiciliary monitoring, digital pathology, and digital radiology.

mHealth, with recent interest in the field of integrating smartphones and tablet technology in healthcare with particular attention to opportunities, risks, abuse, and regulation.

Acceptance of and consensus in the use of robots for assistance and rehabilitation.

Challenges and acceptance of the use of Artificial Intelligence in Digital Radiology and Digital Pathology.

Cybersecurity in the health domain.

He received an MD in Electronic Engineering at Sapienza University, Rome, 1991; a PhD in Telecommunications and Microelectronics Engineering at Tor Vergata University, Rome, 1997; and an Academic Specialization in Cognitive Psychology and Neural Networks at Sapienza University, Rome, 1997.

He obtained a specialization in Medical Physics at Sapienza University, Rome, 2005. Dr. Giansanti was in charge of the Design of VLSI ASICs for DSP in the Civil Field (1991–1997) during his MD and PhD, and he served as a CAE-CAD-CAM system manager and Design Engineer in projects of electronic systems (Boards and VLSI) for the Warfare sector at Elettronica spa (1992–2000), one of the leaders in the military field.

Dr. Giansanti is a Professor at Sapienza and Catholic University in Rome and a tutor of theses. He is a Board Editor and reviewer for several journals. He has 203 publications indexed on Scopus and more than 200 other contributions, including monographs, book chapters, and conference papers.

# Preface

The field of digital healthcare is undergoing a profound transformation, driven by the rapid integration of artificial intelligence (AI), mobile health applications, telemedicine, and wearable technologies into clinical practice. These innovations are demonstrating great potential to enhance patient care, improve workflow efficiency, and support personalized medicine. Digital tools, including AI-driven analytics, chatbots, virtual assistants, and telehealth platforms, are shifting healthcare from traditional approaches toward data-driven, patient-centered, and accessible systems. At the same time, these advancements raise important considerations regarding privacy, security, interoperability, and ethical use of health data. Addressing these challenges is essential to ensure that technological progress aligns with the principles of safe, equitable, and effective healthcare delivery.

This Special Issue provides a scientific forum for international scholars to share insights on digital health innovations. It includes 13 contributions plus the concluding editorial, encompassing original research and review articles that collectively highlight the transformative impact of these technologies across multiple healthcare domains. Research articles explore mobile health, electronic health, virtual reality interventions, AI-assisted patient care, home-based radiology, and other solutions, demonstrating improvements in clinical outcomes, patient engagement, and decision-making. Complementary review articles cover telerehabilitation, voice assistants, chatbots, digital psychotherapy, wearable monitoring, and other digital health solutions offering broader perspectives on current trends, challenges, and future directions in digital health.

I would like to sincerely thank all the authors, reviewers, and contributors whose outstanding work made the reprint of this Special Issue possible. I also extend my gratitude to the editorial team for their dedication and support, and to Managing Editor Vicky Luo for her exceptional dedication, support, and continued guidance. Their combined efforts have been essential in bringing this Special Issue to fruition.

**Daniele Giansanti**
*Guest Editor*

healthcare MDPI

*Editorial*

# The Future of Healthcare Is Digital: Unlocking the Potential of Mobile Health and E-Health Solutions

**Daniele Giansanti**

Centro Tisp, Istituto Superiore di Sanità, 00161 Roma, Italy; daniele.giansanti@iss.it; Tel.: +39-06-49902701

In the era of rapid technological advancement, healthcare is undergoing a profound transformation driven by digital solutions. The integration of artificial intelligence (AI) and conversational agents, such as ChatGPT, is reshaping the way healthcare is delivered, offering innovative opportunities to enhance patient care, streamline workflows, and improve overall efficiency.

The Special Issue "Healthcare Goes Digital: Mobile Health and Electronic Health Technology in the 21st Century" [1] aimed to explore emerging themes, examining their innovative applications, challenges, and prospects. A crucial focus is on both telemedicine [2] and mobile health applications and their impact on healthcare delivery, patient monitoring, and disease management [3]. Another area of interest is wearable health technology [4] and its role in continuously monitoring health metrics, offering new possibilities for personalized medicine. The evolution and effectiveness of telemedicine, particularly with AI-driven diagnostic tools [5] and virtual consultations [6], also form a central part of the discussion today. Furthermore, the integration of AI-driven analytics in electronic health records (EHRs) [7] is crucial for clinical decision-making and interoperability.

Security and privacy concerns in digital healthcare [8], especially regarding AI-driven applications nowadays, are key considerations that must be faced to ensure the responsible deployment of these technologies. Patient engagement through digital platforms, including AI-driven chat interfaces and virtual health assistants, is another significant topic in rapid evolution [9]. Finally, the influence of AI, the Internet of Things (IoT) [10], and other emerging technologies in healthcare is a field in need of special attention, both for its potential and implications.

As digital healthcare continues to evolve, it is crucial to critically assess the potential benefits and challenges of the integration of all this emerging technology.

Thanks to the contribution of numerous international scholars, this Special Issue has collected, in addition to this editorial, 13 studies, including 7 scientific articles [11–17] and 6 reviews [18–23], 5 of which are systematic reviews [19–23].

*Contributions of the Article studies*

Table 1 provides a brief summary of the foci and contributions of the articles published in this Special Issue.

Some studies have explored the intersection of healthcare technology, patient care, and innovative solutions aimed at enhancing both accessibility and outcomes. One notable study by Alzghaibi [11], investigates barriers to the adoption of the Sehaty mobile health application, particularly for patients suffering from chronic diseases. It reveals challenges in technical performance, user interface design, and privacy concerns. This research provides valuable insights for improving mobile health platforms by enhancing stability, user experience, and security to ensure higher user satisfaction and engagement.


https://doi.org/10.3390/healthcare13070802

**Table 1.** Sketch of the articles published in the Special Issue.

| Study/Minititle | Focus | Brief Summary | Contribution |
| --- | --- | --- | --- |
| [11] Sehaty App Usability in Saudi Arabia | Mobile health (mHealth) app adoption and usability | This study investigates the barriers hindering the adoption of the Sehaty app among chronic disease patients in Saudi Arabia. It identifies issues like technical performance, navigation difficulties, privacy concerns, and accessibility challenges. | Provides actionable insights for improving the technical stability, user interface design, and security features of mHealth platforms to enhance user engagement and satisfaction. |
| [12] Cross-Regional Healthcare Choices | Online healthcare services and patient decision-making | The study examines how online medical platform signals (hospital ratings, patient reviews) influence patients' decisions to seek cross-regional treatment. It explores how these signals impact healthcare choices in underserved regions. | Offers insights for improving online healthcare platforms by optimizing hospital ratings and review systems, promoting healthcare equity, and supporting informed decision-making. |
| [13] Community-Acquired Pressure Injuries (CAPIs) in Elderly | Data-driven detection and prevention of pressure injuries | The study analyzes the electronic medical records of elderly patients to identify key factors associated with community-acquired pressure injuries (CAPIs). | Highlights novel indicators that can help detect and prevent CAPIs in community care settings, providing valuable data for clinical practice and improving patient safety. |
| [14] Virtual Reality in Office Hysteroscopy | Use of VR for pain and stress management | This study evaluates the effectiveness of virtual reality (VR) in reducing pain and stress during office hysteroscopy procedures. | Demonstrates that VR can significantly reduce pain during medical procedures, especially in patients with lower baseline stress, contributing to less invasive, patient-centered care. |
| [15] Virtual Music Therapy for College Students | Mental health intervention using virtual music therapy | This study explores the effectiveness of a virtual music therapy program based on positive psychology to enhance mental health among college students during the COVID-19 pandemic. | Shows that positive psychology-based virtual music therapy can significantly reduce stress, anxiety, and depression in college students, especially during stressful times. |
| [16] Large Language Models in Postoperative Care | AI in patient care: Postoperative recommendations | The study compares the performance of LLMs (ChatGPT-3.5, GPT-4, Gemini) in providing postoperative care advice to plastic surgery patients. | Highlights the potential of LLMs in providing accurate, readable, and understandable postoperative care information, emphasizing their role as adjunct tools in patient care. |

**Table 1.** *Cont.*

| Study/Minititle | Focus | Brief Summary | Contribution |
|---|---|---|---|
| [17] Home Radiology Integration | Shifting landscape of diagnostic imaging with home radiology | The study examines the integration of home radiology into healthcare, especially post COVID-19. It explores the experiences and challenges of medical radiology technicians with domiciliary imaging. | Offers insights into the challenges and potential of home radiology, urging further research and collaboration to enhance patient-centric care |

Lu et al. [12], delve into how online healthcare platforms influence patient decision-making. Specifically, their study looks at how hospital ratings and patient reviews shape the choices of patients seeking care across regions. The findings emphasize the need to optimize these systems to promote healthcare equity, thereby improving informed decision-making for underserved populations.

Shafran-Tikva et al. [13] propose a study taking a data-driven approach to preventing pressure injuries in elderly patients by analyzing electronic medical records. It identifies key factors that can help detect and prevent community-acquired pressure injuries, offering practical data that can improve clinical practices and patient safety.

In the field of patient-centered care, the work proposed by Estadella et al. [14] investigates the role of virtual reality (VR) in reducing pain and stress during medical procedures like office hysteroscopy. The study demonstrates that VR can significantly enhance patient comfort and reduce the need for invasive interventions, highlighting the potential of VR to revolutionize procedural care.

For mental health, Han et al. [15] explore the effects of virtual music therapy, based on positive psychology, on the mental health of college students during the COVID-19 pandemic. The findings underscore the effectiveness of such interventions in reducing stress, anxiety, and depression, especially during challenging times.

Artificial Intelligence (AI) also plays a crucial role in patient care, as highlighted by Gomez-Cabello et al. [16]. Their study evaluates the potential of AI models like ChatGPT-3.5 and GPT-4 in providing postoperative care advice to plastic surgery patients. It emphasizes the potential of large language models to deliver accurate and accessible care information, presenting them as valuable adjuncts in patient education.

Lastly, Lepri et al. [17] examine the shift toward home-based radiology services, particularly after the COVID-19 pandemic. The study uncovers the challenges and opportunities faced by medical radiology technicians, highlighting the need for further research and collaboration to integrate AI and improve patient care in a home setting.

Together, these studies shed light on the growing role of technology in enhancing patient care, from mobile health apps and AI integration to innovative pain management and virtual therapy solutions. The insights gained provide a foundation for the continued evolution of healthcare services, ensuring that they remain accessible, patient-centered, and efficient.

*Contribution of the review studies*

Table 2 focuses on the published review studies with a sketch. An overview of the reviews published in this Special Issue highlights the diverse ways in which digital interventions are transforming healthcare across various domains.

One of the most significant advancements is in telerehabilitation for chronic neck pain as highlighted by Valenza-Peña et al. [18]. Their review confirmed the efficacy of virtual consultations and remote exercise programs in reducing pain and improving functional outcomes for patients suffering from chronic neck pain. This demonstrates the growing potential of telerehabilitation to provide effective pain management and rehabilitation, particularly in remote or underserved areas.

**Table 2.** Sketch of the review studies published in the Special Issue.

| Study/Minititle (Type of Review) | Focus | Brief Summary | Contribution |
|---|---|---|---|
| [18] Telerehabilitation for Chronic Neck Pain (REVIEW) | Telerehabilitation interventions in managing chronic neck pain, particularly focusing on pain reduction and improving functional outcomes. | This systematic review and meta-analysis explore the effectiveness of telerehabilitation as a method for managing chronic neck pain, particularly through virtual consultations and remote exercise programs. It evaluates studies that address pain and disability reduction in patients. | The review confirms the efficacy of telerehabilitation in reducing pain and improving disability outcomes in patients with chronic neck pain. Remote interventions such as exercise programs and virtual consultations are highlighted as key contributors to positive outcomes. |
| [19] Voice Assistants in Non-Communicable Diseases (SYSTEMATIC REVIEW) | Investigating the role of voice assistants (VAs) in supporting the management of non-communicable diseases (NCDs) such as diabetes, cardiovascular diseases, and mental health conditions. | This systematic review analyzes studies on the use of voice assistants in managing NCDs. It looks at various aspects such as usability, acceptability, adherence, behavioral outcomes, and overall impact on clinical and quality-of-life outcomes for patients with chronic conditions. | The review emphasizes the potential of voice assistants to enhance patient engagement, improve self-management, and facilitate behavioral changes. However, it identifies challenges such as privacy concerns, speech recognition errors, and barriers to adoption that need to be addressed. |
| [20] Chatbots for Women and Expectant Parents (SYSTEMATIC REVIEW) | The use of interactive conversational agents (chatbots) in supporting women and expectant parents during the preconception, pregnancy, and postnatal periods. | This systematic review synthesizes studies on the application of chatbots in healthcare for women and their families, covering the entire reproductive cycle from preconception to 12 months postpartum. It focuses on chatbots' impacts on health behaviors, knowledge, and service utilization. | The review demonstrates the positive impact of chatbots in improving health knowledge, behaviors, and attitudes, as well as facilitating better access to health information and interactions with healthcare providers during the perinatal period. |
| [21] Digital Psychotherapy for Suicide and Depression (SYSTEMATIC REVIEW) | The effectiveness of digital psychotherapy, particularly Cognitive Behavioral Therapy (CBT), in addressing suicide ideation and depression. | This study investigates the effects of digital psychotherapy on suicide ideation and depression, analyzing randomized controlled trials that compare digital interventions to traditional therapy. It provides a quantitative analysis of the impact on suicide and depression outcomes. | The findings suggest that digital psychotherapy has a significant positive effect on reducing suicide ideation and depression compared to traditional face-to-face therapy, making it a promising alternative for mental healthcare. |

**Table 2.** *Cont.*

| Study/Minititle (Type of Review) | Focus | Brief Summary | Contribution |
|---|---|---|---|
| [22] Smartwatches for Arrhythmia Detection (SYSTEMATIC REVIEW) | The role of smartwatches in detecting and monitoring cardiac arrhythmias, especially atrial fibrillation, and their potential integration into clinical care. | This systematic review gathers evidence on the use of smartwatches for arrhythmia detection, focusing on their ability to monitor heart conditions like atrial fibrillation. It examines various case studies and cohort studies on smartwatch-based arrhythmia detection. | The review highlights the potential of smartwatches as a tool for the early detection and continuous monitoring of arrhythmias, offering the possibility for timely interventions and more effective patient care, particularly for those at risk of heart-related complications. |
| [23] Digital Technologies for Weight Loss (SYSTEMATIC REVIEW) | Evaluating the effectiveness of digital interventions (such as mobile apps, wearables, and online programs) in promoting weight loss and improving lifestyle behaviors related to obesity. | This systematic review investigates digital interventions aimed at promoting weight loss in individuals with overweight or obesity. It includes studies that employ mobile technologies to increase physical activity and improve dietary habits, focusing on their impact on weight management. | The review concludes that digital technologies, particularly those offering personalized feedback, are effective in promoting weight loss and encouraging healthy behaviors in individuals with overweight or obesity, enhancing the overall effectiveness of lifestyle interventions. |

Another key area of digital health innovation is the use of voice assistants (VAs) in managing non-communicable diseases (NCDs) as reported by Bramanti et al. [19]. The systematic review examining the role of VAs in managing illnesses like diabetes, cardiovascular diseases, and mental health conditions found that these technologies enhance patient engagement, improve self-management, and encourage behavioral changes. However, challenges such as privacy concerns and adoption barriers remain, which must be addressed to maximize their potential in healthcare settings.

In maternal and perinatal care, chatbots for women and expectant parents based on Amil et al. [20] have proven to be an invaluable resource. A systematic review of studies on the use of chatbots in supporting women throughout the reproductive cycle showed that these interactive tools significantly improved health knowledge, behaviors, and attitudes. They also facilitated better access to healthcare information and services, offering an effective way to engage expectant parents and women during preconception, pregnancy, and postpartum periods.

The use of digital psychotherapy in addressing suicide ideation and depression has also gained considerable attention as reported in Oh et al. [21]. This systematic review found that digital interventions, particularly Cognitive Behavioral Therapy (CBT), significantly reduced both suicide ideation and depression, providing a promising alternative to traditional face-to-face therapy. This approach offers greater accessibility and convenience, making it an increasingly important option for mental healthcare.

Bogár et al. [22], focused on the field of cardiac care, highlighting that smartwatches for arrhythmia detection [22] have shown to play a crucial role in the early detection and continuous monitoring of cardiac conditions such as atrial fibrillation. The systematic review highlights the potential of these wearable devices to enable timely interventions and improve patient outcomes, particularly for individuals at high risk of heart-related complications.

Lastly Protano et al. [23] demonstrated that digital technologies have also proven effective in promoting weight loss and healthy behaviors [23]. The systematic review of studies on mobile apps, wearables, and online programs for weight management demonstrated their effectiveness in encouraging healthier lifestyles, particularly by increasing physical activity and improving dietary habits. The personalized feedback provided by these digital tools has been shown to enhance weight loss efforts, offering significant benefits for individuals with obesity or overweight conditions.

Together, these reviews underline the transformative role of digital health technologies in modern healthcare. They highlight how virtual interventions, whether through telerehabilitation, voice assistants, chatbots, digital psychotherapy, or wearables, can enhance patient care, improve clinical outcomes, and provide accessible, personalized healthcare solutions across various health conditions.

*Conclusions and future routes*

Based on the contributions presented in this Special Issue, it is evident that healthcare technologies, including mobile health applications, virtual interventions, and digital platforms, are playing a transformative role in improving patient care, access, and overall health outcomes. The articles and reviews provide valuable insights into the challenges, opportunities, and effectiveness of these technologies across various healthcare domains, such as chronic disease management, mental health support, rehabilitation, and the monitoring of cardiovascular conditions [11–17].

Looking ahead, several key areas have been detected for further exploration and development. First, improving the usability, accessibility, and technical stability of mHealth platforms is crucial for ensuring their broader adoption and sustained engagement among patients, particularly those with chronic conditions [11]. In addition, focusing on the challenges related to data privacy, security, and the integration of digital tools into existing healthcare systems will be essential for maximizing their impact on patient care [12].

Future research should continue to focus on optimizing the integration of AI-powered tools, such as voice assistants, chatbots, and large language models, to enhance patient–provider communication, support self-management, and provide personalized care [19–23]. Moreover, the growing role of digital psychotherapy, telerehabilitation, and wearables in mental health and physical rehabilitation underscores the potential for remote healthcare interventions to complement traditional care models and offer more flexible, patient-centered solutions [18,21,22].

Lastly, as the healthcare landscape continues to evolve, it will be essential to address the ethical considerations surrounding the use of AI and digital technologies, ensuring that these tools are used responsibly and in ways that enhance health equity, patient autonomy, and trust in digital healthcare systems [19,23].

In conclusion, the ongoing advancement of digital health technologies promises to revolutionize healthcare delivery and provide more efficient, accessible, and personalized care. However, reaching the full potential of these technologies will require continued innovation, interdisciplinary collaboration, and a commitment to addressing the challenges that accompany their integration into real-world healthcare practices.

**Conflicts of Interest:** The authors declare no conflict of interest.

## References

1. Special Issue: Healthcare Goes Digital: Mobile Health and Electronic Health Technology in the 21st Century. Available online: https://www.mdpi.com/journal/healthcare/special_issues/0P14J89UOQ (accessed on 20 March 2025).
2. Farias, F.A.C.; Dagostini, C.M.; Bicca, Y.A.; Falavigna, V.F.; Falavigna, A. Remote Patient Monitoring: A Systematic Review. *Telemed. J. E Health* **2020**, *26*, 576–583. [CrossRef] [PubMed]

3. Han, M.; Lee, E. Effectiveness of Mobile Health Application Use to Improve Health Behavior Changes: A Systematic Review of Randomized Controlled Trials. *Healthc. Inform. Res.* **2018**, *24*, 207–226. [CrossRef] [PubMed] [PubMed Central]
4. Lu, L.; Zhang, J.; Xie, Y.; Gao, F.; Xu, S.; Wu, X.; Ye, Z. Wearable Health Devices in Health Care: Narrative Systematic Review. *JMIR Mhealth Uhealth* **2020**, *8*, e18907. [CrossRef] [PubMed] [PubMed Central]
5. Esteva, A.; Kuprel, B.; Novoa, R.A.; Ko, J.; Swetter, S.M.; Blau, H.M.; Thrun, S. Dermatologist-level classification of skin cancer with deep neural networks. *Nature* **2017**, *542*, 115–118. [CrossRef] [PubMed]
6. Available online: https://www.nejm.org/doi/full/10.1056/NEJMp2003539 (accessed on 19 March 2025).
7. Rajkomar, A.; Oren, E.; Chen, K.; Dai, A.M.; Hajaj, N.; Hardt, M.; Liu, P.J.; Liu, X.; Marcus, J.; Sun, M.; et al. Scalable and accurate deep learning with electronic health records. *NPJ Digit. Med.* **2018**, *1*, 18. [CrossRef] [PubMed]
8. Available online: https://www.ncbi.nlm.nih.gov/books/NBK233428/ (accessed on 19 March 2025).
9. Kurniawan, M.H.; Handiyani, H.; Nuraini, T.; Hariyati, R.T.S.; Sutrisno, S. A systematic review of artificial intelligence-powered (AI-powered) chatbot intervention for managing chronic illness. *Ann. Med.* **2024**, *56*, 2302980. [CrossRef] [PubMed] [PubMed Central]
10. Al-Rawashdeh, M.; Keikhosrokiani, P.; Belaton, B.; Alawida, M.; Zwiri, A. IoT Adoption and Application for Smart Healthcare: A Systematic Review. *Sensors* **2022**, *22*, 5377. [CrossRef] [PubMed] [PubMed Central]
11. Alzghaibi, H. Barriers to the Utilization of mHealth Applications in Saudi Arabia: Insights from Patients with Chronic Diseases. *Healthcare* **2025**, *13*, 665. [CrossRef] [PubMed]
12. Lu, Y.; Shi, L.; Wang, Z. Patient Mobility in the Digital Era: How Online Service Information from Internet Hospitals Shapes Patients' Cross-Regional Healthcare Choices. *Healthcare* **2025**, *13*, 484. [CrossRef] [PubMed]
13. Shafran-Tikva, S.; Gabay, G.; Kagan, I. Transformative Insights into Community-Acquired Pressure Injuries Among the Elderly: A Big Data Analysis. *Healthcare* **2025**, *13*, 153. [CrossRef] [PubMed]
14. Estadella Tarriel, J.; Perelló Capó, J.; Simó González, M.; Bailón Queiruga, M.; Real Gatius, J.; Gomis-Pastor, M.; Marre, D.; Llurba Olivé, E. Effectiveness of Virtual Reality in Reducing Pain and Stress During Office Hysteroscopy: A Randomized Controlled Trial. *Healthcare* **2025**, *13*, 131. [CrossRef] [PubMed]
15. Han, J.; Lee, H.; Kim, T.; Lee, S. Exploring the Impact of Positive Psychology-Based Virtual Music Therapy on Mental Health in Stressed College Students during COVID-19: A Pilot Investigation. *Healthcare* **2024**, *12*, 1467. [CrossRef] [PubMed]
16. Gomez-Cabello, C.A.; Borna, S.; Pressman, S.M.; Haider, S.A.; Sehgal, A.; Leibovich, B.C.; Forte, A.J. Artificial Intelligence in Postoperative Care: Assessing Large Language Models for Patient Recommendations in Plastic Surgery. *Healthcare* **2024**, *12*, 1083. [CrossRef] [PubMed]
17. Lepri, G.; Oddi, F.; Gulino, R.A.; Giansanti, D. Beyond the Clinic Walls: Examining Radiology Technicians' Experiences in Home-Based Radiography. *Healthcare* **2024**, *12*, 732. [CrossRef] [PubMed]
18. Valenza-Peña, G.; Calvache-Mateo, A.; Valenza, M.C.; Granados-Santiago, M.; Raya-Benítez, J.; Cabrera-Martos, I.; Díaz-Mohedo, E. Effects of Telerehabilitation on Pain and Disability in Patients with Chronic Neck Pain: A Systematic Review and Meta-Analysis. *Healthcare* **2024**, *12*, 796. [CrossRef]
19. Bramanti, A.; Corallo, A.; Clemente, G.; Greco, L.; Garofano, M.; Giordano, M.; Pascarelli, C.; Mitrano, G.; Di Palo, M.P.; Di Spirito, F.; et al. Exploring the Role of Voice Assistants in Managing Noncommunicable Diseases: A Systematic Review on Clinical, Behavioral Outcomes, Quality of Life, and User Experiences. *Healthcare* **2025**, *13*, 517. [CrossRef] [PubMed]
20. Amil, S.; Da, S.-M.-A.-R.; Plaisimond, J.; Roch, G.; Sasseville, M.; Bergeron, F.; Gagnon, M.-P. Interactive Conversational Agents for Perinatal Health: A Mixed Methods Systematic Review. *Healthcare* **2025**, *13*, 363. [CrossRef] [PubMed]
21. Oh, J.; Ho, J.; Lee, S.; Park, J.-H. Effects of Digital Psychotherapy on Suicide: A Systematic Review and Meta-Analysis. *Healthcare* **2024**, *12*, 1435. [CrossRef] [PubMed]
22. Bogár, B.; Pető, D.; Sipos, D.; Füredi, G.; Keszthelyi, A.; Betlehem, J.; Pandur, A.A. Detection of Arrhythmias Using Smartwatches—A Systematic Literature Review. *Healthcare* **2024**, *12*, 892. [CrossRef] [PubMed]
23. Protano, C.; De Giorgi, A.; Valeriani, F.; Mazzeo, E.; Zanni, S.; Cofone, L.; D'Ancona, G.; Hasnaoui, A.; Pindinello, I.; Sabato, M.; et al. Can Digital Technologies Be Useful for Weight Loss in Individuals with Overweight or Obesity? A Systematic Review. *Healthcare* **2024**, *12*, 670. [CrossRef] [PubMed]

healthcare

MDPI

Article

# Patient Mobility in the Digital Era: How Online Service Information from Internet Hospitals Shapes Patients' Cross-Regional Healthcare Choices

**Yingjie Lu, Luli Shi and Zimeng Wang ***

School of Economics and Management, Beijing University of Chemical Technology, Beijing 100029, China; luyingjie982@163.com (Y.L.)
* Correspondence: wzm4533018@163.com; Tel.: +86-010-64434892

**Abstract: Background/Objectives:** Patients in medically underserved regions often seek cross-regional healthcare for high-quality medical services but face significant barriers due to limited information about providers. Internet hospitals address this gap by offering online consultations, remote diagnoses, and public service information. This study examines how such information shapes patients' cross-regional healthcare choices. **Methods:** A binary logistic regression model using signaling theory was employed to evaluate the impact of platform-generated signals (e.g., hospital ratings) and patient-generated signals (e.g., review quantity and polarity) on patients' cross-regional healthcare choices. The experimental data were sourced from a leading Chinese online medical platform, comprising 1901 hospitals and 273,884 patient feedback records. Among these, 216,793 patients (79.16%) sought cross-regional treatment, while 57,091 patients (20.84%) opted for local treatment. **Results:** Platform-generated signals, such as hospital ratings (B = 0.406, $p < 0.01$) and patient-generated signals, including review quantity (B = 0.089, $p < 0.01$) and polarity (B = 0.634, $p < 0.01$), significantly and positively influence patients' cross-regional healthcare choices. Disease severity and local medical resource availability moderated these effects: Patients with severe conditions rely less on hospital ratings (B = −0.365, $p < 0.01$), while those in resource-limited areas depend more on hospital ratings (B = −0.138, $p < 0.01$) and review quantity (B = −0.029, $p < 0.01$) but less on review polarity (B = 0.273, $p < 0.01$). **Conclusions:** These findings offer actionable insights for policymakers and platform developers to optimize online healthcare services, facilitating informed cross-regional healthcare decisions and advancing healthcare equity in the digital era.

**Keywords:** patient mobility; online medical service; cross-regional healthcare choices; signaling theory; China online healthcare platforms

## 1. Introduction

The rapid rise of internet healthcare services has significantly expanded access to high-quality medical resources, especially for patients in medically underserved regions [1]. For individuals unable or unwilling to visit healthcare facilities in person, internet healthcare offers efficient services such as online consultations and remote diagnostics, effectively reducing the individual's time and financial burdens [2–4]. Moreover, the importance of internet healthcare cannot be overlooked for patients planning to seek in-person treatment. With the widespread adoption of internet technology, the accessibility of medical service information and doctor–patient communication has been significantly enhanced. Recent studies have demonstrated that Internet healthcare has not only transformed traditional face-to-face communication models but also reduced information asymmetry by providing patients with more comprehensive access to medical service information [5]. This shift has empowered patients with greater autonomy and decision-making capabilities, thereby promoting a more patient-centered approach to healthcare communication and engagement.

However, in traditional healthcare settings, patients often face significant challenges in assessing the capabilities and quality of services offered by hospitals, which limits their ability to make informed decisions. This issue is especially challenging for patients seeking care in distant locations. The lack of information about out-of-area hospitals creates uncertainty about whether traveling for treatment is worthwhile, complicating their decision-making. The emergence of Internet healthcare services has the potential to address this challenge by providing patients with a critical source of information. Through access to publicly available online service information, patients can evaluate the performance, reputation, and quality of healthcare providers, enabling them to make more informed health-related decisions.

However, while the existing research on online medical services has primarily focused on online doctor–patient interactions, such as behaviors, characteristics, motivations, and benefits, there remains a significant gap in understanding how publicly available online service information influences patients' cross-regional healthcare choices. Specifically, little is known about which types of online information are most impactful in reducing information asymmetry and guiding patients' decisions to seek care outside their local regions. This study aims to fill this gap by exploring the role of publicly available online service information, provided by internet hospitals via online medical platforms, in reducing information asymmetry for cross-regional medical decisions. Specifically, it seeks to identify which types of information have the most significant impact on these decisions. Signaling theory, which addresses the challenges of information asymmetry, offers a robust theoretical framework for this investigation. Information asymmetry arises when one party (e.g., healthcare providers) possesses more information than another party (e.g., patients). To bridge this gap, signaling theory posits the informed party can convey credible signals to reduce uncertainty and enhance trust. Online service information from Internet hospitals acts as these signals, enabling patients to assess the quality and reliability of healthcare providers. By applying signaling theory, this study examines how these signals alleviate the consequences of information asymmetry and facilitate informed decision-making in cross-regional healthcare contexts. Consequently, the core research questions of this study are as follows:

*How does the online service information provided by internet healthcare platforms influence patients' cross-regional healthcare choices, and more precisely, which types of online signals play a critical role in shaping these decisions?*

By developing an analytical framework grounded in signaling theory, this research identifies key types of signals and evaluates their influence on patients' cross-regional healthcare choices. The insights from this study will enhance our understanding of how internet healthcare platforms influence patient mobility. They will also contribute to improving policy development and platform design in the digital healthcare era.

## 2. Literature Review and Hypothesis Development

### 2.1. Patient Cross-Regional Mobility

The cross-regional mobility of patients for medical treatment is a widespread global phenomenon that is particularly prevalent in regions such as the European Union (EU), the United Kingdom, and China [2–4,6–8]. To provide a broader perspective, similar mobility patterns and challenges have been reported in the Gulf Cooperation Council (GCC) countries, where disparities in healthcare quality and accessibility play a crucial role in shaping patient decisions [9]. The existing studies widely recognize the uneven distribution of medical resources as a core factor driving this phenomenon [4,10]. A survey in the EU reported that 71% of patients pursued cross-border care due to unavailable treatments in their home country, whereas 53% sought higher-quality services [6]. These findings suggest that the lack of local medical resources and the desire for higher-quality medical services are the primary drivers of cross-regional mobility.

The cross-regional healthcare-seeking behavior of patients is influenced by a combination of individual characteristics and structural factors based on Andersen's behavioral model of health services [4,8]. Individual factors include demographics (e.g., age, gender, education), socioeconomic status (e.g., income, health beliefs), and disease-related attributes (e.g., severity) [2,4,11–15]. Structural factors refer primarily to factors within the regional medical system, including medical resource availability, service quality, and medical insurance coverage [12]. The recent research has further expanded Andersen's model by categorizing factors that influence cross-regional medical choices into "availability" (e.g., the sufficiency of hospitals, available beds, and medical professionals), "affordability" (e.g., insurance coverage and reimbursement policies, income levels), "accessibility" (e.g., geographical distance, transportation), and "economic level" (e.g., financial ability to afford travel expenses) [12,13]. Additionally, patients may also consider their familiarity with the target region and their perception of medical quality when selecting cross-regional treatment [13,14,16]. Overall, cross-regional healthcare choices are influenced by multifaceted interactions of individual, systemic, and policy-related factors [2,11,17].

Despite these studies exploring the multidimensional and complex influencing factors of cross-regional patient mobility, research indicates that patients often face challenges in making rational decisions due to factors such as limited access to information, the unreliability or unavailability of data, and individual capability constraints [12,18]. First, patients seeking cross-regional medical care face significant challenges due to restricted access to essential information [18]. Without the support of familiar local networks and guidance systems, they struggle to obtain comprehensive and accurate details about medical institutions in other regions, including service quality, processes, and treatment outcomes. The absence of clear information decreases their ability to make informed choices, frequently resulting in the selection of suboptimal healthcare options [19]. Second, patients are often confronted with flawed information that is overloaded, untrustworthy, and poorly presented, making it difficult to assess the quality of healthcare providers effectively [12]. Despite evidence that comparative data on various aspects of available hospitals can help patients better choose medical providers, this information is rarely applied in real-life situations. Patients may perceive this information as irrelevant or too complex to understand, be unwilling to dedicate further time to comparing options, or lack the capacity to judge complex information. Finally, individual capability constraints are critical factors that limit patients' ability to make rational decisions. Rational healthcare choices require patients to possess high levels of health literacy (including the ability to access, process, and understand health information) and numeracy skills (the ability to apply numerical information in health management) [12]. However, many patients lack these essential competencies, which makes the complex decision-making process difficult for them when selecting medical institutions.

Therefore, addressing the challenges of limited information accessibility, clarity, and trustworthiness is essential for empowering patients to make more rational and informed decisions. To achieve this, we must focus on improving the availability of reliable data and presenting it in user-friendly formats. By doing so, we not only empower individuals to make better informed decisions but also facilitate the optimization of patient mobility and ensure equitable access to high-quality healthcare across regions.

### 2.2. Signaling Theory for Online Service Information from Internet Hospitals

Signaling theory is a widely adopted analytical framework for understanding how consumers, confronted with information asymmetry, evaluate the quality of products prior to purchase. Consumers typically rely on various signals, such as product introductions or word-of-mouth recommendations, to infer product quality, establish trust, reduce perceived risk, and ultimately influence their purchasing decisions. Especially for goods characterized by high levels of information asymmetry, such as experience goods and credence goods, consumers often cannot evaluate quality solely on the basis of observable characteristics and thus must rely heavily on external signals to make informed judgments about product quality.

When patients consider seeking medical treatment in distant hospitals, they often cannot visit the hospital in person. Instead, they gather information about these hospitals from various sources to evaluate their medical services. On the one hand, patients can obtain internal signals provided by hospitals from their official websites, promotional materials, and news reports. However, such information is typically concise and homogeneous and lacks comparative data based on uniform standards, which poses significant challenges for patients in making comparative decisions among multiple hospitals. On the other hand, patients may turn to external signals, such as reviews shared by family and friends or word-of-mouth recommendations from local social media. Unfortunately, given that distant hospitals are relatively unfamiliar to patients and that friends or family may not have comprehensive knowledge of the target hospital, these external signals are often scarce, making decision-making even more difficult.

In this context, internet hospitals offer a unique solution by providing online medical service information. This serves as a valuable external signal about their services that is both comprehensive and easily accessible and can significantly reduce the cost of searching for information and alleviate information asymmetry when hospitals are chosen for cross-regional medical treatment [20,21]. The external signals provided by internet hospitals can be categorized into platform-generated signals and patient-generated signals [22,23]. Platform-generated signals include comprehensive evaluations, rankings, certifications, and recommendations provided by the online platform itself, which can offer patients an intuitive understanding of a hospital's overall medical capabilities. Patient-generated signals, on the other hand, consist of feedback and reviews from individuals who have previously utilized the hospital's medical services. These signals reflect the hospital's actual performance and reputation from the perspective of its patients, thus providing reliable insights into service quality and patient satisfaction (reflecting the actual patient experience and the hospital's reputation) [22,24–26].

#### 2.2.1. Platform-Generated Signals

Platform-generated signals, derived from the aggregation of diverse hospital-related metrics by online medical platforms, play a critical role in assisting patients with cross-regional medical decisions. These signals combine internal attributes of hospitals—such as grade, size, certifications, specialized departments, medical equipment, and doctor teams—with historical service data available on the platform, including patient interaction records, consultation transcripts, and offline follow-up visits [20,21,24,25]. By consolidating these metrics into comprehensive evaluations, rankings, and recommendations, platforms provide patients with an objective, accessible, and intuitive comparison of hospitals, thereby reducing cognitive overload and facilitating informed decision-making, especially for patients seeking healthcare in unfamiliar regions. Numerous prior studies have highlighted the significance of platform-generated signals in influencing patient behavior. Metrics such as comprehensive recommendations, overall ratings, and rankings have been shown to effectively attract patients, increase online consultation volumes, and enhance doctor performance [27]. These findings suggest that patients rely heavily on such signals when assessing the credibility and quality of hospitals.

When patients consider cross-regional medical visits and turn to online medical platforms for information, platform-generated signals, such as comprehensive ratings and recommendations, play a critical role in shaping patients' perceptions of hospital credibility [20]. These signals provide an accessible, objective, and reliable basis for evaluating hospitals, reducing the inherent uncertainty and perceived risks associated with cross-regional medical decisions. Furthermore, drawing on health behavior models, it is evident that perceived benefits, barriers, and self-efficacy play a critical role in shaping health-related decisions. Platform-generated signals, such as comprehensive ratings and recommendations, align with these constructs by offering patients clear and actionable information, which strengthens their confidence and reduces uncertainty in cross-regional medical decision-making. Based on the above, it is reasonable to hypothesize that platform-generated signals—such as comprehensive recommendations, aggregated evaluations, and ratings—serve as critical indicators of hospital credibility. These signals significantly influence patients' cross-regional medical decisions. Thus, we propose the following hypothesis:

**H1:** *Platform-generated signals, such as comprehensive recommendations, evaluations, and ratings, have a significant positive effect on patients' decisions about cross-regional medical decisions.*

2.2.2. Patient-Generated Signals

Patient-generated signals stem from a feedback mechanism, where individuals who have experienced a service provider's quality can offer their insights to others who lack such experience [20]. In the context of online medical platforms, these platforms allow patients to share their consultation experience with other patients and provide valuable information to those who lack first-hand experience with a hospital's services. Such feedback acts as a critical external signal, empowering potential patients to gain knowledge about hospitals, evaluate the quality of their services, and ultimately influence their decision-making processes [28]. From a trust theory perspective, patient-generated signals contribute to the establishment of trust between potential patients and hospitals, as the aggregation of patient experiences can foster a sense of reliability and credibility. Patient-generated signals encompass two fundamental dimensions, namely, the quantity of patient reviews and the polarity of patient reviews, which reflect a hospital's influence and reputation, respectively.

(1) Review quantity

The review quantity, which represents the total amount of patient-generated feedback, is a critical indicator of a hospital's influence and popularity. A high review volume signals that the hospital has a large service audience, indicating its widespread acceptance and utilization by patients. When potential patients observe a substantial number of reviews, they may infer that the hospital's services are in demand and trusted by others, which positively influences their perception of its service quality. From a trust theory perspective, a high volume of reviews enhances the perceived credibility of the hospital, as it suggests that the hospital has been widely evaluated by a wide range of patients. Empirical studies support this notion, showing that a greater volume of online reviews is positively associated with increased consultation volume in online healthcare settings. For patients considering cross-regional medical visits, a hospital with a high review volume conveys a sense of reliability and service acceptance, thereby increasing their confidence in making cross-regional medical treatment decisions. Hence, the following hypothesis is proposed:

**H2:** *The quantity of patient reviews, as an indicator of a hospital's influence, positively impacts patients' willingness to choose cross-regional medical treatment.*

(2) Review polarity

The review polarity, which represents the overall positivity of patient-generated feedback, is a critical indicator of a hospital's reputation and perceived word-of-mouth regarding its services. High review polarity, characterized by favorable ratings, positive comments, and expressions of gratitude, reflects a high level of patient satisfaction and trust in the hospital's services [29]. When potential patients observe consistently positive feedback, they are likely to infer that the hospital provides high-quality and reliable services, thereby reinforcing its reputation and perceived value [30]. Empirical studies have demonstrated that higher polarity in patient reviews is significantly associated with increased patient trust and appointment volumes in online healthcare settings. For patients considering cross-regional medical visits, who often face greater uncertainty and additional challenges in choosing a nonlocal hospital, review polarity plays an even more decisive role. A hospital with high review polarity conveys a sense of exceptional service quality and trustworthiness, thereby increasing the patient's willingness to seek treatment from such a hospital.

**H3:** *The polarity of patient reviews, as an indicator of a hospital's reputation, positively impacts patients' willingness to choose cross-regional medical treatment.*

### 2.3. The Moderating Role of Individual Differences

The previous research has suggested that personal characteristics play a significant role in determining how users interact with information technology and information systems, including in the context of online medical platforms. This study examines two aspects of the individual differences among patients that can affect their cross-regional healthcare choices: disease severity [22,31–33] and medical resource availability [34].

#### 2.3.1. Disease Severity

Disease severity significantly influences patients' reliance on external signals during medical decision-making [22]. Critically ill patients face greater risks associated with inappropriate treatment or misdiagnosis, making the decision-making process more complex and cautious. These patients often seek more reliable information to guide their choices [22]. Online platforms provide patients with access to external signals, such as hospital ratings, patient feedback, and other indicators of quality and expertise, which are crucial in reducing decision-making uncertainty, particularly for severe cases [31,33]. For critically ill patients considering cross-regional healthcare, these signals are invaluable in alleviating perceived risks, enhancing their confidence in making such decisions, and providing psychological reassurance, thereby minimizing the uncertainties associated with cross-regional healthcare choices.

(1) Disease severity and hospital rating

First, the platform-generated signals, such as hospital ratings, serve as an authoritative reflection of a hospital's overall performance and competence. These signals are especially influential for patients with severe illnesses, who prioritize the credibility and authority of information to minimize treatment risks and guide their decisions. Critically ill patients are more likely to depend on such signals to make decisions about cross-regional healthcare. Therefore, we propose the following hypothesis:

**H4a:** *Disease severity positively moderates the effect of platform-generated signals (e.g., hospital ratings) on patients' decisions to seek cross-regional healthcare. Specifically, patients with more severe illnesses are more likely to be influenced by platform-generated signals and, consequently, choose cross-regional healthcare.*

(2) Disease severity and patient review quantity

Second, the quantity of patient reviews serves as a signal of the hospital's popularity, influence, and capacity to treat similar cases. Severely ill patients often perceive a larger number of reviews as a reflection of the hospital's extensive experience and reliability, which provides them with a sense of security through the "herd effect". This effect may further reassure critically ill patients, enhancing their confidence in making cross-regional healthcare choices. Therefore, we propose the following hypothesis:

**H4b:** *Disease severity positively moderates the effect of patient review quantity on cross-regional healthcare choices. Specifically, patients with more severe illnesses are likely to rely more heavily on the quantity of patient reviews when making decisions about cross-regional healthcare.*

(3) Disease severity and patient review polarity

Third, the polarity of patient reviews provides deeper insights into a hospital's medical capabilities, service quality, and treatment effectiveness, which are particularly critical for patients facing high-risk conditions. For severely ill patients considering cross-regional visits, review polarity is crucial for assessing the potential risks and benefits associated with diagnosis and treatment. These patients are more likely to prioritize the polarity of reviews as an essential extrinsic signal when evaluating cross-regional healthcare options. In contrast, patients with less severe conditions are generally less sensitive to review polarity, as their decisions may be driven more by convenience and cost rather than perceived treatment risks. Therefore, we propose the following hypothesis:

**H4c:** *Disease severity positively moderates the effect of patient review polarity on patients' cross-regional healthcare choices. Specifically, patients with more severe illnesses are likely to rely more heavily on the polarity of patient reviews when making decisions about cross-regional healthcare.*

#### 2.3.2. Medical Resource Availability

In medically underserved areas, the scarcity of available medical resources significantly increases patients' reliance on external information signals when making cross-regional healthcare choices [34]. Patients in these regions often encounter limited access to high-quality medical resources and lack personal experience or exposure to such services, which leads to greater dependence on external signals to assess hospital quality. As a result, they are more likely to rely heavily on online signals, such as hospital ratings, reviews, and rankings provided by online medical platforms. These signals are perceived as credible and authoritative sources of information, especially when contrasted with the limited availability of local medical resources. This contrast further amplifies the impact of such signals on patients' decisions to seek cross-regional healthcare.

(1) Medical resource availability and hospital rating

In regions with limited medical resources, patients exhibit a stronger dependence on platform-generated signals, such as hospital recommendations based on comparative rankings and perceived credibility. The scarcity of high-quality local options amplifies the authority of these signals, making them a critical guide for patients lacking firsthand experience with advanced healthcare. Compared with urban patients, those from medically underserved areas are more inclined to rely on these recommendations, which significantly influences their willingness to seek cross-regional healthcare. Thus, we propose the following hypothesis:

**H5a:** *The availability of medical resources negatively moderates the effect of platform-generated signals, such as hospital ratings, on cross-regional healthcare choices. Specifically, patients in medically underserved areas are more likely to rely on hospital ratings when making cross-regional healthcare choices.*

(2) Medical resource availability and patient review quantity

Patients in medically underserved areas often lack firsthand personal or peer experience and exposure to high-quality healthcare, making them more dependent on the experiences of others to guide their decisions. The quantity of patient feedback on online platforms serves as an indicator of hospital influence and reliability, which helps reduce the perceived risks associated with seeking care in unfamiliar regions. For these patients, particularly those from medically underserved areas, a greater volume of peer reviews significantly enhances their level of trust, encouraging them to seek care in hospitals outside their immediate area and thereby enhancing their confidence in cross-regional healthcare choices. Thus, we propose the following hypothesis:

**H5b:** *The availability of medical resources negatively moderates the effect of patient review quantity on patients' cross-regional healthcare choices. Specifically, the quantity of peer patient reviews has a more positive effect on the willingness of patients from medically underserved areas to seek cross-regional healthcare from distant hospitals than do urban patients.*

(3) Medical resource availability and patient review polarity

In addition to the quantity of reviews, the polarity of patient feedback becomes particularly valuable for patients in medically underserved areas. Owing to insufficient exposure to high-quality medical services and lower medical literacy, these patients rely more heavily on the polarity of feedback from other patients to evaluate the real medical capabilities of hospitals. Especially when considering cross-regional healthcare choices, positive online reputations of distant hospitals help effectively alleviate patients' uncertainty about the potential risks associated with cross-regional healthcare, thereby enhancing their confidence in seeking treatment outside their local area. Therefore, we propose the following hypothesis:

**H5c:** *The availability of medical resources negatively moderates the impact of patient review polarity on patients' cross-regional healthcare choices. Specifically, the polarity of peer patient reviews has a more positive effect on the willingness of patients from medically underserved areas to seek cross-regional healthcare from distant hospitals than do urban patients.*

## 3. Materials and Methods

### 3.1. Research Context and Data Collection

One of the most popular online health platforms for Chinese patients, "Good Doctor Online", was chosen as the data source. This platform hosts over 10,000 registered hospitals, offering a variety of online medical services to patients, including text-based consultations, telephone consultations, online inquiries, and offline navigation services. Each hospital has a dedicated profile page on the platform, providing detailed information, including hospital qualifications, departments, areas of expertise, and the number of doctors. Additionally, the profiles include records of the hospital's online service activities, such as patient visits, consultation volumes, the total number of patients served online, as well as paid and free medical services. Based on these records, the platform generates overall ratings and recommendations for patients to consider when selecting suitable hospitals.

Patients can browse hospital profiles of interest on the basis of their medical conditions, gather information about available services, and consult doctors for basic advice. However, for certain medical conditions unsuitable for online diagnosis or for those preferring in-person care, patients can use the platform's basic consultation features to communicate with the hospital and arrange offline visits for diagnosis, tests, or treatment. In such cases, hospitals also offer online appointment services on the platform to facilitate patients' offline visits. After visiting the hospital, they are encouraged to leave feedback and ratings regarding their experience. This feedback system not only helps future patients make informed choices but also allows patients to continue interacting with the hospital through the platform for follow-up consultations and discussions about ongoing treatment and recovery.

We collected empirical data from the website from 17 July 2006, to 31 August 2023, based on data availability. Our initial dataset comprised 10,190 hospitals registered and providing services on the platform, with a total of 613,282 patient evaluations and feedback records following offline consultations. However, private hospitals were excluded from the analysis due to the extremely limited availability of data, which would otherwise compromise the sample size and diversity necessary for a comprehensive analysis. Additionally, patient records with missing critical information, such as diagnoses, treatment processes, or outcome assessments, were excluded to mitigate potential biases arising from incomplete data, which could otherwise distort the study results. Taking these considerations into account, we conducted data preprocessing and ultimately retained records for 1901 hospitals, along with 273,884 pieces of feedback from patients who had evaluated these hospitals.

The data available for empirical analysis in this study comprise two primary sources. The first part is derived from hospital profile information, including institutional attributes such as the hospital level, and online service metrics, including hospital ratings. The second source originates from the patient evaluation system, which includes the quantity and polarity of reviews patients have provided about the hospitals they visit, as well as individual attribute information of the patients themselves, such as the type of illness they experience, its severity, and their residential area. Considering the potential risk to privacy and confidentiality, we only used the information that was available to the general public. No user identification data, such as names and ID numbers, were used to ensure that there was no risk of sensitive information disclosure.

### 3.2. Method

A binary logistic regression analysis was conducted to identify significant factors from online medical platforms that influence patients' decisions to seek cross-regional treatment at hospitals in other locations. Binary logistic regression is particularly suitable for this analysis because the dependent variable, cross-regional healthcare choice, is binary (1 for choosing cross-regional treatment, 0 otherwise). It allows for the estimation of the probability of this decision based on various predictor variables, including platform-generated and patient-generated signals. Moreover, this model can handle both continuous and categorical predictors, which is essential given the diverse nature of the signals examined in this study. Additionally, logistic regression allows for the interpretation of odds ratios that quantify the strength of the relationship between predictors and the outcome, providing insights into the relative importance of each independent variable in influencing patients' decisions. In the empirical model, cross-regional healthcare choice (CRH) serves as the dependent variable, whereas three extrinsic signals reflecting the quality of medical services provided by internet hospitals are used as independent variables: one platform-generated signal, hospital rating, and two patient-generated signals, review quantity and review polarity, as represented in Equation (1):

$$\text{Logit(CRH)} = \alpha_0 + \alpha_1 * \text{Hosptial\_level} + \alpha_2 * \text{Hospital\_rating} + \alpha_3 * \text{Review\_quantity} + \alpha_4 * \text{Review\_polarity} + \varepsilon \quad (1)$$

The dependent variable indicates whether patients who participate in the online medical platform choose cross-regional treatment. It is measured as a binary variable, with a value of 1 indicating the choice of cross-regional treatment and a value of 0 indicating local treatment. *Hospital_rating* (*HR*) serves as an independent variable representing a platform-generated comprehensive evaluation of a hospital's medical service capabilities and online service performance. This rating is derived from a weighted scoring system that considers multiple factors, including medical quality, service attitude, and patient satisfaction. Additionally, the platform may incorporate other metrics such as service volume, service depth, response timeliness, and response satisfaction. The weights for these components are determined based on their relative importance, which is calibrated through expert consultation and platform-specific algorithms. *Review_quantity* (*RQ*) serves as an independent variable reflecting the hospital's online influence, which is measured by counting the number of feedback entries and reviews explicitly linked to patients' completed offline visits, as verified through the platform's tracking system. *Review_polarity* (*RP*) serves as an independent variable reflecting the hospital's word-of-mouth reputation. It is measured by aggregating sentiment-weighted patient reviews. The sentiment weights are assigned as follows: positive sentiments are assigned a weight of 1, and negative sentiments are assigned a weight of −1. The aggregation process involves summing the sentiment-weighted review lengths to compute the overall polarity score for a given hospital. The final review polarity score is then normalized to account for differences in the number of reviews across hospitals. In addition, this study introduces the level of the hospital (*Hospital_level*) as a control variable that may influence patients' cross-regional healthcare choices. Hospitals in China are classified into a 3-tier system based on their ability to provide medical care, education, and research. Accordingly, *Hospital_level* (*HL*) is measured as a dummy variable with a value of 1 for tertiary hospitals and a value of 0 for other hospitals.

Furthermore, this study incorporates two moderator variables, defined as variables that influence the strength or direction of the relationship between independent and dependent variables, namely, *Disease_severity* (*DS*) and *Medical_resources* (*MR*), to examine the moderating effects of patients' illness severity and medical resource availability in their location on their decision to seek cross-regional treatment. The moderator variable *DS* is measured using a dummy variable, with a value of 1 representing severe illness and 0 representing mild illness. The moderator variable *MR* is measured as a dummy variable, with a value of 1 indicating abundant medical resources and a value of 0 indicating inadequate medical resources, according to the China Health Statistics Yearbook. With the inclusion of these moderator variables, the model equations are formulated as follows:

$$\begin{aligned} \text{Logit}(CRH) = \beta_0 &+ \beta_1 * Hospital\_level + \beta_2 * Hospital\_rating + \beta_3 \\ &* Review\_quantity + \beta_4 * Review\_polarity + \beta_5 \\ &* Disease\_severity + \beta_6 * Disease\_severity \\ &* Hospital\_rating + \beta_7 * Disease\_severity \\ &* Review\_quantity + \beta_8 * Disease\_severity \\ &* Review\_polarity + \varepsilon \end{aligned} \quad (2)$$

$$\begin{aligned}\text{Logit}(CRH) = \gamma_0 + \; & \gamma_1 * Hospital\_level + \gamma_2 * Hospital\_rating + \gamma_3 \\ & * Review\_quantity + \gamma_4 * Review\_polarity \\ & + \gamma_5\ Medical\_resources + \gamma_6 * Medical\_resources \\ & * Hospital\_rating + \gamma_7 * Medical\_resources \\ & * Review\_quantity + \gamma_8 * Medical\_resources \\ & * Review\_polarity + \varepsilon\end{aligned} \quad (3)$$

## 4. Results

### 4.1. Preliminary Analysis

Table 1 presents the descriptive statistics of the independent and moderator variables. The patients were categorized into two groups: the cross-regional treatment group and the local treatment group. The cross-regional treatment group comprises 216,793 patients, accounting for 79.16% of the total population, whereas the local treatment group includes 57,091 patients, accounting for 20.84% of the total population.

**Table 1.** Descriptive statistics of the independent variables and moderator variables.

| Variable | Total (n = 273,884) | | | | Cross-Regional (n = 216,793) | | | | Local (n = 57,091) | | | |
|---|---|---|---|---|---|---|---|---|---|---|---|---|
| | Min | Max | Mean | S.D. | Min | Max | Mean | S.D. | Min | Max | Mean | S.D. |
| *HL* | 0 | 1 | 0.98 | 0.12 | 0 | 1 | 0.99 | 0.08 | 0 | 1 | 0.96 | 0.20 |
| *HR* | 1 | 5 | 4.31 | 0.52 | 1 | 5 | 4.37 | 0.50 | 2.6 | 5 | 4.09 | 0.52 |
| *RQ* | 2.92 | 51.22 | 31.92 | 12.42 | 2.92 | 51.22 | 34.58 | 11.70 | 2.92 | 46.90 | 21.84 | 9.55 |
| *RP* | 0 | 1 | 0.33 | 0.16 | 0 | 1 | 0.33 | 0.16 | 0 | 1 | 0.32 | 0.15 |
| *DS* | 0 | 1 | 0.36 | 0.48 | 0 | 1 | 0.40 | 0.49 | 0 | 1 | 0.23 | 0.42 |
| *MR* | 0 | 1 | 0.50 | 0.50 | 0 | 1 | 0.45 | 0.50 | 0 | 1 | 0.71 | 0.46 |

Note: S.D. = Standard Deviation.

On average, the hospitals visited by patients in the cross-regional treatment group have a higher level than those visited by patients in the local treatment group (88.60 vs. 11.40). Compared with the local treatment group, the cross-regional treatment group presented higher average values for hospital ratings provided by online platforms, the quantity of patient reviews, and the polarity of these reviews (4.37 vs. 4.09; 34.58 vs. 21.84; 0.33 vs. 0.31). Moreover, for the two moderator variables, patients in the cross-regional treatment group presented higher levels of disease severity but had lower average values for the availability of medical resources in their regions than patients in the local treatment group did (0.40 vs. 0.23; 0.45 vs. 0.71).

Table 2 displays the correlation matrix encompassing all the measured variables, which includes the dependent variable, the independent variables, and the moderator variables. The results show that the correlations among the variables are relatively low, suggesting the absence of significant multicollinearity concerns.

**Table 2.** Correlation between the dependent variable (CRH), the independent variables (HL, HR, RP, and RQ) and the moderator variables (DS and MR).

| Variable | (1) | (2) | (3) | (4) | (5) | (6) | (7) |
|---|---|---|---|---|---|---|---|
| (1) *HL* | 1.000 | | | | | | |
| (2) *HR* | 0.048 ** | 1.000 | | | | | |
| (3) *RQ* | 0.186 ** | 0.329 ** | 1.000 | | | | |
| (4) *RP* | −0.055 ** | 0.082 ** | 0.030 ** | 1.000 | | | |
| (5) *DS* | 0.073 ** | 0.112 ** | 0.276 ** | 0.048 ** | 1.000 | | |
| (6) *MR* | 0.006 ** | 0.032 ** | −0.007 ** | 0.035 ** | −0.008 ** | 1.000 | |
| (7) *CRH* | 0.120 ** | 0.220 ** | 0.417 ** | 0.037 ** | 0.143 ** | −0.208 ** | 1.000 |

** Correlation is significant at the 0.01 level (two-tailed).

To further validate this observation, we calculated the variance inflation factor (VIF) for all explanatory variables. As shown in Table 3, the VIF values were all below 2 (Mean VIF = 1.08), confirming that there is no substantial multicollinearity in our model.

**Table 3.** Variance inflation factor (VIF) calculation for the independent variables (HL, HR, RP, and RQ) and the moderator variables (DS and MR).

| Variable | VIF | 1/VIF |
|---|---|---|
| *RQ* | 1.23 | 0.810 |
| *HR* | 1.13 | 0.885 |
| *DS* | 1.09 | 0.921 |
| *HL* | 1.04 | 0.961 |
| *RP* | 1.01 | 0.987 |
| *MR* | 1.00 | 0.997 |
| Mean VIF | 1.08 | |

*4.2. Hypotheses Tests*

A logistic regression model was constructed to test all of the hypotheses. The basic model regressed the dependent variable CRH on the three independent variables *HR*, *RQ*, and *RP* to test the effects of the platform-generated signals and patient-generated signals indicating the quality of the online medical services provided by internet hospitals on patients' cross-regional healthcare choices.

Table 4 presents the results of the logistic regression analysis. We found that all three independent variables are significant predictors of cross-regional healthcare choice. The detailed analyses are as follows. First, the coefficient of the independent variable *HR* is significantly positive (B = 0.406, $p < 0.01$), indicating that the online ratings for internet hospitals have a positive effect on patients' decisions about cross-regional medical visits. Thus, Hypothesis 1 is supported. Second, the coefficient of the independent variable *RQ* is significantly positive (B = 0.089, $p < 0.01$), indicating that the volume of patient reviews has a positive effect on patients' willingness to choose cross-regional medical treatment. Thus, Hypothesis 2 is supported. Finally, the coefficient of the independent variable *RP* is significantly positive (B = 0.634, $p < 0.01$), indicating that the polarity of patient reviews has a positive effect on patients' willingness to choose cross-regional medical treatment. Thus, Hypothesis 3 is supported. The likelihood-ratio chi-square statistic ($LR\chi^2$) for the model is 52,725.12, indicating that the independent variables in the model have a strong explanatory power for the dependent variable, and the model fits the data well. The Prob > $LR\chi^2$ value of 0.000, which is far below 0.05, suggests that the model is statistically significant and the independent variables have a significant impact on the dependent variable. Additionally, McFadden's $R^2$ value of 0.188 suggests that the model explains approximately 18.8% of the variation in the dependent variable.

Next, the moderator variable *DS* and the interaction terms between this moderator and the three independent variables were incorporated into the baseline model to examine how the severity of a patient's illness moderates the relationship between the external signals provided by internet hospitals and patients' willingness to choose cross-regional medical treatment. Table 5 presents the results of the moderating effects of *DS*. First, the coefficient of the interaction term between *HR* and *DS* was significantly negative (B = −0.365, $p < 0.01$), which is the opposite of the main effect of *HR*. This finding indicates that the impact of platform-generated signals on patients' cross-regional healthcare choices is significantly weaker for patients with high-risk illnesses than for those with low-risk illnesses. Hence, H4a was not supported. Second, the coefficient of the interaction term between *RQ* and *DS* was significantly positive (B = 0.004, $p < 0.01$), which is consistent with the main effect of *RQ*. This suggests that the volume of patient reviews has a more positive effect on patients' willingness to choose cross-regional medical treatment in high-risk patients than in low-risk illnesses. Hence, H4b was supported. Third, the coefficient of the interaction term between *RP* and *DS* was significantly positive (B = 0.337, $p < 0.01$), which is consistent with the main effect of *RQ*. This finding indicates that the polarity of patient reviews has a more positive effect on patients' willingness to choose cross-regional medical treatment in high-risk patients than in low-risk patients. Hence, H4c was supported. The $LR\chi^2$ value for this model is 53,374.42, indicating strong explanatory power. The Prob > $LR\chi^2$ value of 0.000 confirms that the model is statistically significant. Furthermore, McFadden's $R^2$ value of 0.190 suggests that the model explains approximately 19.0% of the variation in the dependent variable.

**Table 4.** Results of logistic regression analysis examining the impact of three independent variables (HL, HR, RP, and RQ) on the dependent variable (CRH).

| Variable | Coefficient | Std. Err. | z | $p > \|z\|$ | [95% Conf. Interval] | |
|---|---|---|---|---|---|---|
| *HL* | 0.496 | 0.036 | 13.82 | 0.000 | 0.426 | 0.566 |
| *HR* | 0.406 | 0.011 | 38.25 | 0.000 | 0.385 | 0.427 |
| *RQ* | 0.089 | 0.001 | 170.3 | 0.000 | 0.088 | 0.090 |
| *RP* | 0.634 | 0.034 | 18.46 | 0.000 | 0.567 | 0.701 |
| _cons | −3.578 | 0.056 | −63.45 | 0.000 | −3.689 | −3.468 |
| Model Evaluation | | | | | | |
| $LR\chi^2$ | | | | 52,725.12 | | |
| Prob > $LR\chi^2$ | | | | 0.000 | | |
| McFadden's $R^2$ | | | | 0.188 | | |

**Table 5.** Results of logistic regression analysis examining the moderating effects of disease severity.

| Variable | Coefficient | Std. Err. | z | $p > \|z\|$ | [95% Conf. Interval] | |
|---|---|---|---|---|---|---|
| *HL* | 0.480 | 0.036 | 13.290 | 0.000 | 0.409 | 0.551 |
| *HR* | 0.501 | 0.012 | 40.580 | 0.000 | 0.477 | 0.525 |
| *RQ* | 0.086 | 0.001 | 135.360 | 0.000 | 0.085 | 0.088 |
| *RP* | 0.528 | 0.040 | 13.170 | 0.000 | 0.449 | 0.606 |
| *DS* | 1.579 | 0.100 | 15.840 | 0.000 | 1.384 | 1.775 |
| *HR* × *DS* | −0.365 | 0.024 | −15.010 | 0.000 | −0.413 | −0.317 |
| *RQ* × *DS* | 0.004 | 0.001 | 3.110 | 0.002 | 0.001 | 0.006 |
| *RP* × *DS* | 0.337 | 0.078 | 4.310 | 0.000 | 0.184 | 0.491 |
| *_cons* | −3.924 | 0.063 | −62.540 | 0.000 | −4.047 | −3.801 |
| Model Evaluation | | | | | | |
| $LR\chi^2$ | | | | 53,374.42 | | |
| Prob > $LR\chi^2$ | | | | 0.000 | | |
| McFadden's $R^2$ | | | | 0.1904 | | |

To further clarify the moderating role of disease severity, we have included Figure 1, which presents the interaction effects of DS with HR, RQ, and RP. As shown in Figure 1, the relationships between these variables vary significantly across different levels of disease severity.

Finally, the moderator variable *MR* and the interaction terms between this moderator and the three independent variables were incorporated into the baseline model to examine how the availability of medical resources in a patient's location moderates the relationship between the external signals provided by internet hospitals and patients' willingness to choose cross-regional medical treatment. Table 6 presents the results of the moderating effects of *MR*. First, the coefficient of the interaction term between *HR* and *MR* was significantly negative (B = −0.138, $p < 0.01$), which is the opposite of the main effect of *HR*. This finding indicates that the impact of platform-generated signals on patients' cross-regional healthcare choices was weaker for patients from regions with abundant medical resources. In other words, patients from medically underdeveloped regions rely more heavily on platform-generated signals. Hence, H5a was supported. Second, the coefficient of the interaction term between *RQ* and *MR* was also significantly negative (B = −0.029, $p < 0.01$), which is the opposite of the main effect of *RQ*. This suggests that the volume of patient reviews has a less positive effect on the willingness of patients from regions with abundant medical resources to seek cross-regional medical treatment. Conversely, patients from medically underdeveloped regions place greater importance on the quantity of reviews provided by other patients. Hence, H5b was supported. Third, the coefficient of the interaction term between *RP* and *MR* was significantly positive (B = 0.273, $p < 0.01$), which is consistent with the main effect of *RP*. This finding indicates that the polarity of patient reviews has a stronger positive effect on the willingness of patients from regions with abundant medical resources to choose cross-regional medical treatment. As a result, H5c was not supported. The $LR\chi^2$ value for this model is 69,901.26, indicating strong explanatory power. The Prob > $LR\chi^2$ value of 0.000 confirms the model's statistical significance. Moreover, McFadden's $R^2$ value of 0.249 suggests that the model explains approximately 24.9% of the variation in the dependent variable.

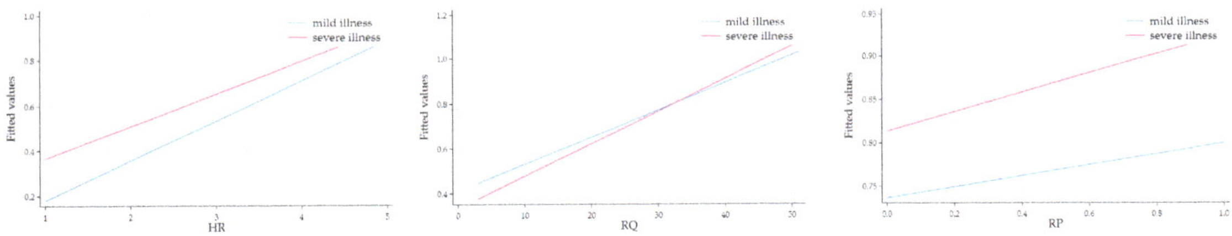


(a) (b) (c)

**Figure 1.** The interaction plots for the moderating effects of disease severity. (**a**) The interaction plot for the moderating effects of DS with HR; (**b**) The interaction plot for the moderating effects of DS with RQ; (**c**) The interaction plot for the moderating effects of DS with RP.

**Table 6.** Results of logistic regression analysis examining the moderating effects of medical resource availability.

| Variable | Coefficient | Std. Err. | z | $p > \lvert z \rvert$ | [95% Conf. | Interval] |
|---|---|---|---|---|---|---|
| *HL* | 0.567 | 0.038 | 15.050 | 0.000 | 0.493 | 0.641 |
| *HR* | 0.554 | 0.020 | 28.380 | 0.000 | 0.516 | 0.592 |
| *RQ* | 0.117 | 0.001 | 108.440 | 0.000 | 0.115 | 0.119 |
| *RP* | 0.635 | 0.061 | 10.330 | 0.000 | 0.514 | 0.755 |
| *MR* | −0.288 | 0.096 | −2.990 | 0.003 | −0.477 | −0.100 |
| *HR* * *MR* | −0.138 | 0.024 | −5.840 | 0.000 | −0.185 | −0.092 |
| *RQ* * *MR* | −0.029 | 0.001 | −22.940 | 0.000 | −0.031 | −0.026 |
| *RP* * *MR* | 0.273 | 0.075 | 3.640 | 0.000 | 0.126 | 0.420 |
| *_cons* | −4.044 | 0.087 | −46.360 | 0.000 | −4.215 | −3.873 |
| Model Evaluation | | | | | | |
| $LR\chi^2$ | | | | 69,901.26 | | |
| Prob > $LR\chi^2$ | | | | 0.000 | | |
| McFadden's $R^2$ | | | | 0.249 | | |

To further clarify the moderating role of medical resource availability, we have included Figure 2, which presents the interaction effects of MR with HR, RQ, and RP. As shown in Figure 2, the relationships between these variables vary significantly across different levels of medical resource availability.

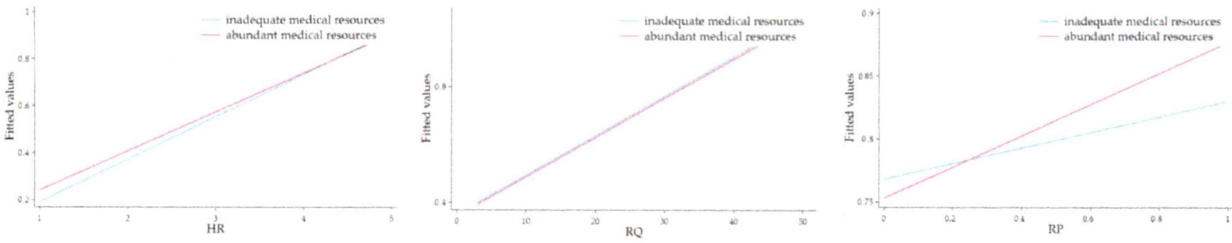


(a) (b) (c)

**Figure 2.** The interaction plots for the moderating effects of medical resource availability. (**a**) The interaction plot for the moderating effects of MR with HR; (**b**) The interaction plot for the moderating effects of MR with RQ; (**c**) The interaction plot for the moderating effects of MR with RP.

## 5. Discussion

First, the findings of this study demonstrate that online service information from internet hospitals positively influences patients' decisions regarding cross-regional healthcare. Online medical services offer patients a new channel through which to understand the service capabilities and quality of hospitals. This is particularly valuable for patients considering cross-regional treatment but who are anxious due to a lack of knowledge about hospitals in other areas. By effectively bridging the information gap, these platforms enable patients to gain a deeper understanding of how specific hospitals can meet their healthcare needs and address their concerns. Consequently, the availability of detailed online medical information from internet hospitals increases patients' confidence in the target hospitals for cross-regional treatment, ultimately increasing the likelihood of their decision to seek such treatment.

Second, this study identified some critical signals from online medical services provided by internet hospitals that reflect their ability to deliver high-quality healthcare. These signals, which can be categorized as platform-generated or patient-generated, play a significant role in influencing patients' cross-regional healthcare choices. Platform-generated signals, such as hospital ratings, serve as credibility indicators. Higher online ratings are often interpreted by patients as evidence of the hospital's competence and expertise. This perception enhances their trust and confidence, increasing the likelihood of selecting these hospitals for treatment. As noted by Victoor et al. [12], such signals are particularly valuable in assisting patients who may lack comprehensive information or the cognitive ability to evaluate all aspects of healthcare providers systematically. Simplified cues like ratings serve as effective decision-making aids, especially for patients with limited health literacy or numeracy. Patient-generated signals include the quantity and polarity of reviews and provide further insights into the hospital's influence and reputation. A large volume of reviews suggest that the hospital is widely recognized and influential, which helps alleviate patients' anxiety and uncertainty about its service capabilities. This aligns with the previous studies [12], which indicate that patients rely heavily on others' previous care experiences when making medical decisions, especially in the absence of easily accessible information. Moreover, the polarity of reviews reflects a hospital's reputation and serves as social proof of its trustworthiness. Positive feedback from previous patients creates a sense of assurance and strengthens patients' confidence in the hospital's ability to deliver quality care. As Shah et al. [22] highlight, positive online word-of-mouth (WOM) not only enhances patients' trust but also directly influences their decision-making. In conclusion, these signals have been shown to significantly shape patients' trust and preferences when healthcare providers are selected across regions.

Third, we further explored the moderating role of disease severity and obtained some interesting findings. Specifically, patients with less severe conditions are more likely to rely on platform-generated signals, such as high online ratings of hospitals. They are likely to use this indicator as a primary reference for deciding whether to seek treatment locally or at an out-of-region hospital. In contrast, patients with more severe conditions place greater emphasis on patient-generated signals, such as the volume and polarity of patient reviews. In other words, the greater the number of reviews or the more positive the reviews from other patients are, the more likely these severely ill patients are to consider these hospitals for their cross-regional medical care. These differences suggest that disease severity significantly impacts patients' reliance on information sources and decision-making behavior when considering cross-regional medical treatment. Possible reasons for this include the following: First, patients' attitudes toward risk directly affect their trust in and reliance on various information sources. Severely ill patients, with heightened risk perceptions, tend to be more cautious in their decision-making process. They prefer to avoid the potential misjudgment risks associated with platform recommendations and instead rely more on authentic feedback from other patients. Such patient-generated signals are often perceived as more realistic, directly reflecting hospitals' actual capabilities and service quality, thus making them more credible. Conversely, patients with mild conditions perceive lower health risks and are more willing to accept a certain level of uncertainty. As a result, they are less sensitive to the authenticity of signals and are more likely to trust straightforward, authoritative signals, such as platform recommendations. For these patients, platform-generated signals, which are typically based on systematic evaluations, are considered comprehensive and sufficient to facilitate quick and efficient decision-making. Second, patients with varying levels of disease severity present distinct information requirements. While platform-generated signals are authoritative, they may be perceived by severely ill patients as too generalized, lacking relevance to their specific and complex treatment needs. As a result, severely ill patients exhibit reduced reliance on platform-generated signals and seek more personalized and detailed information, which is often gathered from other patients' reviews or alternative online and offline channels. In contrast, patients with mild conditions find platform recommendations sufficient, as these provide simple and clear guidance, enabling them to make decisions with minimal effort. Finally, from the perspective of time and effort, patients with mild conditions, owing to the lower severity of their illness, are more likely to accept platform recommendations to save time and effort without conducting extensive analyses of other signals. In contrast, severely ill patients facing greater health risks are more willing to invest considerable effort to gather and analyze a wider range of signals, such as specific feedback from other patients, to ensure they make the most informed and optimal decision possible. This aligns with the view proposed by Shah et al. [22], who argued that patients with severe conditions are more motivated to expend greater efforts and seek a broader range of information sources to ensure that they make well-informed decisions that optimize their outcomes.

Finally, we focused on the moderating role of medical resource availability and obtained some interesting findings. This study revealed that patients in regions with scarce medical resources tend to rely more heavily on platform-generated signals, such as hospital ratings, when hospitals are selected for cross-regional treatment. This reliance is partly driven by the limited spatial accessibility of offline medical resources in these regions. As Guo et al. [35] highlighted, geographic distance directly influences the availability and accessibility of medical resources, making online channels a critical tool for patients in remote or underserved areas to overcome these barriers. Additionally, these patients place greater importance on one aspect of patient-generated signals: the volume of patient reviews, as an indicator of the hospital's influence, making them more inclined to choose such hospitals for cross-regional visits. However, a contrasting result was observed: compared with patients in areas with scarce medical resources, those in regions with more abundant medical resources tend to prioritize another aspect of patient-generated signals: the sentiment polarity of patient reviews, as an indicator of the hospital's reputation, thus making them more likely to select these hospitals for cross-regional medical care. These differences highlight the significant impact of medical resource availability on patients' decision-making behavior regarding cross-regional medical care, which can be explained from several perspectives. First, patients from regions with scarce medical resources prioritize the practicality of signals. They tend to rely on comprehensive information such as platform ratings and the volume of reviews, as these signals quickly reflect a hospital's credibility and influence. This helps them reduce the cost and risk of making cross-regional healthcare choices. In contrast, patients from areas with abundant medical resources focus more on the quality of signals, especially the polarity of reviews, as they have more options and are more inclined to pursue higher-quality medical services and optimize their treatment experiences. Second, patients in areas with scarce medical resources, due to their limited experience with diverse medical options, exhibit greater trust in platform-generated signals and give more attention to hospital influence reflected by the amount of patient feedback. These signals are perceived as authoritative and reliable, enabling them to filter potential medical options efficiently. This aligns with the observation by Guo et al. [35] that patients in remote areas may rely on online channels to compensate for the lack of local familiarity with medical resources. Conversely, patients in areas with abundant medical resources, with better access to high-quality healthcare and greater experience in evaluating medical services, are more inclined to trust the authentic experiences reflected in patient reviews. They may perceive platform recommendations as overly commercialized or generalized, making them less influential in their decision-making. Finally, psychological and social factors play critical roles. Patients in areas with scarce medical resources rely more on the sense of security provided by group consensus. They tend to use platform recommendations and review volumes to gauge collective agreement (e.g., "hospitals chosen by many are likely reliable") to reduce the psychological burden of making the wrong choice. Conversely, patients in areas with abundant medical resources, benefiting from a wider range of choices, exhibit more individualized decision-making. They emphasize personal experiences, prioritizing the online reputation of hospitals as reflected in patient reviews to identify hospitals that offer greater value and enhanced experiences.

## 6. Implications

This study contributes to the field of internet healthcare by introducing a novel perspective on how online service information provided by internet hospitals influences patients' offline cross-regional healthcare choices. Unlike the previous studies that focused primarily on online doctor–patient interactions, including behaviors, characteristics, motivations, and benefits, this study highlights the role of platform-generated signals and patient-generated signals in reducing information asymmetry for cross-regional medical decisions. Furthermore, by leveraging signaling theory, the study develops a tailored analytical model that identifies and categorizes critical signals, offering a systematic framework to understand their differential impacts on patients' decisions on the basis of disease severity and local medical resource availability. These insights expand our understanding of the intersection between digital information environments and offline healthcare behaviors, enriching the theoretical discourse on patient decision-making in the digital era.

This study has significant practical implications for designers and managers of online medical platforms and internet hospitals providing online medical services. By identifying the critical role of platform-generated signals (e.g., hospital ratings) and patient-generated signals (e.g., the quantity and polarity of patient reviews) in shaping cross-regional healthcare choices, online platform providers can optimize signal presentation strategies and tailor recommendations to meet the diverse needs of patients, particularly considering factors such as disease severity and local medical resource availability. For instance, platforms can improve the reliability of hospital ratings by implementing multi-source rating systems that aggregate data from patients, medical professionals, and certifications by medical authorities. Additionally, platforms could incorporate verification mechanisms to detect and filter out biased, fake, or fraudulent information, thereby enhancing the overall credibility of the rating system. Furthermore, platforms could introduce features such as personalized recommendation filters based on patient demographics (e.g., age, gender, and medical history) and disease-specific support tools (e.g., symptom checkers or virtual consultations for chronic conditions) to better serve diverse patient groups. For internet hospitals, these insights highlight the importance of enhancing online signals to build patient trust, such as improving the credibility of hospital ratings and showcasing high-quality patient reviews. This, in turn, increases the likelihood of attracting potential cross-regional patients and converting them into actual clients, thereby increasing cross-regional patient mobility. Furthermore, this study provides valuable practical guidance for policy-makers and healthcare administrators to address regional disparities in medical resources by leveraging digital platforms to improve access to reliable and trustworthy information, ultimately promoting equity and efficiency in cross-regional healthcare services. These practical contributions collectively empower stakeholders to enhance patient decision-making, optimize platform design, and foster a more equitable healthcare ecosystem in the digital era.

Furthermore, the findings provide actionable insights for policymakers and healthcare administrators to enhance the effectiveness and equity of digital healthcare platforms through specific policy interventions. First, to ensure equitable access to digital healthcare services, policies should incentivize collaborations between local governments and digital healthcare platforms, focusing on improving internet infrastructure in rural and underserved areas and providing subsidies for disadvantaged populations. Second, regulatory standards should be established to ensure the consistency, reliability, and accuracy of platform-generated information, such as hospital ratings and patient reviews. Finally, policies promoting transparency in patient-generated content can help mitigate the risks of biased or misleading information. These policy interventions enhance trust, expand access, and optimize digital healthcare platforms, enabling informed and equitable cross-regional healthcare decisions in the digital era. Such strategies are particularly relevant for addressing global health challenges, such as pandemics or chronic disease management, where cross-regional collaboration and resource sharing play a critical role. By applying these insights, low- and middle-income countries, where digital healthcare adoption is accelerating, can prioritize infrastructure development and data accuracy to bridge gaps in healthcare accessibility, promote equitable outcomes, and foster resilience in healthcare systems worldwide.

While this study provides valuable insights into the impact of online service information on cross-regional healthcare choices, certain limitations must be acknowledged. One significant limitation is the potential presence of false, manipulated, or biased reviews, which could distort perceptions and lead to misleading conclusions. Although the use of large-scale aggregated data minimizes these effects, future research should focus on developing robust methodologies, such as advanced text analysis and semantic understanding techniques, to detect and filter biased or false information. These efforts will enhance the ethical and practical validity of conclusions based on online health information. Additionally, future studies could explore the generalizability of the findings across different cultural and institutional contexts, particularly in low- and middle-income countries where digital healthcare adoption is rapidly growing.

**Author Contributions:** Conceptualization, Y.L.; methodology, L.S.; formal analysis, L.S.; data curation, L.S.; writing—original draft preparation, L.S.; writing—review and editing, Y.L. and Z.W.; visualization, Z.W.; supervision, Y.L. and Z.W.; project administration, Y.L.; funding acquisition, Y.L. All authors have read and agreed to the published version of the manuscript.

**Funding:** This research was funded by the National Social Science Fund of China, grant number 20BTQ080.

**Institutional Review Board Statement:** Not applicable.

**Informed Consent Statement:** Not applicable.

**Data Availability Statement:** The data presented in this study are available on request from the corresponding author. The data are not publicly available due to ethical and privacy restrictions.

**Conflicts of Interest:** The authors declare no conflicts of interest.

## References

1. Dong, X.; Wang, Y. The geography of healthcare: Mapping patient flow and medical resource allocation in China. *Econ. Hum. Biol.* **2024**, *55*, 101431. [CrossRef]
2. Zhang, J.G.; Wang, H.; Gu, X.F.; Wang, X.Y.; Wang, W.J.; Du, L.B.; Cao, H.L.; Zhang, X.; Shi, J.H.; Zhao, Y.Q.; et al. China Working Group on Colorectal Cancer Survey. Status and associated factors of cross-regional healthcare-seeking among patients with advanced colorectal cancer in China: A multicenter cross-sectional study. *Ann. Transl. Med.* **2022**, *10*, 342. [CrossRef]
3. Li, L.; Cui, X.; Feng, W. Enhancing Patient Satisfaction in Cross-Regional Healthcare: A Cross-Sectional Study in the Knowledge-Based Healthcare Landscape. *J. Knowl. Econ.* **2023**, *15*, 14172–14198. [CrossRef]
4. Yan, X.; Shan, L.; HE, S.; Zhang, J. Cross-city patient mobility and healthcare equity and efficiency: Evidence from Hefei, China. *Travel Behav. Soc.* **2022**, *28*, 1–12. [CrossRef]
5. Song, M.; Elson, J.; Bastola, D. Digital Age Transformation in Patient-Physician Communication: 25-Year Narrative Review (1999–2023). *J. Med. Int. Res.* **2025**, *27*, e60512. [CrossRef] [PubMed]
6. Brekke, K.R.; Levaggi, R.; Siciliani, L.; Straume, O.R. Patient mobility and health care quality when regions and patients differ in income. *J. Health Econ.* **2016**, *50*, 372–387. [CrossRef] [PubMed]
7. Brenna, E.; Spandonaro, F. Regional incentives and patient cross-border mobility: Evidence from the Italian experience. *Int. J. Health Policy Manag.* **2015**, *4*, 363–372. [CrossRef] [PubMed]
8. Wang, X.; Nie, X. The uneven distribution of medical resources for severe diseases in China: An analysis of the disparity in inter-city patient mobility. *Appl. Geogr.* **2024**, *165*, 103226. [CrossRef]
9. Alsubahi, N.; Pavlova, M.; Alzahrani, A.A.; Ahmad, A.; Groot, W. Healthcare Quality from the Perspective of Patients in Gulf Cooperation Council Countries: A Systematic Literature Review. *Healthcare* **2024**, *12*, 315. [CrossRef] [PubMed]
10. Yang, J.; Yan, B.; Fan, S.; Ni, Z.; Yan, X.; Xiao, G. Cross-provincial inpatient mobility patterns and their determinants in China. *BMC Health Serv. Res.* **2024**, *24*, 1004. [CrossRef]
11. Zhang, B.; Wang, H.; Zhang, H.; Tian, G.; Zhang, T.; Shi, Q.; Liu, J.; Xu, J.; Liu, J.; Wu, Q.; et al. The influence of cross-regional medical treatment on total medical expenses, medical insurance payments, and out-of-pocket expenses of patients with malignant tumors in Chinese low-income areas. *Cost Eff. Resour. Alloc. C/E* **2022**, *20*, 35. [CrossRef]
12. Victoor, A.; Delnoij, D.; Friele, R.; Rademakers, J.J. Determinants of patient choice of healthcare providers: A scoping review. *BMC Health Serv. Res.* **2012**, *12*, 272. [CrossRef]
13. Yang, Y.; Wang, Y. Analysis of the Characteristics of Cross-Regional Patient Groups and Differences in Hospital Service Utilization in Beijing. *Int. J. Environ. Res. Public Health* **2022**, *6*, 3227. [CrossRef]
14. Nante, N.; Guarducci, G.; Lorenzini, C.; Messina, G.; Carle, F.; Carbone, S.; Urbani, A. Inter-Regional Hospital Patients' Mobility in Italy. *Healthcare* **2021**, *9*, 1182. [CrossRef] [PubMed]
15. Xiang, B.; Hong, M.; Guo, F.; Wei, W. Spatial structure and mechanism of cross-city patient mobility network in the Yangtze River economic belt of China. *J. Urban Manag.* **2024**. [CrossRef]
16. Balia, S.; Brau, R.; Moro, D. Choice of hospital and long-distances: Evidence from Italy. *Reg. Sci. Urban Econ.* **2020**, *81*, 103502. [CrossRef]
17. Ricci, A.; Barzan, E.; Longo, F. How to identify the drivers of patient inter-regional mobility in beveridgean systems? Critical review and assessment matrix for policy design & managerial interventions. *Health Serv. Manag. Res.* **2020**, *34*, 258–268. [CrossRef]
18. Qiu, C.; Zhang, Y.; Wang, X.; Gu, D. Trust-Based Research: Influencing Factors of Patients' Medical Choice Behavior in the Online Medical Community. *Healthcare* **2022**, *10*, 938. [CrossRef] [PubMed]

19. Alrashdi, I. Evaluation of quality of healthcare: To what extent can we rely on patient expectations and preferences. *Oman Med. J.* **2012**, *27*, 448–449. [CrossRef] [PubMed]
20. Shah, A.M.; Muhammad, W.; Lee, K.; Naqvi, R.A. Examining Different Factors in Web-Based Patients' Decision-Making Process: Systematic Review on Digital Platforms for Clinical Decision Support System. *Int. J. Environ. Res. Public Health* **2021**, *18*, 11226. [CrossRef] [PubMed]
21. Khurana, S.; Qiu, L.; Kumar, S. When a Doctor Knows, It Shows: An Empirical Analysis of Doctors' Responses in a Q&A Forum of an Online Healthcare Portal. *Inf. Syst. Res.* **2019**, *30*, 872–891. [CrossRef]
22. Shah, A.M.; Yan, X.; Shah, S.A.A.; Shah, S.J.; Mamirkulova, G. Exploring the impact of online information signals in leveraging the economic returns of physicians. *J. Biomed. Inform.* **2019**, *98*, 103272. [CrossRef]
23. Yang, H.; Guo, X.; Wu, T.; Ju, X. Exploring the effects of patient-generated and system-generated information on patients' online search, evaluation and decision. *Electron. Commer. Res. Appl.* **2015**, *14*, 192–203. [CrossRef]
24. Wu, B. Patient Continued Use of Online Health Care Communities: Web Mining of Patient-Doctor Communication. *J. Med. Internet Res.* **2018**, *20*, e126. [CrossRef] [PubMed]
25. Rauf, A.; Muhammad, N.; Mahmood, H.; Yen, Y.Y. The influence of healthcare service quality on patients' satisfaction in urban areas: The case of Pakistan. *Heliyon* **2024**, *10*, e37506. [CrossRef] [PubMed]
26. Chang, C.S.; Chen, S.Y.; Lan, Y.T. Service quality, trust, and patient satisfaction in interpersonal-based medical service encounters. *BMC Health Serv. Res.* **2013**, *13*, 22. [CrossRef] [PubMed]
27. Hanauer, D.A.; Zheng, K.; Singer, D.C.; Gebremariam, A.; Davis, M.M. Public Awareness, Perception, and Use of Online Physician Rating Sites. *JAMA* **2014**, *311*, 734–735. [CrossRef] [PubMed]
28. Chen, L.; Baird, A.; Straub, D. A Linguistic Signaling Model of Social Support Exchange in Online Health Communities. *Decis. Support Syst.* **2019**, *130*, 113233. [CrossRef]
29. Michael, S. Job Market Signaling. *Q. J. Econ.* **1973**, *3*, 355–374. [CrossRef]
30. Mira, J.J.; Lorenzo, S.; Navarro, I. Hospital Reputation and Perceptions of Patient Safety. *Med. Princ. Pract. Int. J. Kuwait Univ. Health Sci. Cent.* **2014**, *23*, 92–94. [CrossRef]
31. Li J, Tang J, Yen D C; Liu, X. Disease risk and its moderating effect on the e-consultation market offline and online signals. *Inf. Technol. People* **2019**, *32*, 1065–1084. [CrossRef]
32. Gautam, S.; Galgali, S.; Mishra, A. Patients' Perception Towards Periodontal Therapy: A Cross-Sectional Survey. *J. Appl. Dent. Med. Sci.* **2016**, *2*, 4.
33. Li, D.; Hu, Y.; Pfaff, H.; Wang, L.; Deng, L.; Lu, C.; Xia, S.; Cheng, S.; Zhu, X.; Wu, X. Determinants of Patients' Intention to Use the Online Inquiry Services Provided by Internet Hospitals: Empirical Evidence From China. *J. Med. Internet Res.* **2020**, *22*, e22716. [CrossRef] [PubMed]
34. Khan, S.I.; Ani, J.F.; Rani, B.; Apon, S.J.; Rashid, F.; Yead, T.I.; Begum, M.R.; Chowdhury, S. Healthcare-seeking behavior for infectious diseases in a community in Bangladesh. *Int. J. Adv. Med. Health Res.* **2018**, *5*, 52. [CrossRef]
35. Guo, S.; Dang, Y.; Vogel, D.; She, B. The Effect of Offline Medical Resource Distribution on Online Physician-Patient Interaction: Empirical Study with Online and Offline Data. *JMIR Form. Res.* **2023**, *7*, e43533. [CrossRef] [PubMed]

*healthcare*

MDPI

*Article*

# Barriers to the Utilization of mHealth Applications in Saudi Arabia: Insights from Patients with Chronic Diseases

**Haitham Alzghaibi**

Department of Health Informatics, College of Applied Medical Sciences, Qassim University, Buraydah 52571, Saudi Arabia; halzghaibi@qu.edu.sa

**Abstract:** Background: Mobile health (mHealth) applications play a crucial role in enhancing healthcare accessibility, patient engagement, and chronic disease management. However, technical, usability, accessibility, and privacy-related barriers continue to hinder their widespread adoption. The Sehaty app, a government-managed mHealth platform in Saudi Arabia, is widely used for scheduling medical appointments, accessing health records, and communicating with healthcare providers. Understanding the challenges associated with its utilization is essential for optimizing its functionality and improving user experience. Aim: This study aims to identify and evaluate the key barriers affecting the adoption and usability of the Sehaty mHealth application among patients with chronic conditions in Saudi Arabia. Specifically, it examines challenges related to technical performance, usability, accessibility, privacy, and security and their impact on user satisfaction and engagement. Methods: A cross-sectional study was conducted using a structured questionnaire distributed to 344 participants selected through purposive sampling to ensure the inclusion of active Sehaty users with chronic conditions. The questionnaire assessed 10 primary usability barriers, including technical issues, navigation difficulties, privacy concerns, and accessibility limitations. Descriptive statistics and correlation analyses were performed to evaluate the prevalence and interrelationships of these barriers. Results: The findings indicate that technical barriers, including frequent application crashes, slow responsiveness, and system instability, significantly hinder user satisfaction. Usability challenges, such as difficulties in navigation and task completion, further impede engagement. Moreover, privacy and security concerns emerged as significant deterrents, with users expressing apprehensions about data safety and transparency. Accessibility barriers, particularly for older adults and individuals with disabilities, were associated with insufficient support and training, making the app less user-friendly for these populations. The study highlights the interconnected nature of usability challenges, suggesting that improvements in technical stability and interface design could lead to enhanced user confidence, engagement, and overall satisfaction. Conclusions: Addressing these barriers requires targeted technical enhancements, user-centered design improvements, and strengthened data security measures to promote trust and engagement. Additionally, implementing comprehensive user support systems and accessibility features is essential to ensuring equitable access to mHealth services. While the study's generalizability is limited by its focus on a single government-managed platform, its findings offer valuable insights applicable to broader mHealth initiatives. Future research should incorporate longitudinal studies to assess the long-term impact of usability improvements on mHealth adoption and healthcare outcomes.

**Keywords:** mHealth; patients' perspectives; digital health; Saudi Arabia; chronic diseases

## 1. Introduction

Mobile health (mHealth) applications have emerged as transformative tools in healthcare, offering enhanced access to medical information, real-time monitoring, and seamless communication with healthcare providers [1–5]. Despite their potential, the adoption and sustained use of mHealth apps face substantial challenges spanning technical, usability, financial, and psychological domains. These barriers limit the effectiveness and accessibility of these technologies, particularly among diverse patient populations [5–7].

A significant barrier to mHealth adoption is usability. Many patients struggle with complex interfaces and insufficient design considerations, particularly elderly users who may have limited technological literacy, visual impairments, or dexterity issues [4,8]. The time commitment required to learn and navigate these applications further discourages engagement, especially among individuals with busy schedules or low motivation [8].

Digital literacy is another critical factor influencing mHealth adoption. A considerable proportion of users are unaware of these applications or lack the technical skills to use them effectively [8,9]. This digital divide is particularly pronounced among older adults and underserved populations with limited access to technology and digital education [9,10]. Without targeted digital literacy initiatives, these groups remain excluded from the benefits of mHealth solutions.

Privacy and security concerns also deter patients from using mHealth apps. Users often express apprehension regarding unauthorized access to sensitive health data, particularly when dealing with stigmatized conditions such as mental health disorders or HIV/AIDS [1,8]. Many applications lack transparent privacy policies and robust security features, leading to decreased trust among potential users [1].

Another significant challenge is the lack of seamless integration with existing healthcare systems. Many mHealth apps function in isolation, lacking interoperability with electronic health records (EHRs) or healthcare provider systems [8,9]. Patients often have to manually input data, creating additional burdens and reducing engagement [1,11,12].

Financial constraints further impede widespread adoption. While some applications are free, others require subscription fees or in-app purchases that may be unaffordable for certain users [12,13]. Hidden costs within "free" apps, along with the need for high-speed internet and modern mobile devices, add an indirect financial burden, particularly for individuals in low-income settings [4].

The regulatory landscape surrounding mHealth applications remains fragmented and inconsistent across regions. Patients often question accountability in their healthcare management when using these tools, whether responsibility lies with app developers or healthcare providers [1,4]. Ethical concerns related to informed consent, data ownership, and patient autonomy further complicate widespread implementation [1].

Motivation plays a pivotal role in mHealth adoption. Many individuals do not engage consistently with these applications due to a perceived lack of immediate benefits [8]. Time constraints further exacerbate this issue, as busy schedules make it challenging to learn new technologies or regularly input health data [8].

Infrastructure limitations also hinder the effective use of mHealth applications. Rural and remote areas often lack reliable internet connectivity, preventing users from fully utilizing teleconsultations and real-time monitoring features [9]. Poor internet access, outdated mobile devices, and compatibility issues with different operating systems further limit accessibility [1].

### *1.1. The Sehhaty App: A Case Study in Saudi Arabia*

The Sehhaty app, developed by the Saudi Ministry of Health (MoH), exemplifies the potential of mHealth applications in transforming healthcare delivery [14]. The Sehaty application (Version 1.3), a government-managed mHealth platform, aligns with this vision by providing users with the ability to schedule medical appointments, access EHRs, monitor test results, and communicate with healthcare professionals remotely. Given its widespread adoption, a comprehensive examination of the usability challenges and adoption barriers associated with Sehaty is crucial to optimizing its effectiveness and ensuring it meets the diverse needs of its users [7,14,15]. Sehhaty played a critical role in Saudi Arabia's COVID-19 response, facilitating over 24 million testing appointments and administering more than 61 million vaccine doses [16]. Saudi Arabia has prioritized digital health innovations as a key component of its Vision 2030 strategy, which seeks to modernize healthcare services through the integration of advanced digital platforms and telemedicine solutions [16].

With over 24 million users, approximately 68.5% of Saudi Arabia's population, the Sehhaty app is integral to the country's digital health transformation aligned with Saudi Vision 2030 [16]. However, barriers to its utilization persist, including usability concerns, digital literacy gaps, and integration challenges. Understanding these obstacles is essential for optimizing the app's functionality and ensuring equitable healthcare access across the Kingdom [7,17].

### *1.2. Global Perspectives on mHealth Implementation*

mHealth has emerged as a transformative tool in healthcare, enhancing patient engagement and improving care delivery. In Europe and the United States, its adoption is supported by strong regulatory frameworks, government initiatives, and advanced digital infrastructure. Policies such as the HITECH Act (United States), DiGA (Germany), and EHDS (Europe) facilitate the integration and reimbursement of digital health tools, fostering widespread implementation [18]. A notable example is the Netherlands' "The Box" project, which provides cardiac patients with mHealth devices post-discharge, improving remote monitoring and outpatient care. Despite these advancements, challenges remain, including data privacy concerns, interoperability issues, digital literacy gaps, and socioeconomic disparities that hinder equitable access. Addressing these barriers is essential to fully leverage mHealth's potential in modern healthcare systems [18,19]. Similarly, in Sub-Saharan Africa, mHealth systems have contributed to reducing data collection costs, elderly care expenses, and maternal and perinatal mortality [20].

However, implementation challenges vary across countries. Technical barriers, such as usability issues, system integration failures, and data security concerns, persist. Ensuring user-friendly design and interoperability with existing health systems remains a major challenge. Limited internet connectivity, particularly in rural areas, also constrains the effectiveness of these solutions [1–3,5,9,20].

Socioeconomic and cultural factors further influence adoption. Limited access to mobile devices, language barriers, and variations in digital literacy hinder widespread use [20,21]. Cultural attitudes toward technology and healthcare practices also shape acceptance levels [21]. Financial constraints, including the absence of sustainable business models and limited insurance coverage for mHealth services, exacerbate implementation difficulties, particularly in low-income nations [20].

Regulatory and policy inconsistencies present additional challenges. Many countries lack clear digital health regulations, leading to uncertainties in implementation and data governance issues [22–24]. The integration of mHealth into national healthcare systems remains a complex process, often requiring parallel reporting structures and specialized workforce training [24].

To address these challenges, several strategies have been proposed. Strengthening government coordination mechanisms, integrating vertical data systems into broader health information frameworks, and increasing transparency in mHealth funding and activities, are crucial. Channeling resources through national institutional frameworks while supporting capacity-building initiatives can further enhance mHealth adoption. Additionally, prioritizing user-centered design is essential to ensure that mHealth interventions meet the diverse needs of target populations [20].

While mHealth presents significant opportunities for improving healthcare accessibility and delivery, its successful implementation requires addressing a complex set of technical, socioeconomic, and systemic barriers. Tailoring solutions to local contexts, fostering multi-sectoral collaborations, and investing in digital health literacy initiatives are critical for maximizing the potential of mHealth. As digital healthcare continues to evolve, ongoing research and policy interventions will be essential in overcoming persistent challenges and ensuring the effective integration of mHealth applications into global healthcare systems.

### *1.3. Aim of Study*

To explore the barriers to the implementation of the mHealth application in Saudi Arabia.

What this study adds:

- The research classifies obstacles into 10 factors comprising 45 operationalized items, providing a comprehensive framework for evaluating problems in mobile health applications.
- It underscores the interconnection of hurdles, such as technical difficulties and usability challenges, highlighting the necessity for comprehensive solutions.
- The research delineates accessibility obstacles faced by elderly individuals and marginalized populations, recommending targeted design enhancements to mitigate the digital gap.
- It offers region-specific data for Saudi Arabia, linking enhancements in mobile health applications with national healthcare objectives under Vision 2030.

## 2. Methods

### *2.1. Study Design*

This research utilized a cross-sectional design focusing on patients who have utilized the Sehaty app in Saudi Arabia. The cross-sectional approach facilitated a temporal assessment of the barriers encountered by app users at a designated moment.

### *2.2. Population and Sampling*

The study focused on patients with chronic diseases who frequently use the Sehaty app in Saudi Arabia. To ensure the inclusion of individuals actively engaged in managing their health through the app, a purposive sampling method was employed. This approach allowed the study to gather insights from participants with firsthand experience using Sehaty for chronic disease management. Eligibility criteria required participants to have been diagnosed with at least one chronic disease, such as diabetes, hypertension, or cardiovascular conditions, and to demonstrate consistent engagement with the app for accessing healthcare services, scheduling appointments, or monitoring their health. Patients with infrequent app usage or limited digital health literacy were excluded to maintain a focus on those who rely on Sehaty as a primary health resource. In total, 344 responses were collected, serving as the foundation for subsequent data analysis.

### *2.3. Data Collection Instrument*

This study employed a structured questionnaire to assess the barriers to the utilization of the Sehaty mobile health application. The questionnaire was developed based on an extensive review of the literature, identifying 10 primary variables recognized as key challenges in mHealth adoption. These variables included Technical Barriers (e.g., system crashes, slow responsiveness, and frequent bugs), Usability Barriers (e.g., ease of navigation, task completion time, and interface complexity), Support and Training Barriers (e.g., availability of user support and clarity of instructions), Accessibility Barriers (e.g., usability for individuals with disabilities and readability of text), and Privacy and Security Barriers (e.g., concerns about data security and trust in information handling). Other key variables assessed were Communication and Interaction Barriers (e.g., ability to contact healthcare providers and responsiveness of messaging features), Functionality Barriers (e.g., availability of essential features and accuracy of medical data), User Satisfaction Barriers (e.g., overall confidence in using the app and perceived usefulness), Cost and Accessibility Barriers (e.g., internet access, device compatibility, and app memory requirements), and Time and Productivity Barriers (e.g., efficiency of app tasks and additional steps required for healthcare management).

Each of these variables was operationalized through 4 to 5 items, resulting in a total of 45 structured items in the questionnaire. To supplement the quantitative data, an open-ended question was included to allow participants to elaborate on specific barriers they encountered while using the Sehaty app. This qualitative component provided contextual depth, helping to identify emerging user concerns that may not have been fully captured by the structured survey items.

The questionnaire was divided into four main sections to ensure clarity and comprehensiveness. The first section included an assurance letter outlining the purpose and scope of the study. Participants were informed that their participation was voluntary and that the estimated time required to complete the questionnaire was 10–15 min. The letter also assured respondents of data confidentiality and security, emphasizing that all responses would be anonymized and used exclusively for research purposes.

The second section focused on demographic information, capturing key characteristics, such as age, gender, level of education, frequency of Sehaty app usage, and digital health literacy levels. This section allowed for the analysis of potential variations in usability perceptions across different user groups. The third section comprised 45 Likert scale items, measuring the 10 usability and barrier-related variables. Participants were asked to rate their level of agreement with each statement on a 5-point Likert scale (1 = Strongly Disagree, 5 = Strongly Agree). This section provided quantitative insights into the specific usability challenges that influenced the adoption and effectiveness of the Sehaty application. The fourth and final section featured an open-ended question, allowing participants to describe additional usability barriers or challenges they faced while using Sehaty. This qualitative component enriched the dataset by capturing user experiences and concerns that may not have been fully reflected in the structured items.

Pilot Study

Before launching the full-scale data collection, the questionnaire underwent a pilot study to test its reliability, validity, and clarity. A total of 13 participants, representative of the target population, were recruited to complete the questionnaire and provide feedback on its clarity, comprehensiveness, and ease of understanding.

Several key aspects were evaluated during the pilot study. Item clarity and wording were assessed to ensure that all questions were clearly phrased and easily understood. The relevance of the questions was reviewed to confirm that the questionnaire effectively captured the intended barriers to Sehaty app usage. Additionally, the time required for completion was measured to prevent respondent fatigue while maintaining a comprehensive assessment.

To ensure internal consistency and reliability, Cronbach's alpha was calculated for each of the 10 variables. All variables demonstrated acceptable reliability levels ($\alpha > 0.70$), confirming the internal coherence of the scale. Furthermore, the questionnaire underwent face and content validity assessments by experts in digital health and usability research, who ensured the instrument adequately covered all relevant usability dimensions. Based on the feedback received, minor modifications were made to improve question clarity and optimize item wording before the full-scale implementation.

### *2.4. Data Collection and Analysis Procedure*

Data analysis was conducted using SPSS v29 and R software (Version 4.3.0) to ensure a comprehensive examination of the study's findings. Descriptive statistics, including frequencies, percentages, and means, were computed for each of the 45 items to summarize participants' responses. This analysis provided insights into the prevalence and intensity of perceived barriers to the utilization of mobile health applications.

To assess the reliability of the questionnaire, Cronbach's alpha was calculated for both the entire instrument and the 10 key variables, each representing distinct dimensions of barriers to Sehaty app utilization. The results confirmed that the questionnaire demonstrated strong internal consistency, making it suitable for further statistical analysis. Additionally, inferential statistics were applied to examine statistically significant differences in participants' responses across various demographic groups. Correlation analyses were conducted to explore relationships among the main variables, offering deeper insights into the interconnected nature of barriers to mobile health application utilization.

R software (Version 4.3.0) was employed for data visualization, particularly in representing correlations among the 10 primary variables (themes). Graphical representations provided a clearer understanding of the relationships between usability, accessibility, privacy, technical challenges, and other barriers, highlighting potential areas requiring further intervention. In addition to quantitative analysis, qualitative responses from open-ended questions were analyzed using a thematic approach. Responses were coded and categorized into distinct themes, with frequencies calculated to determine the most commonly reported barriers. This thematic analysis provided valuable contextual insights, complementing the quantitative findings and identifying specific user concerns that may not have been captured through structured survey items.

To ensure the validity and reliability of the findings, collinearity diagnostics were also conducted. Variance inflation factor (VIF) and Tolerance values were computed to assess potential collinearity among independent variables. The results indicated that all VIF values were below 10 and Tolerance values exceeded 0.1, confirming that collinearity was not a significant concern. Therefore, all variables were retained in the analysis without modification.

## 3. Results

As seen in Table 1, the questionnaire's reliability was evaluated using Cronbach's alpha, demonstrating robust internal consistency among all variables and the overall instrument. The Cronbach's alpha values for individual variables varied from 0.76 (Functionality Barriers) to 0.92 (Accessibility Barriers), demonstrating strong reliability for each item subset. The questionnaire exhibited exceptional reliability, evidenced by a Cronbach's alpha of 0.95, affirming that the tool is highly dependable for assessing barriers to the use of the Sehaty app. The results indicate that the questionnaire is reliable and effectively captures participants' perceptions across several aspects.

**Table 1.** Scale reliability using Cronbach's alpha test.

| Variables | Number of Items | Cronbach's Alpha |
|---|---|---|
| Technical Barriers | 5 | 0.85 |
| Usability Barriers | 5 | 0.88 |
| Accessibility Barriers | 4 | 0.92 |
| Support and Training Barriers | 5 | 0.85 |
| Privacy and Security Barriers | 4 | 0.89 |
| Communication and Interaction Barriers | 4 | 0.90 |
| Functionality Barriers | 4 | 0.76 |
| User Satisfaction Barriers | 5 | 0.83 |
| Cost and Accessibility Barriers | 5 | 0.83 |
| Time and Productivity Barriers | 4 | 0.89 |
| Entire questionnaire | 45 | 0.95 |

Figure 1 presents the demographic distribution of participants categorized by app usage frequency, smartphone experience, age, education level, and purpose of using mHealth applications, illustrating key trends in mHealth adoption across different user groups. The data indicate that younger adults, particularly those aged 26–35 years (105 participants, 25.1%), represent the largest group of mHealth users, followed by those in the 18–25 years category (79 participants, 20.2%). The frequency of app usage also varies, with a significant proportion of users engaging with the Sehaty app daily or weekly (144 users, 34.1%), reflecting a high reliance on digital healthcare services. Similarly, smartphone experience data reveal that most participants have been using smartphones for over 6 years (190 participants, 71%), demonstrating a well-established familiarity with mobile technology. In contrast, only 31 participants (11%) reported having 1 to 3 years of smartphone experience, suggesting that digital literacy is generally high within this sample.

Education level further influences mHealth adoption, as the majority of users hold a bachelor's degree (82 participants, 29.8%), followed by those with a master's degree (78 participants, 28.3%), while a smaller segment of respondents have only a high school diploma (54 participants, 14.7%). This trend aligns with previous research, suggesting that higher education levels correspond with greater engagement in digital health solutions. The purpose of using mHealth applications varies, with the most common reason being appointment booking (79 users, 39.5%), followed by accessing test results (29 users, 29.5%), while fewer participants used it for teleconsultation or health record management. These findings highlight the increasing role of mHealth applications in enhancing healthcare accessibility and efficiency. They also emphasize the need for user-friendly interfaces and improved usability features, ensuring that digital healthcare tools remain accessible and efficient for diverse user demographics, particularly those with lower digital literacy levels.

Figure 2 illustrates the demographic distribution of participants categorized by gender, health condition, and preferred language for mHealth applications, providing insights into the user characteristics and language preferences that may influence mHealth adoption and engagement. The first chart presents the gender distribution, revealing that the majority of participants were male (194 participants, 56.4%), while females constituted 150 participants (43.6%). This suggests a relatively balanced gender representation among the respondents, though with a slightly higher proportion of male users. The second chart illustrates the distribution of health conditions among participants, with hypertension being the most commonly reported condition (210 participants, 61%), followed by diabetes (134 participants, 39%). These findings indicate that a significant portion of Sehaty users rely on the application for managing chronic diseases, reinforcing the importance of mHealth platforms in supporting long-term disease management.

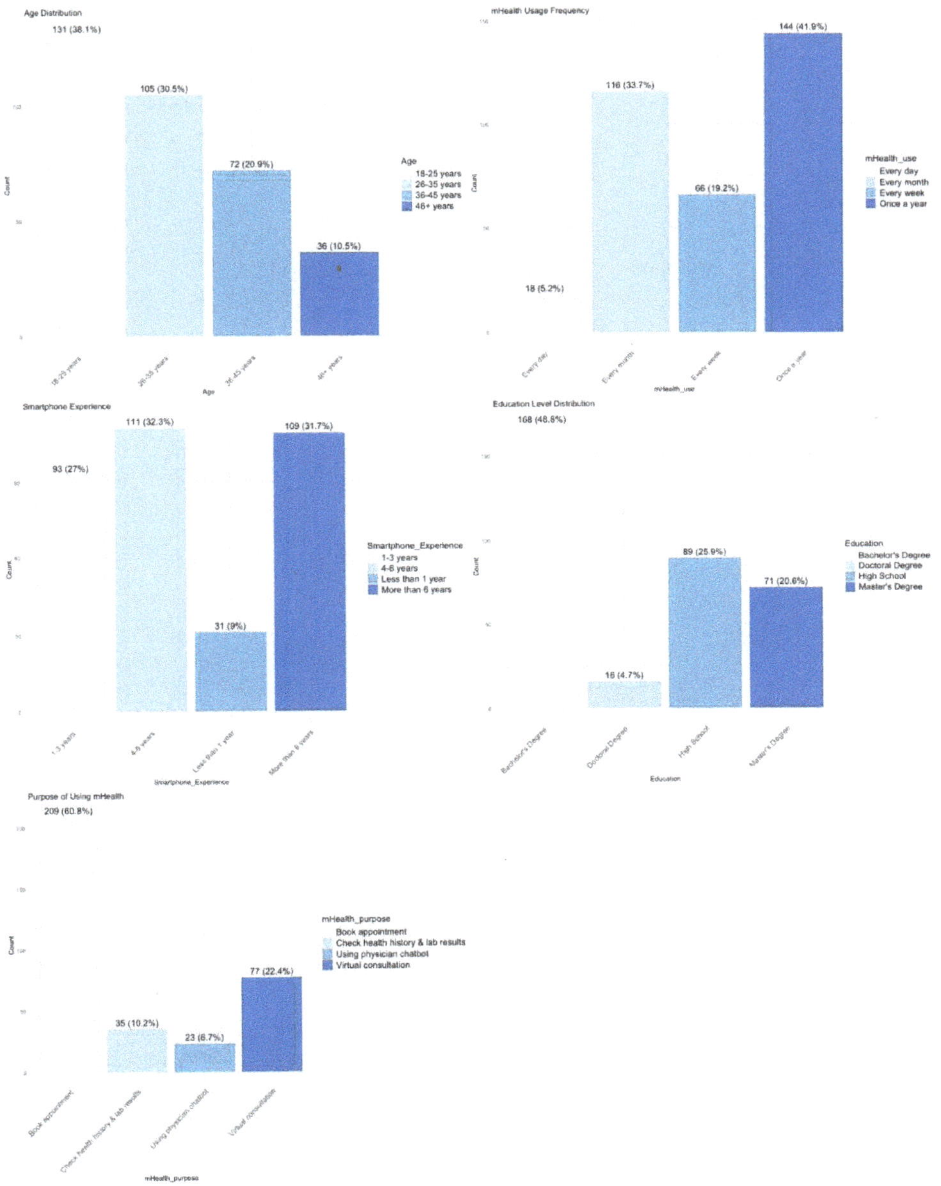


**Figure 1.** Patient demographic distribution by app usage, smartphone experience, age, education, and purpose of mHealth use.

The third chart highlights the preferred language for mHealth applications, demonstrating a strong preference for Arabic (210 participants, 61%), compared to English (134 participants, 39%). This emphasizes the need for mHealth platforms to prioritize Arabic language support, ensuring that content, navigation, and user assistance are fully accessible to Arabic-speaking users. The overall findings suggest that gender, health conditions, and language preferences play a crucial role in shaping mHealth usability and adoption. Ensuring that digital health services cater to linguistic diversity and chronic disease management needs could enhance engagement and effectiveness for a broader user base.

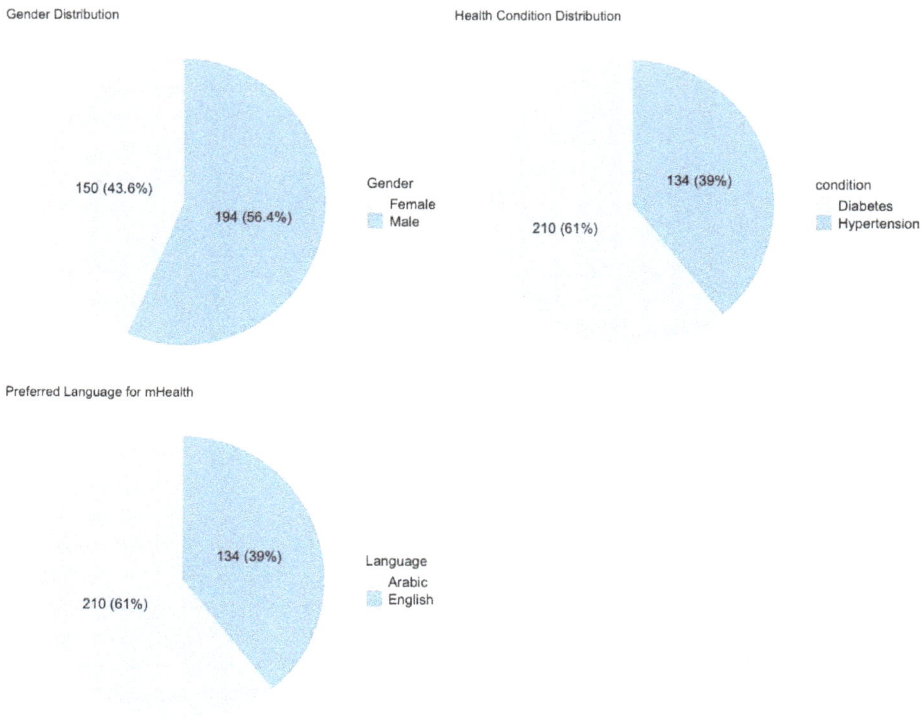


**Figure 2.** Patient demographic distribution by gender, condition, and the app language used.

Table 2 presents key findings on the challenges users face in utilizing the Sehaty application, with a particular focus on technical and usability issues. The most significant technical barrier identified was frequent crashes and application instability, which received the highest mean score (mean = 4.02). Users also reported difficulties in locating information within the application (mean = 3.84), indicating navigation challenges, while layout design was comparatively less criticized (mean = 2.09).

Issues related to support, accessibility, and privacy were also notable. Many participants highlighted a lack of instructional support or training for application use (mean = 2.22), while accessibility concerns, particularly among older users, emerged as a significant barrier (mean = 3.79). Additionally, privacy concerns regarding data security and transparency were prominent, with the statement "The application does not provide enough information about how my data is used" receiving a mean score of 3.93.

Challenges in communication and interaction further impacted the user experience. Messaging and chat features were particularly problematic (mean = 4.01), while functionality and user satisfaction barriers pointed to key areas needing improvement. Users reported difficulties in tracking health data effectively (mean = 4.02) and expressed low confidence in using the application (mean = 3.96). Although cost concerns were minimal (mean = 2.01), consistent internet access was highlighted as a significant obstacle (mean = 3.99). Overall, these findings underscore the need for enhanced usability, better support and training, improved accessibility features, and greater transparency in data security to comprehensively address these barriers.

**Table 2.** Barriers distribution with percentages and mean.

| Items | Strongly Disagree | Disagree | Neutral | Agree | Strongly Agree | Mean |
|---|---|---|---|---|---|---|
| Technical Barriers | | | | | | |
| The application often crashes or stops working while I am using it. | 27 (7.85%) | 26 (7.56%) | 21 (6.1%) | 113 (32.85%) | 157 (45.64%) | 4.02 |
| The application is slow and unresponsive. | 107 (31.1%) | 136 (39.53%) | 17 (4.94%) | 48 (13.95%) | 36 (10.47%) | 2.32 |
| The application often fails to connect to the internet. | 141 (40.99%) | 135 (39.24%) | 21 (6.1%) | 23 (6.69%) | 24 (6.98%) | 2.02 |
| I experience frequent bugs or errors while using the application. | 99 (28.78%) | 135 (39.24%) | 33 (9.59%) | 45 (13.08%) | 32 (9.3%) | 2.37 |
| The application doesn't work well on my device (phone, tablet, etc.). | 117 (34.01%) | 138 (40.12%) | 22 (6.4%) | 30 (8.72%) | 37 (10.76%) | 2.22 |
| Usability Barriers | | | | | | |
| The application is difficult to use without help. | 95 (27.62%) | 120 (34.88%) | 40 (11.63%) | 52 (15.12%) | 37 (10.76%) | 2.4 |
| I find it hard to navigate through the different features of the application. | 105 (30.52%) | 114 (33.14%) | 42 (12.21%) | 50 (14.53%) | 33 (9.59%) | 2.29 |
| It takes too long to complete tasks, like booking appointments or viewing records, in the application. | 110 (31.98%) | 122 (35.47%) | 35 (10.17%) | 45 (13.08%) | 32 (9.3%) | 2.36 |
| The application's layout is confusing and not user-friendly. | 124 (36.05%) | 132 (38.37%) | 31 (9.01%) | 38 (11.05%) | 19 (5.52%) | 2.09 |
| I often struggle to find the information I need within the application. | 25 (7.27%) | 68 (19.77%) | 20 (5.81%) | 110 (31.98%) | 121 (35.17%) | 3.84 |
| Support and Training Barriers | | | | | | |
| I did not receive any instructions or training on how to use the application. | 95 (27.62%) | 110 (31.98%) | 48 (13.95%) | 45 (13.08%) | 46 (13.37%) | 2.22 |
| There is no help or support available when I have issues with the application. | 100 (29.07%) | 103 (29.94%) | 50 (14.53%) | 42 (12.21%) | 49 (14.24%) | 2.17 |
| The instructions provided in the application are not clear or helpful. | 94 (27.33%) | 111 (32.27%) | 49 (14.24%) | 50 (14.53%) | 40 (11.63%) | 2.24 |
| I do not know how to get assistance if the application doesn't work. | 101 (29.36%) | 109 (31.69%) | 41 (11.92%) | 48 (13.95%) | 45 (13.08%) | 2.22 |
| Accessibility Barriers | | | | | | |
| The application is not accessible for people with disabilities (e.g., visual, hearing impairments). | 105 (30.52%) | 118 (34.3%) | 27 (7.85%) | 50 (14.53%) | 44 (12.79%) | 2.17 |
| The font size and layout of the application make it difficult to read or use. | 28 (8.14%) | 55 (15.99%) | 29 (8.43%) | 140 (40.7%) | 92 (26.74%) | 3.88 |
| The application is difficult to use for older people. | 32 (9.3%) | 58 (16.86%) | 30 (8.72%) | 130 (37.79%) | 94 (27.33%) | 3.79 |
| I find it difficult to input information into the application. | 110 (31.98%) | 112 (32.56%) | 45 (13.08%) | 47 (13.66%) | 30 (8.72%) | 2.37 |

**Table 2.** *Cont.*

| Items | Strongly Disagree | Disagree | Neutral | Agree | Strongly Agree | Mean |
|---|---|---|---|---|---|---|
| Privacy and Security Barriers | | | | | | |
| I am concerned about the privacy of my personal and medical information in the application. | 40 (11.63%) | 39 (11.34%) | 36 (10.47%) | 99 (28.78%) | 130 (37.79%) | 3.9 |
| I am worried that unauthorized people could access my data through the application. | 98 (28.49%) | 108 (31.4%) | 37 (10.76%) | 43 (12.5%) | 58 (16.86%) | 2.44 |
| The application does not provide enough information about how my data is used. | 38 (11.05%) | 40 (11.63%) | 40 (11.63%) | 92 (26.74%) | 134 (38.95%) | 3.93 |
| I do not trust the security of the application when it comes to protecting my medical records. | 34 (12.01%) | 37 (13.07%) | 35 (12.37%) | 128 (45.23%) | 49 (17.31%) | 3.93 |
| Communication and Interaction Barriers | | | | | | |
| The application makes it difficult to communicate with my healthcare providers. | 125 (36.34%) | 110 (31.98%) | 55 (15.99%) | 35 (10.17%) | 19 (5.52%) | 2.1 |
| I do not receive timely responses from my healthcare provider through the application. | 96 (27.91%) | 99 (28.78%) | 48 (13.95%) | 64 (18.6%) | 37 (10.76%) | 2.41 |
| I find it challenging to use the messaging or chat features in the application. | 32 (9.22%) | 33 (9.51%) | 40 (11.53%) | 110 (31.7%) | 132 (38.04%) | 4.01 |
| The application does not allow me to interact effectively with my doctor or healthcare team. | 121 (35.17%) | 108 (31.4%) | 52 (15.12%) | 35 (10.17%) | 28 (8.14%) | 2.26 |
| Functionality Barriers | | | | | | |
| The application lacks important features I need (e.g., scheduling appointments, viewing prescriptions). | 105 (30.52%) | 123 (35.76%) | 45 (13.08%) | 45 (13.08%) | 26 (7.56%) | 2.25 |
| The application does not provide updated or accurate medical information. | 110 (31.98%) | 113 (32.85%) | 39 (11.34%) | 40 (11.63%) | 42 (12.21%) | 2.29 |
| I find it hard to track my health or medical data using the application. | 35 (11.67%) | 48 (16%) | 42 (14%) | 112 (37.33%) | 63 (21%) | 4.02 |
| The application doesn't integrate well with other health services I use. | 125 (33.69%) | 140 (37.74%) | 48 (12.94%) | 28 (7.55%) | 30 (8.09%) | 2.2 |
| User Satisfaction Barriers | | | | | | |
| I do not feel confident using the application. | 21 (6.48%) | 50 (15.43%) | 24 (7.41%) | 115 (35.49%) | 114 (35.19%) | 3.96 |
| I don't find the application helpful for managing my health. | 22 (6.79%) | 46 (14.2%) | 25 (7.72%) | 116 (35.8%) | 115 (35.49%) | 4.01 |
| The application is not improving my experience with healthcare. | 130 (37.79%) | 135 (39.24%) | 42 (12.21%) | 26 (7.56%) | 11 (3.2%) | 2.18 |

**Table 2.** *Cont.*

| Items | Strongly Disagree | Disagree | Neutral | Agree | Strongly Agree | Mean |
|---|---|---|---|---|---|---|
| I would prefer to manage my healthcare without using this application. | 31 (10.2%) | 32 (10.53%) | 26 (8.55%) | 108 (35.53%) | 107 (35.2%) | 3.94 |
| I would not recommend this application to others. | 112 (32.56%) | 117 (34.01%) | 41 (11.92%) | 64 (18.6%) | 10 (2.91%) | 2.29 |
| Cost and Accessibility Barriers | | | | | | |
| The application is too expensive or requires paid features to access important services. | 97 (28.2%) | 102 (29.65%) | 38 (11.05%) | 55 (15.99%) | 52 (15.12%) | 2.01 |
| I cannot use the application because I don't have consistent access to the internet. | 102 (29.65%) | 104 (30.23%) | 35 (10.17%) | 48 (13.95%) | 55 (15.99%) | 3.99 |
| My device (phone, tablet) is too old or incompatible with the application. | 98 (28.49%) | 97 (28.2%) | 39 (11.34%) | 50 (14.53%) | 60 (17.44%) | 2.33 |
| The application requires too much data or memory on my device. | 99 (28.78%) | 98 (28.49%) | 35 (10.17%) | 52 (15.12%) | 60 (17.44%) | 3.83 |
| Time and Productivity Barriers | | | | | | |
| It takes too long to accomplish tasks in the application compared to other methods. | 110 (31.98%) | 106 (30.81%) | 40 (11.63%) | 38 (11.05%) | 50 (14.53%) | 3.89 |
| The application adds unnecessary steps to managing my healthcare. | 104 (30.23%) | 103 (29.94%) | 38 (11.05%) | 39 (11.34%) | 60 (17.44%) | 2.29 |
| Using the application does not save me time when managing my health. | 108 (31.4%) | 112 (32.56%) | 42 (12.21%) | 42 (12.21%) | 40 (11.63%) | 3.91 |
| The application slows down my ability to book appointments or access services. | 107 (31.1%) | 105 (30.52%) | 39 (11.34%) | 50 (14.53%) | 43 (12.5%) | 3.84 |

The correlation analysis, as illustrated in Figure 3, reveals moderate correlations between accessibility and support barriers, as well as between time and productivity constraints and cost-related barriers. These findings suggest that accessibility challenges often stem from insufficient training or support, while time management inefficiencies are closely linked to broader accessibility limitations. In contrast, weak correlations between factors such as cost and technical barriers indicate that certain challenges may operate independently. These results underscore the need for a comprehensive approach to application enhancement, with a focus on technical reliability, usability, security, and accessibility to improve user satisfaction and effectively mitigate barriers.

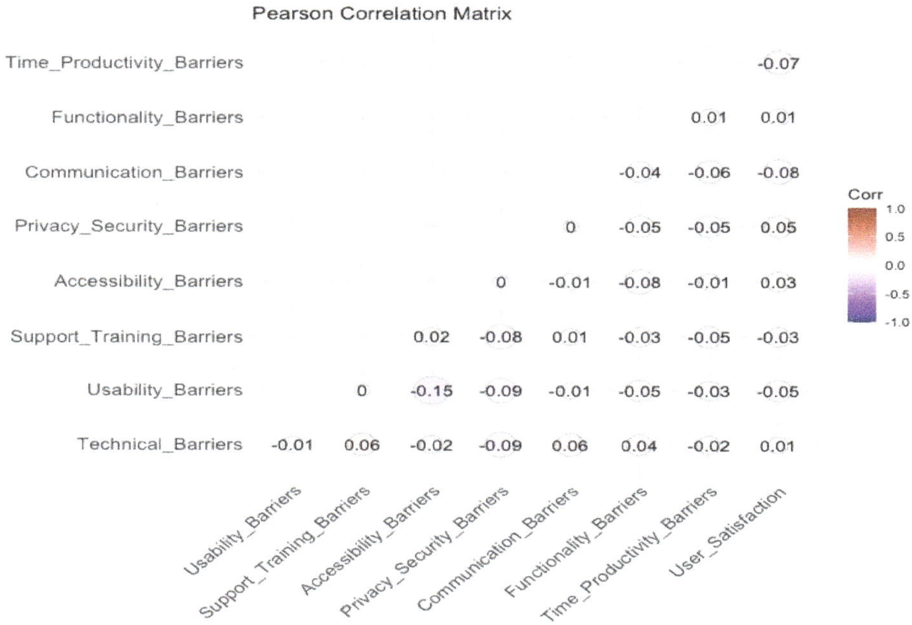


**Figure 3.** Correlation between main variables.

Further examination of the correlation analysis highlights significant relationships among the primary barriers faced by users. Notably, strong correlations were observed among technical, usability, and functionality barriers, indicating that technical issues, such as crashes and system instability, have a direct negative impact on the user experience and essential application features. Additionally, user satisfaction was significantly associated with privacy and security concerns, emphasizing the crucial role of data protection and transparency in fostering user trust and confidence.

These findings reinforce the interconnected nature of user challenges, suggesting that addressing one issue, such as enhancing technical stability or improving accessibility, can lead to broader improvements across multiple aspects of the user experience.

As illustrated in Figure 4, the analysis of statistical differences across demographic factors and perceived barriers reveals that most comparisons do not exhibit statistically significant variation. The majority of p-values exceed the conventional threshold of 0.05, indicating that demographic characteristics, such as gender, age, education, language, and smartphone experience, do not significantly influence participants' perceptions of the identified barriers. However, a statistically significant difference was observed in the relationship between gender and communication barriers ($p = 0.018$), suggesting that males and females experience communication-related challenges in distinct ways.

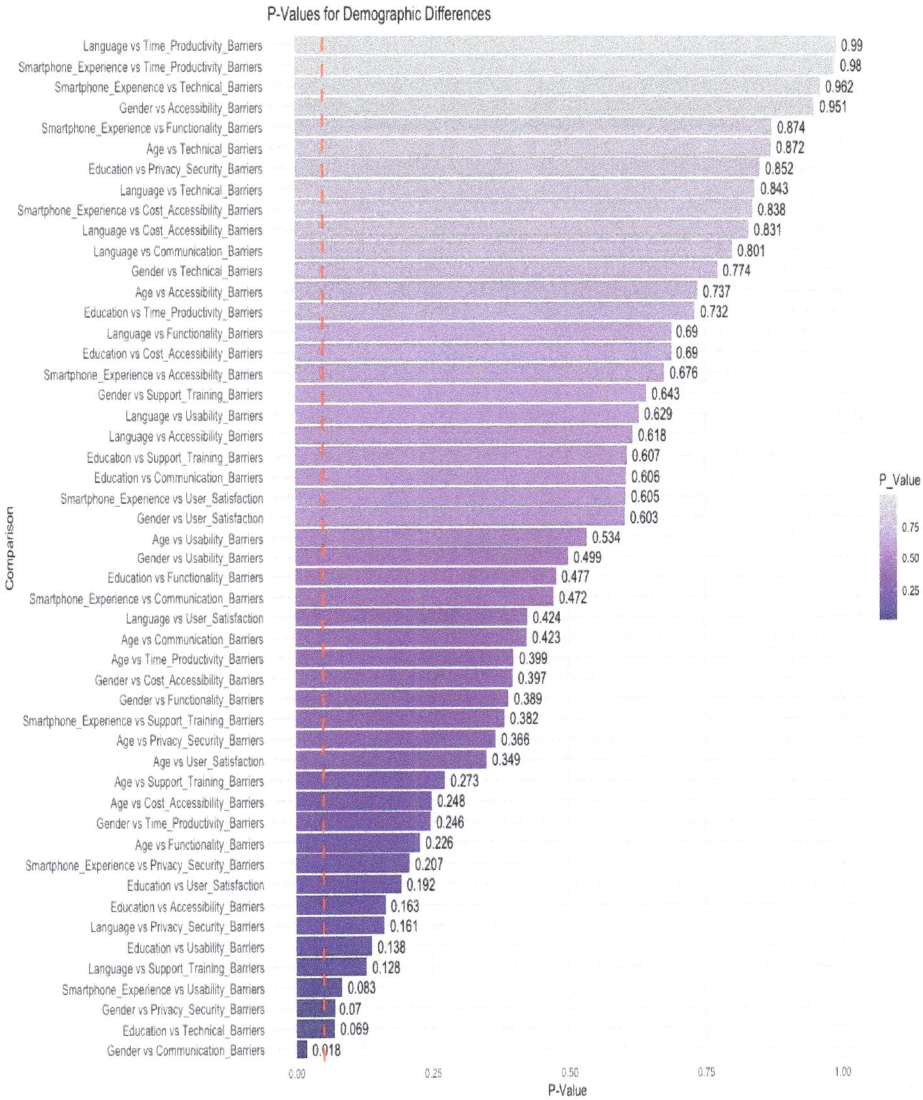


**Figure 4.** *p*-values for demographic differences.

Additionally, while not reaching statistical significance, the relationships between education and technical barriers ($p = 0.069$) and smartphone experience and usability barriers ($p = 0.083$) approached significance, indicating potential trends that warrant further investigation. In contrast, comparisons such as language and time productivity barriers ($p = 0.991$) and smartphone experience and time productivity barriers ($p = 0.989$) yielded high *p*-values, suggesting that perceptions of time and productivity barriers remain consistent across participant groups.

The limited number of statistically significant differences suggests that the potential bias introduced by convenience sampling is minimal. If significant bias were present, greater disparities among demographic subgroups would be expected. The consistency of responses across various categories strengthens the study's validity, indicating that demographic differences do not substantially influence the overall findings. However, the notable disparity in gender-based communication barriers highlights the need for further exploration, potentially through qualitative studies or larger, more diverse sample sizes, to better understand gender-specific communication challenges in mHealth applications.

The qualitative analysis of open-ended responses identified 12 key themes related to the challenges patients face when using mHealth applications, including telehealth, virtual consultations, and follow-up services (see Figure 5). The most frequently mentioned themes were Technical Issues and Access and Equity, each cited in 15 responses (12.1%). Patients frequently expressed dissatisfaction with recurrent application failures, prolonged loading times, and unreliable internet connectivity. Similarly, concerns regarding equitable access, including unstable internet connections and language barriers, were prominent, emphasizing the need for improved infrastructure and inclusive application design.

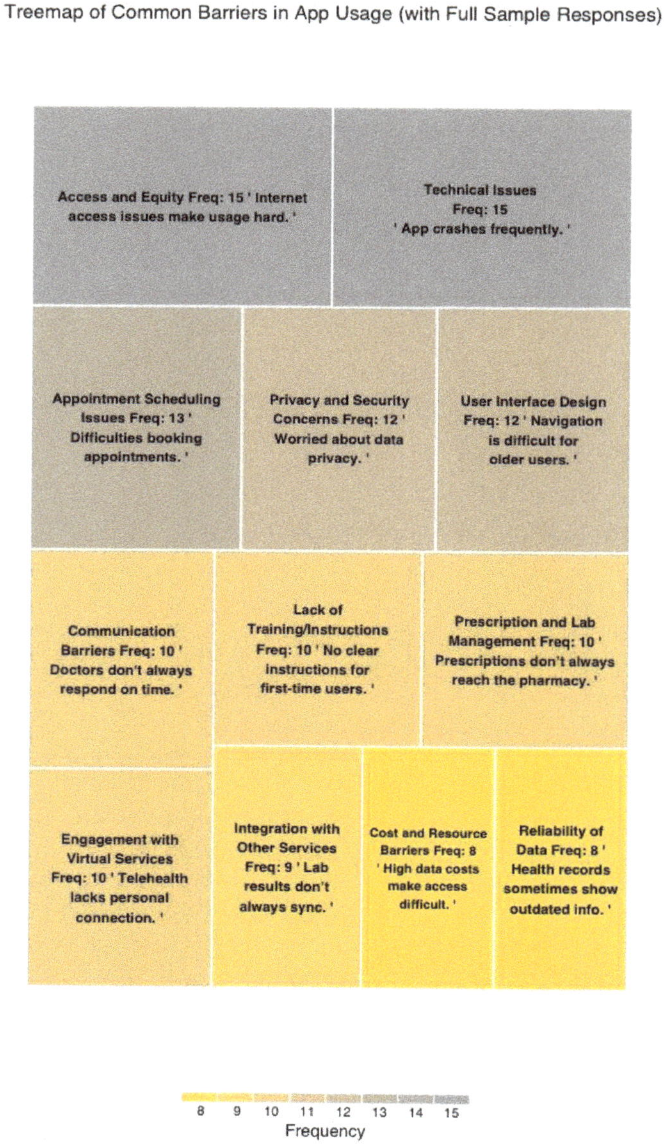


**Figure 5.** Responses to open-ended question: what other barriers you face when using Sehatty app.

Other notable themes included Privacy and Security Concerns (12 responses, 9.7%) and Appointment Scheduling Issues (13 responses, 10.5%). Participants raised concerns about the storage and protection of their medical data, as well as difficulties in securing available appointment slots and obtaining timely booking confirmations. Additionally, themes such as User Interface Design (12 responses, 9.7%) and Engagement with Virtual Services (10 responses, 8.1%) highlighted challenges in navigating the application and a reluctance to fully adopt virtual consultations due to a perceived lack of human interaction.

Less frequently mentioned but still significant themes included Cost and Resource Barriers (8 responses, 6.5%) and Reliability of Data (8 responses, 6.5%), reflecting concerns about affordability and occasional inaccuracies in health records. These findings provide valuable insights into the barriers that patients face, underscoring opportunities for enhancing application design, functionality, and accessibility to improve the overall mHealth experience.

## 4. Discussion

The findings of this study reveal significant barriers to the utilization of the Sehaty app among patients with chronic diseases in Saudi Arabia, with technical and usability issues emerging as the most critical challenges. Frequent app crashes, slow responsiveness, and navigation difficulties were identified as primary obstacles, contributing to user dissatisfaction and reduced engagement. These findings align with the work of Giebel, Abels [9], who identified technical instability as a major deterrent to digital health adoption, negatively impacting user trust and engagement. Similarly, usability concerns, particularly difficulties in locating essential features and the complexity of the user interface, support the observations of Zhou, Bao [8], who emphasized the role of poor design and navigation challenges in limiting mHealth adoption. Comparable results were reported by Nurgalieva, O'Callaghan [25], who highlighted security and privacy concerns as additional obstacles in mHealth use, leading to diminished patient confidence.

The findings of this study align with prior research on the usability of the Sehaty application while also revealing important differences in user experiences. Similar to Ali [26], the results indicate that although many users found Sehaty easy to use, a significant portion remained neutral, suggesting that usability challenges persist, particularly in terms of navigation and accessibility. Banwas, Ajina [27] further reinforce this observation, highlighting that urban users reported higher ease of use and satisfaction, whereas provincial users faced greater challenges, likely due to differences in digital literacy and access to high-speed internet. Additionally, Dawood and Alkadi [17] provide a comparative assessment of Sehhaty's usability and reliability, demonstrating that while the application performed moderately well, users remained skeptical about its ability to fully replace traditional in-person healthcare services. This finding is consistent with the usability barriers identified in the present study, particularly regarding technical instability, slow responsiveness, and navigation difficulties, which may undermine user confidence in mHealth solutions. While Ali [26] noted that Tawakkalna was perceived as more user-friendly than Sehaty, the present study, along with Banwas, Ajina [27], emphasizes that Sehaty's usability varies across different user demographics, with urban users reporting a more favorable experience compared to those in underserved areas.

A similar trend is observed in European mHealth research, where studies have noted that a lack of user-friendly technology and simple user interfaces remains a major barrier to adoption. For example, Stefanicka-Wojtas and Kurpas [28] identified that even in well-developed healthcare ecosystems, digital health platforms often struggle with accessibility issues, leading to disparities in user experiences across different demographic groups. Similarly, Hassanaly and Dufour [23] found that mHealth applications in Europe suffer from usability challenges related to interface complexity and inconsistent user experiences, particularly for older adults and individuals with limited digital proficiency. Collectively, these findings highlight the need for targeted usability improvements, including enhanced interface design, system stability, and accessibility features, to ensure that Sehaty effectively meets the needs of diverse user populations.

Beyond technical challenges, privacy and security concerns emerged as significant barriers, as participants expressed apprehension regarding data safety and transparency. This is consistent with findings from Kansiime, Atusingwize [1], who highlighted privacy concerns as a major impediment to mHealth adoption, particularly when users lack clarity about data collection and usage policies. A systematic review by Alhammad, Alajlani [29] further corroborates these concerns, emphasizing that data confidentiality issues significantly impact user trust and willingness to engage with mHealth solutions. Another systematic review conducted in the United States identified legal challenges, particularly privacy regulations, as a significant barrier to mHealth adoption. The study emphasized that stringent compliance requirements not only complicate implementation but also hinder the scalability and widespread integration of digital healthcare solutions [23]. Moreover, a study conducted in Europe by Iwaya, Ahmad [30] highlighted that inadequately implemented security protocols not only jeopardize patient data but also erode trust in digital healthcare applications.

Accessibility barriers were also evident, particularly among older adults and individuals with disabilities, reflecting challenges in interface design, navigation, and ease of use. These findings are consistent with Byambasuren, Byambasuren, Beller [10], who noted that underserved populations, including the elderly, often struggle with mHealth adoption due to insufficient accessibility features and limited technical support. The study by Liu, Lu [31] supports this, suggesting that self-efficacy and privacy concerns influence digital health adoption, particularly for users with lower digital literacy. Enhancing accessibility through larger fonts, simplified navigation, voice assistance, and multilingual support could significantly improve usability for diverse user groups.

Interestingly, cost was not identified as a major barrier, contrasting with findings from studies conducted in low-income settings, where financial constraints hinder mHealth adoption. This discrepancy may be attributed to the subsidized nature of the Sehaty app and its alignment with Saudi Arabia's Vision 2030 initiative, which aims to expand digital healthcare access. However, time-related barriers, such as inefficiencies in task completion, redundant workflows, and slow processing speeds, were frequently reported, echoing the concerns raised by [11], who found that poorly optimized mHealth applications fail to streamline healthcare management tasks. This finding aligns with the study by Alenoghena, Onumanyi [32], which discusses how technological limitations, including weak internet infrastructure, can hinder the efficiency of digital health solutions.

These findings underscore the interconnected nature of user challenges, where improvements in technical stability and usability could also enhance time efficiency and overall user satisfaction. Additionally, further research could explore the intersection of security measures, usability enhancements, and accessibility improvements to create a more comprehensive approach to overcoming mHealth adoption barriers. With the global expansion of digital health solutions, addressing and mitigating barriers to mHealth adoption is critical to ensuring their effective integration into healthcare systems. As governments and healthcare providers increasingly incorporate digital health technologies, the findings of this study provide valuable insights for the development of user-centered, secure, and accessible mHealth platforms. In the post-pandemic era, where reliance on telehealth services has significantly increased, overcoming usability and security challenges has become more essential than ever. By informing future policy and design improvements, this research can contribute to advancing digital health equity, ensuring that mHealth solutions effectively serve diverse populations and enhance healthcare delivery at scale.

To enhance the practical applicability of the proposed improvements, a structured approach is recommended, categorizing them into short-term, mid-term, and long-term strategies to ensure systematic and sustainable enhancements. Short-term strategies should prioritize addressing critical technical issues, including reducing application crashes, improving system responsiveness, and optimizing navigation through immediate software updates and user interface refinements. Mid-term strategies should focus on enhancing data privacy measures, expanding accessibility features for individuals with disabilities, and implementing comprehensive user training programs to improve digital literacy and engagement. Long-term strategies should involve leveraging advanced analytics to monitor user behavior, integrating AI-driven personalization to enhance usability, and conducting regular user experience assessments to facilitate continuous improvements. By adopting a phased and strategic approach, the Sehaty app can achieve progressive enhancements, ultimately leading to higher user adoption, improved engagement, and long-term satisfaction in the evolving digital healthcare landscape.

### 4.1. Strengths and Limitations

This study offers several strengths. It provides a comprehensive evaluation of barriers to mHealth application adoption, focusing on the Sehaty app, a widely used digital health platform in Saudi Arabia. By examining technical, usability, privacy, accessibility, and time-related constraints, the study presents a holistic perspective on user challenges. Additionally, the inclusion of diverse demographic groups, including older adults and individuals with disabilities, enhances the study's applicability to marginalized populations. The use of a systematic questionnaire ensures consistency across participants, while the application of statistical analysis, including correlation assessments, adds depth to the findings.

Nonetheless, some limitations should be acknowledged. The study's reliance on self-reported data may introduce response bias, as participants' subjective experiences may not fully reflect objective assessments of app performance. Furthermore, the cross-sectional design limits the ability to establish causal relationships between perceived barriers and app adoption patterns. While the sample size is substantial, it may not fully represent all patient demographics, particularly those in rural or underserved regions. Additionally, the findings are specific to the Sehaty app and may not be generalizable to other mHealth platforms in different cultural or healthcare contexts.

### 4.2. Future Research Directions

Future research could address these limitations by adopting longitudinal study designs to assess changes in user experiences over time. Incorporating objective performance metrics, such as application log data and error reports, could complement self-reported insights and provide a more accurate representation of usability challenges. Furthermore, comparative analyses across various mHealth platforms could offer broader insights into best practices for enhancing digital health adoption. Given the gender-based differences observed in communication barriers, future studies could also explore these disparities through qualitative methods or larger, more diverse samples to better understand how communication preferences and challenges vary across user groups.

## 5. Conclusions

The findings of this study emphasize the critical need for targeted improvements in technical stability, usability, security, and accessibility to enhance the adoption and effectiveness of the Sehaty app. While technical and usability issues emerged as the most prominent barriers, privacy concerns, accessibility limitations, and time-related inefficiencies also significantly affected user experiences. The study highlights the interconnected nature of these challenges, suggesting that enhancing key aspects of the application, such as stability, navigation, and security, could have positive ripple effects on user confidence, engagement, and overall satisfaction.

To address these challenges, the study proposes actionable recommendations for improving accessibility and security, including integrating assistive technologies for users with disabilities, enhancing data transparency and security protocols, and streamlining navigation and task completion workflows. Additionally, future research should incorporate longitudinal studies to assess the long-term impact of these improvements on user adoption and satisfaction. A user-centered design approach, incorporating accessibility enhancements, robust security measures, and optimized workflows, is essential for maximizing the impact of digital health initiatives and ensuring equitable healthcare access in Saudi Arabia.

**Funding:** This project was fully funded by the Deanship of Graduate Studies and Scientific Research at Qassim University, grant number QU-APC-2025.

**Institutional Review Board Statement:** All methods in this study were performed in accordance with the declaration of Helsinki and was approved by the Institutional Review Board (IRB) of Qassim University No. 23-19-02 (Approval date: 19 February 2023). All the participants provided informed consent to participate. In the case of the questionnaire-based study, all participants were informed of the voluntary nature, confidentiality, and aim of the study and the nature of their participation before they participated in the study.

**Informed Consent Statement:** Informed consent was obtained from all subjects involved in the study.

**Data Availability Statement:** The datasets used and analyzed during the current study are available from the corresponding author on reasonable request.

**Acknowledgments:** The researchers would like to thank the Deanship of Graduate Studies and Scientific Research at Qassim University for financial support (QU-APC-2025).

**Conflicts of Interest:** The authors declare that they have no competing interests.

## References

1. Kansiime, W.K.; Atusingwize, E.; Ndejjo, R.; Balinda, E.; Ntanda, M.; Mugambe, R.K.; Musoke, D. Barriers and benefits of mHealth for community health workers in integrated community case management of childhood diseases in Banda Parish, Kampala, Uganda: A cross-sectional study. *BMC Primary Care* **2024**, *25*, 173. [CrossRef] [PubMed]
2. Inampudi, S.; Rajkumar, E.; Gopi, A.; Vany Mol, K.S.; Sruthi, K.S. Barriers to implementation of digital transformation in the Indian health sector: A systematic review. *Humanit. Soc. Sci. Commun.* **2024**, *11*, 632. [CrossRef]
3. Deniz-Garcia, A.; Fabelo, H.; Rodriguez-Almeida, A.J.; Zamora-Zamorano, G.; Castro-Fernandez, M.; Alberiche Ruano, M.d.P.; Solvoll, T.; Granja, C.; Schopf, T.R.; Callico, G.M.; et al. Quality, Usability, and Effectiveness of mHealth Apps and the Role of Artificial Intelligence: Current Scenario and Challenges. *J. Med. Internet Res.* **2023**, *25*, e44030. [CrossRef] [PubMed]
4. Giebel, G.D.; Speckemeier, C.; Abels, C.; Plescher, F.; Börchers, K.; Wasem, J.; Blase, N.; Neusser, S. Problems and Barriers Related to the Use of Digital Health Applications: Scoping Review. *J. Med. Internet Res.* **2023**, *25*, e43808. [CrossRef]
5. Hengst, T.M.; Lechner, L.; Dohmen, D.; Bolman, C.A. The facilitators and barriers of mHealth adoption and use among people with a low socio-economic position: A scoping review. *Digit. Health* **2023**, *9*, 20552076231198702. [CrossRef] [PubMed]
6. Oudbier, S.J.; Souget-Ruff, S.P.; Chen, B.S.J.; Ziesemer, K.A.; Meij, H.J.; Smets, E.M.A. Implementation barriers and facilitators of remote monitoring, remote consultation and digital care platforms through the eyes of healthcare professionals: A review of reviews. *BMJ Open* **2024**, *14*, e075833. [CrossRef]
7. Almulhem, J.A. Factors, barriers, and recommendations related to mobile health acceptance among the elderly in Saudi Arabia: A qualitative study. *Healthcare* **2023**, *11*, 3024. [CrossRef]
8. Zhou, L.; Bao, J.; Watzlaf, V.; Parmanto, B. Barriers to and Facilitators of the Use of Mobile Health Apps From a Security Perspective: Mixed-Methods Study. *JMIR Mhealth Uhealth* **2019**, *7*, e11223. [CrossRef]

9. Giebel, G.D.; Abels, C.; Plescher, F.; Speckemeier, C.; Schrader, N.F.; Börchers, K.; Wasem, J.; Neusser, S.; Blase, N. Problems and Barriers Related to the Use of mHealth Apps From the Perspective of Patients: Focus Group and Interview Study. *J. Med. Internet Res.* **2024**, *26*, e49982. [CrossRef]
10. Byambasuren, O.; Beller, E.; Hoffmann, T.; Glasziou, P. Barriers to and Facilitators of the Prescription of mHealth Apps in Australian General Practice: Qualitative Study. *JMIR Mhealth Uhealth* **2020**, *8*, e17447. [CrossRef]
11. Abelson, J.S.; Kaufman, E.; Symer, M.; Peters, A.; Charlson, M.; Yeo, H. Barriers and benefits to using mobile health technology after operation: A qualitative study. *Surgery* **2017**, *162*, 605–611. [CrossRef] [PubMed]
12. Auza-Santiváñez, J.C.; Díaz, J.A.C.; Cruz, O.A.V.; Robles-Nina, S.M.; Escalante, C.S.; Huanca, B.A. mHealth in health systems: Barriers to implementation. *Health Leadersh. Qual. Life* **2022**, *1*, 7. [CrossRef]
13. Zakerabasali, S.; Ayyoubzadeh, S.M.; Baniasadi, T.; Yazdani, A.; Abhari, S. Mobile Health Technology and Healthcare Providers: Systemic Barriers to Adoption. *Healthc. Inform. Res.* **2021**, *27*, 267–278. [CrossRef] [PubMed]
14. MoH; Sehhaty Platform. Saudi Arabia: Ministry of Health Saudi Arabia. 2024. Available online: https://www.moh.gov.sa/en/eServices/Sehhaty/Pages/default.aspx (accessed on 1 January 2020).
15. *Health Care in the Kingdom of Saudi Arabia*; Saudi Arabia Ministry of Health: Riyadh, Saudi Arabia, 2024.
16. Alkhalifah, J.M.; Seddiq, W.; Alshehri, B.F.; Alhaluli, A.H.; Alessa, M.M.; Alsulais, N.M. The role of the COVID-19 pandemic in expediting digital health-care transformation: Saudi Arabia's experience. *Inform. Med. Unlocked* **2022**, *33*, 101097. [CrossRef] [PubMed]
17. Dawood, A.M.; Alkadi, K.S. Evaluating usability of telehealth sehhaty application used in Saudi Arabia during COVID-19. In *Advances in Informatics, Management and Technology in Healthcare*; IOS Press: Amsterdam, The Netherlands, 2022; pp. 285–288.
18. Folkvord, F.; Bol, N.; Stazi, G.; Peschke, L.; Lupiáñez-Villanueva, F. Preferences in the Willingness to Download an mHealth App: Discrete Choice Experimental Study in Spain, Germany, and the Netherlands. *JMIR Form. Res.* **2023**, *7*, e48335. [CrossRef]
19. Klaver, N.S.; van de Klundert, J.; van den Broek, R.J.G.M.; Askari, M. Relationship Between Perceived Risks of Using mHealth Applications and the Intention to Use Them Among Older Adults in the Netherlands: Cross-sectional Study. *JMIR Mhealth Uhealth* **2021**, *9*, e26845. [CrossRef]
20. Aboye, G.T.; Simegn, G.L.; Aerts, J.-M. Assessment of the Barriers and Enablers of the Use of mHealth Systems in Sub-Saharan Africa According to the Perceptions of Patients, Physicians, and Health Care Executives in Ethiopia: Qualitative Study. *J. Med. Internet Res.* **2024**, *26*, e50337. [CrossRef]
21. Patel, V.L.; Shortliffe, E.H. Designing and implementing mHealth technology: The challenge of meeting the needs of diverse communities. *BMJ Health Care Inform.* **2023**, *30*, e100813. [CrossRef]
22. Tarricone, R.; Petracca, F.; Ciani, O.; Cucciniello, M. Distinguishing features in the assessment of mHealth apps. *Expert Rev. Pharmacoecon. Outcomes Res.* **2021**, *21*, 521–526. [CrossRef]
23. Hassanaly, P.; Dufour, J.C. Analysis of the Regulatory, Legal, and Medical Conditions for the Prescription of Mobile Health Applications in the United States, The European Union, and France. *Med. Devices Evid. Res.* **2021**, *14*, 389–409. [CrossRef]
24. Alfawzan, N.; Christen, M.; Spitale, G.; Biller-Andorno, N. Privacy, Data Sharing, and Data Security Policies of Women's mHealth Apps: Scoping Review and Content Analysis. *JMIR Mhealth Uhealth* **2022**, *10*, e33735. [CrossRef] [PubMed]
25. Nurgalieva, L.; O'Callaghan, D.; Doherty, G. Security and Privacy of mHealth Applications: A Scoping Review. *IEEE Access* **2020**, *8*, 104247–104268. [CrossRef]
26. Ali, M.A. Usage and usability of health mobile applications during COVID-19 in Saudi Arabia-a case of Tawakkalna and Sehaty application. *Int. J. eBusiness eGov. Stud.* **2022**, *14*, 411–431.
27. Banwas, S.S.; Ajina, M.A.; Alsultan, A.A. The Impact of Using Smart Applications,"Sehaty Application", on Health Care AT Primary Care CENTER in Al-Qurayyat Region. *Int. J. Health Sci.* **2023**, *7*, 1306–1323. [CrossRef]
28. Stefanicka-Wojtas, D.; Kurpas, D. eHealth and mHealth in Chronic Diseases-Identification of Barriers, Existing Solutions, and Promoters Based on a Survey of EU Stakeholders Involved in Regions4PerMed (H2020). *J. Pers. Med.* **2022**, *12*, 467. [CrossRef]
29. Alhammad, N.; Alajlani, M.; Abd-alrazaq, A.; Epiphaniou, G.; Arvanitis, T. Patients' Perspectives on the Data Confidentiality, Privacy, and Security of mHealth Apps: Systematic Review. *J. Med. Internet Res.* **2024**, *26*, e50715. [CrossRef]
30. Iwaya, L.H.; Ahmad, A.; Babar, M.A. Security and Privacy for mHealth and uHealth Systems: A Systematic Mapping Study. *IEEE Access* **2020**, *8*, 150081–150112. [CrossRef]
31. Liu, Y.; Lu, X.; Zhao, G.; Li, C.; Shi, J. Adoption of mobile health services using the unified theory of acceptance and use of technology model: Self-efficacy and privacy concerns. *Front. Psychol.* **2022**, *13*, 944976. [CrossRef]
32. Alenoghena, C.O.; Onumanyi, A.J.; Ohize, H.O.; Adejo, A.O.; Oligbi, M.; Ali, S.I.; Okoh, S.A. eHealth: A Survey of Architectures, Developments in mHealth, Security Concerns and Solutions. *Int. J. Environ. Res. Public Health* **2022**, *19*, 13071. [CrossRef]

*healthcare*

MDPI

*Article*

# Transformative Insights into Community-Acquired Pressure Injuries Among the Elderly: A Big Data Analysis

**Sigal Shafran-Tikva [1,2,*,†], Gillie Gabay [3,†] and Ilya Kagan [4]**

1 Jerusalem College of Technology, Health Informatics, Givat Mordechai, Jerusalem 91160, Israel
2 Research & Innovation Center, Hadassah University Medical Center, Jerusalem 91120, Israel
3 Multi-Disciplinary Studies, Achva Academic College, Shikmim 79800, Israel; gillie.gabay@gmail.com
4 Nursing Department, Ashkelon Academic College, Shikmim 78211, Israel; kagani@gmail.com
* Correspondence: tsigal@hadassah.org.il; Tel.: +972-508573578
† These authors contributed equally to this work.

**Abstract:** Purpose: To investigate community-acquired pressure injuries (CAPIs) in older people by utilizing big data. Design: Retrospective data curation and analysis of inpatient data from two general medical centers between 1 January 2016 and 31 December 2018. Methods: Nursing assessments from 44,449 electronic medical records of patients admitted to internal medicine departments were retrieved, organized, coded by data engineers, and analyzed by data scientists. Potential explanatory patient characteristics tested were gender, age, admission indices, nursing assessments including CAPIs, CAPI type and location, vital signs, and the results of lab tests within the first 36 h of admission. Findings: Most CAPIs were located in the buttocks (56.9%), followed by the sacrum (11.8%), ankle (10.8%), trochanter (5.1%), and leg (3.9%). Tissue associated with CAPIs was described as necrotic, serotic, bloody, granolithic, epithelial, and infected. There were 31% of first-degree CAPIs, 41% second-degree, and 18% third-degree. Previously unacknowledged patient characteristics associated with CAPIs are as follows: age, oxygen use, intestinal function, the touch senses of heat and pain, albumin, RDW (red cell distribution width), and systolic blood pressure. Conclusions: The novel indicators for CAPIs underscore the importance of data-driven approaches in detecting and preventing CAPIs in community care. These markers can detect and prevent pressure ulcers in the community, particularly among the elderly. Relevance for Clinical Practice: Nursing management is called upon to integrate information about novel patient characteristics associated with CAPI into clinical practice. Assimilating the insights from this hospital nursing-led study into community nursing will enhance the safety and quality of care for the elderly.

**Keywords:** big data; community-acquired pressure injuries; hospital; indicators; informatics; nursing clinical data; nursing homes

## 1. Introduction

The increase in life expectancy and the expected growth of the elderly population requires nurses to exploit data from various sources and healthcare facilities to improve the quality of care for the elderly in long-term care settings. Nursing informatics, which integrates nursing science with analytical science, can identify patients at risk and manage and communicate data in the evolving healthcare environment [1]. For example, employing predictive algorithms to identify high-risk situations can reduce readmissions and improve elderly patient outcomes [2]. The current study focuses on pressure injuries (PIs).

PIs are localized damage to the skin and/or underlying soft tissue due to intense and/or prolonged pressure, possibly in combination with shearing or from the use of a medical device. They are a frequent complication in patients with comorbidities and are associated with a higher risk of mortality [3]. Indeed, PIs are acknowledged to be one of the most significant signs of mistreatment and insufficient safety in the elderly [4,5]. Importantly, the associated morbidity, mortality, psychological distress, and vast annual expense due to hospital care may be preventable [6–10].

In this context, previous studies have long associated PIs with low-quality care and adverse health outcomes, especially among bedridden patients [5,11]. Several advisory panels have concluded that addressing PIs is a high priority [5,12].

PIs in the home or nursing home are a common consequence of lack of mobility support, insufficient methods of prevention, or poor understanding of skin breakdown and its consequences [5,13]. PIs on admission refer to PIs that are acquired in the community and are identified on hospitalization [14]. Such events are very common [5,12,15], with 77% of patients admitted to the hospitals presenting with community-acquired pressure injuries (CAPIs), even though only 21.4% were receiving homecare services for these PIs prior to their admission [4]. It should be noted that another study reported the prevalence of CAPIs as 7.4%, of which 76.1% were admitted from the community and 23.9% were admitted from long-term care institutions [16]. Still, other reports estimate the prevalence of CAPIs between 3.3% and 11.1% [4,17]. Accumulated data from long-term care, nursing homes, and rehabilitation facilities indicate a value ranging between 0.40 and 0.77 per 1000 adults [16,18]. Most CAPIs (58%) are superficial (Stage 1 or 2), 15% are deep-tissue PIs, and 22% are full-thickness PIs (Stage 3, 4, or unstageable). The most common anatomic locations for PIs are reported to be the ears (29%) and the feet (12%) [18].

A recent meta-analysis described the difficulty of prevention and treatment of PIs, whose continuous impact on clinical outcomes has a considerable cost [19]. This has led to growing efforts to prevent and treat PIs in hospitals. One study described a decision support model for the prevention of CAPIs in veterans with a spinal cord injury [20]. However, while nurses are responsible for the risk assessment of PIs in hospitals where they can use electronic health records to predict issues, the community lacks valid decision support tools for PIs, and there is a paucity of research into the prevention of PIs in the community [21,22]. Similarly, there is little information about CAPI-associated patient characteristics that could be useful for prevention [4,8,13,16,18,19,22–24].

A review of the last decade of literature indicates that the development of CAPIs is associated with a complex interplay of factors, but there remains a lack of understanding of the components and outcomes associated with effective care of CAPIs in the community [25]. Notably, most efforts to prevent PIs relate to events in acute care settings, and no study on CAPIs in the last decade has included socioeconomic factors [25]. There is, therefore, a consensus that developing comprehensive strategies to mitigate the occurrence and impact of CAPIs would be of great use [25]. This nurse-led research project used a big data analysis approach to examine the prevalence of CAPIs and identify predisposing characteristics among elderly patients admitted to hospitals from community nursing homes. To the best of our knowledge, this is the first study to use big data to identify risk factors for CAPIs based on hospital clinical data and nurse assessments.

## 2. Methods

### 2.1. Study Design

This was a retrospective study of elderly hospitalized adults discharged from internal medicine wards. Data were collected from electronic medical records from various departments in two general Israeli medical centers (900 and 350 beds) over 3 years (from

1 January 2016 through to 31 December 2018). The data were anonymized to satisfy regulations protecting patient privacy and to reduce the ethical challenges, but this made it impossible to analyze CAPI by socioeconomic status [26]. Patients with a comorbidity known to be associated with the indicated diagnosis (e.g., metastatic cancer) were excluded. The database of hospital records provided a diverse and large collection of mostly structured patient clinical data, including prior disease information, blood test results, descriptions of procedures, and patients' assessment by nurses upon admission.

### 2.2. Study Variables

A dataset was created for this study using a predetermined code for PIs to identify patients with CAPIs at admission. Patients arrived at the medical centers from community nursing facilities or nursing homes. The presence of CAPIs was ascertained by the first skin assessment after hospitalization from the emergency department and/or within 36 h of admission to an internal medicine department. While the standard timeframe for CAPI identification is 24 h, preliminary analysis revealed no significant differences in the results after 24 or 36 h post-admission. Therefore, following expert consultation, the assessment window was extended to 36 h to reflect actual clinical practice while maintaining assessment validity.

Potential explanatory variables included the following: demographics (gender and age); clinical indicators (oxygen use, intestinal function, sensory impairments, e.g., heat and pain perception) and vital signs; laboratory results (albumin levels, red cell distribution width (RDW), and systolic blood pressure).

Patients readmitted within seven days of discharge ($n$ = 2831, 6.3%) were excluded to avoid confounding hospital-acquired pressure injuries with CAPIs. This exclusion criterion was implemented because patients with recent hospitalizations have an altered risk profile due to their recent exposure to the hospital environment, and any pressure injuries identified upon readmission may have originated during their previous hospital stay rather than in the community setting.

Additionally, incomplete skin assessments (46.6% of records) were excluded. Comparisons of included and excluded cases showed no significant differences in demographic or clinical characteristics, suggesting random missingness. Due to the critical nature of the skin assessment data, imputation was not applied.

We avoided imputation because the skin assessment data were considered crucial to the primary outcome measure. Potential selection bias was examined by comparing the demographic and clinical characteristics (age, gender, and admission indicators) of the included and excluded cases.

### 2.3. Data Analysis

This study employed state-of-the-art big data analysis of patients with CAPIs upon admission to the hospitals and during their hospitalization in internal medicine, cardiology, hematology, and oncology departments. Data were retrieved and then organized and coded by data engineers to a data cloud dedicated to this study. They were then analyzed by data scientists to identify indicators for CAPIs that could be used for prevention and early treatment in the community, thereby avoiding hospitalization.

Categorical variables are presented by frequencies and percentages, with medians and interquartile ranges (IQR) used for continuous variables. Chi-squared tests were conducted on categorical variables, with Kruskal–Wallis tests used for continuous variables. Logistic regression was used to calculate the unadjusted odds ratio (OR), with a 95% confidence interval (CI) for CAPIs. A multivariate model for estimating the adjusted ORs of the clinical variables for CAPIs was assessed using logistic regression with a 95% CI. Data were collected and analyzed using Python software (version 3.6) and the Stats Models package (version 0.12.1). The categorical variables were recorded using dummy coding since one category for each was used as a reference category. An example is the binary categorical variables such as "mobility," where 0 stands for "no impairment" and 1 implies "impairment." For polytomous variables with greater than two categories, their levels are contrasted in the logistic regression model.

This ensured the proper inclusion and interpretation of these variables in the multivariate model.

Multivariate logistic regression was used to assess the relationship between the explanatory variables and CAPIs. Variables with clinical relevance and statistical significance in univariate analysis were included in the final model. Adjusted odds ratios (ORs) with 95% confidence intervals (CIs) quantified the strength of associations. The final model included pseudo-$R^2$ (0.3244) as a measure of goodness-of-fit. Pseudo-$R^2$ is used in logistic regression to assess the explanatory power of the model. While it is not directly comparable to $R^2$ in linear regression, it provides a relative measure of how well the model explains the variability in the outcome. Analyses were performed using Python (version 3.6) and the StatsModels library (version 0.12.1).

## 3. Findings

A total of 44,495 medical records of hospitalized patients admitted to hospitals in the 3-year period were analyzed. We excluded 2831 (6.3%) for readmissions and 20,745 (46.6%) for lacking full skin assessments. In the process of admission to the emergency department, 2448 (5.5%) patients were diagnosed with CAPIs, of whom 1178 were female (48%) and 1270 male (52%), with an age range between 71 and 80 years. Nearly half (49.8%) of the patients were hospitalized for seven or more days. Table 1 presents the demographics, including gender, age, admission indicators, nursing assessments reported by nurses, vital signs, and the results of lab tests conducted within 36 h of admission.

**Table 1.** Study population.

| Sub Population | Events | % |
|---|---|---|
| Positive Skin Assessment (Within 36 h) | 2448 | 5.5% |
| Negative Skin Assessment (Within 36 h) | 18,471 | 41.5% |
| Readmission | 2831 | 6.3% |
| Missing Skin Assessment | 20,745 | 46.6% |
| Total Basic Population | 44,495 | |

The prevalence of CAPI was analyzed by considering the location, attributes, and degree/stage. Most CAPIs were located in the buttocks (56.9%), followed by the sacrum (11.8%), ankle (10.8%), trochanter (5.1%), and leg (3.9%). Tissue associated with CAPIs was described as necrotic, serotic, bloody, granolithic, epithelial, and infected. The most common grade of CAPIs (41%) was second-degree, with 31% rated as first-degree and 18% as third-degree. Table 2 presents the type, degree, and location of the observed CAPIs.

The results of regression analysis designed to identify indicators of CAPI are presented after adjustment for extreme and missing values. Most variables were categorical, except for individual continuous variables (e.g., age, number of CAPIs). Multivariate logistic regression was used to estimate the adjusted OR of the clinical variables for CAPIs. Table 3 presents variables that were significantly associated with CAPIs.

**Table 2.** Distribution of CAPIs based on assessment at admission ($n$ = 2448).

| Variable | | Missing | * Number of Patients and % |
|---|---|---|---|
| Ulcer area | | 174 | Less than 15 patients |
| | Trochanter | | 126 (5.1) |
| | Ear | | Less than 15 |
| | Abdomen | | Less than 15 |
| | Back | | 15 (0.6) |
| | Chest | | Less than 15 |
| | Arm | | Less than 15 |
| | Foot | | 19 (0.8) |
| | Shoulder | | Less than 15 |
| | Face | | Less than 15 |
| | Genitalia | | Less than 15 |
| | Sacrum | | 290 (11.8) |
| | Buttock | | 1393 (56.9) |
| | Spine | | Less than 15 |
| | Ankle | | 265 (10.8) |
| | Neck | | Less than 15 |
| | Leg | | 96 (3.9) |
| Degree of pressure injury | 1 | 254 | 681 (31.0) |
| | 2 | | 901 (41.1) |
| | 3 | | 396 (18.0) |
| | 4 | | 216 (9.8) |
| Necrotic Tissue | No | | 2253 (92.0) |
| | Yes | | 195 (8.0) |
| Serotic Tissue | No | | 2222 (90.8) |
| | Yes | | 226 (9.2) |
| Bloody Tissue | No | | 2383 (97.3) |
| | Yes | | 65 (2.7) |
| Granolithic Tissue | No | | 2266 (92.6) |
| | Yes | | 182 (7.4) |
| Epithelial Tissue | No | | 1996 (81.5) |
| | Yes | | 452 (18.5) |
| Infected Tissue | No | | 2285 (93.3) |
| | Yes | | 163 (6.7) |

* In big data analysis less than 15 is considered marginal and is not reported.

These results reveal significant variability in the effect sizes of different predictors. For example, mobility exhibited the highest adjusted OR (6.263), indicating a very strong association with CAPIs. Conversely, variables like age and systolic blood pressure had smaller adjusted ORs, suggesting weaker, though still significant, relationships. These findings emphasize the multifactorial nature of CAPIs and highlight actionable areas for intervention, such as improving mobility and monitoring albumin levels in at-risk patients.

**Table 3.** Patient characteristics associated with CAPI on admission.

| Characteristics | Adjusted *OR* | Adjusted *OR CI* | Adjusted *p*-Value | Unadjusted *OR* | Unadjusted *OR CI* |
|---|---|---|---|---|---|
| Age on admission | 1.0102 | [1.01, 1.01] | 0.0000 | 1.039 | [1.04, 1.04] |
| Multi-pharmacy | 1.0132 | [1.01, 1.02] | 0.0001 | 1.0224 | [1.02, 1.03] |
| Albumin level (lab) | 0.9459 | [0.94, 0.95] | 0.0000 | 0.9167 | [0.91, 0.92] |
| Red cell Distribution Width | 1.0623 | [1.04, 1.09] | 0.0000 | 1.1141 | [1.1, 1.13] |
| Systolic blood pressure | 0.9952 | [0.99, 1.0] | 0.0008 | 0.9871 | [0.99, 0.99] |
| Intestinal functions | 1.9262 | [1.62, 2.29] | 0.0000 | 10.1404 | [9.2, 11.17] |
| Eating habits | 1.6759 | [1.41, 1.99] | 0.0000 | 9.0266 | [8.23, 9.9] |
| Mobility | 6.263 | [5.0, 7.84] | 0.0000 | 20.3565 | [17.71, 23.4] |
| Conscious state | 1.1814 | [1.0, 1.39] | 0.0477 | 6.6144 | [5.97, 7.33] |
| Assessment of Senses | 1.8584 | [1.56, 2.21] | 0.0000 | 3.6194 | [3.23, 4.05] |

Notes: Pseudo $R^2 = 0.3244$; First skin assessment within 36 h from admission.

## 4. Discussion

This study used big data to identify risk factors for CAPIs based on hospital clinical data and nurse assessments. The results of this big data study shed light on the characteristics and risks associated with CAPIs among elderly patients who arrived at the hospitals from nursing homes. The findings represent valuable insights that can be used to guide nursing practice in the community and inform future research and implementation strategies. Since CAPIs are often underreported in the community and there is consequently inadequate follow-up [27], our identification of new characteristics and risk factors associated with CAPIs provides an essential foundation for the development of preventive measures in community care [4,8,16,18,21–24]. A recent review of studies on CAPIs published over the last decade indicates that the development of PIs has been associated with a complex interplay of factors, although there remains a lack of understanding of the components associated with PI care in the community [25].

Risk factors previously considered to be associated with CAPIs include older age, impaired mobility, multiple comorbidities, and malnutrition [28,29]. A piezoelectric motion sensor, which provides a movement score based on the mean number of movements per hour, was used to assess patient mobility [30].

Interestingly, our findings identify polypharmacy as a key contributor to CAPIs. Polypharmacy is defined as the use of multiple medicines, which is a common practice in the older population and is associated with multimorbidity and adverse outcomes, including mortality, falls, adverse drug reactions, increased length of stay in hospital, and readmission to hospital soon after discharge [30]. Additional newly revealed contributing factors to CAPIs were poor albumin levels, RDW, systolic blood pressure, and poor intestinal function. Our results also suggest new locations for the development of CAPIs, namely in the buttocks (56.9%), sacrum (11.8%), ankle (10.8%), trochanter (5.1%), and leg (3.9%) (Figure 1). Tissue descriptions associated with CAPIs were necrotic, serotic, bloody, granolithic, epithelial, and infected. This new information can facilitate the ability of nurses to detect and manage PIs in the community.

Our results identify a strong hospital–community linkage, which introduces the potential for data-driven preventive measures and aligns with the principles of nursing informatics, where evidence-based practices are translated from data analysis to improve patient outcomes. Information about patients from nursing homes, gathered during hospital admissions, can enable community nurses to prevent morbidity and complications in elderly patients. The integration of data between hospital and community settings becomes ever more crucial, especially with the trend towards shorter hospitalizations and the provision of more care in the community.

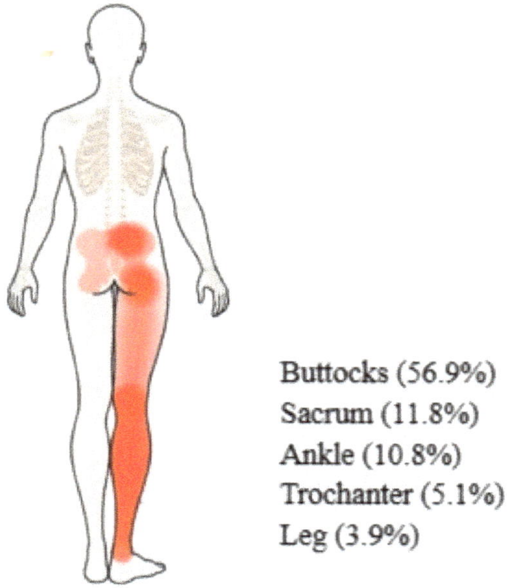


**Figure 1.** CAPI Distribution.

Without targeted efforts to prevent CAPIs, there is a risk of repeated cycles of deterioration and readmission. Our results recommend informing clinical practice in community care based on big data analysis of high-quality evidence from hospital nurses who prioritize the prevention of CAPIs in the elderly. Community settings for the elderly have long been alerted to the need to provide safer care to patients through proactive diagnosis and treatment [30].

### *4.1. Managerial Implications*

The insights from this study support those within the existing literature, such as the report by Friedman et al. [31] that elderly individuals with lower scores for daily activities had the highest rate of CAPIs. The vital role of nurses in preventive care and promoting quality of care makes an essential contribution to the economic and administrative aspects of community healthcare [19]. Nurses, armed with data they record and manage, can integrate effective preventive innovations, thereby enhancing patient safety and overall care quality [32]. The results of our study reinforce the pivotal role of nurses as the primary repository of patient knowledge and data, both in community settings and hospitals [33,34].

Previous studies have introduced various applications (Apps) for the prevention and treatment of PIs in acute care, which classify PIs through image processing on mobile devices [35]. The user uploads a photograph of the PI into the App, and the image is then processed to evaluate the probable stage of the PI based on an implemented algorithm, which then suggests cleaning procedures and provides the recommended treatment for the tissue type [36]. Since PIs are more common at home and in nursing homes where insufficient knowledge may hinder real-time care [4,13], we suggest that it may be useful to transform the informatics presented in this study into an AI-based App for community nursing care of PIs [1,37].

### 4.2. Study Limitation

The big data utilized in this study were obtained from two medical centers (900 and 350 beds, respectively) in Israel, which limits generalizations and calls for repetition. While these centers serve diverse populations and receive referrals from multiple community settings, we acknowledge that patterns of CAPIs may differ in other contexts, particularly in rural areas or smaller healthcare facilities with different resource levels and patient populations. In addition, the centers included in our study are major referral hospitals that may receive more complex cases and thereby affect the observed patterns and severity of CAPIs. Future multi-center studies incorporating a broader range of hospital types and geographical locations would be valuable to validate our findings across different healthcare settings and patient populations.

The exclusion of 46.6% of records due to incomplete skin assessments also represents a potential limitation. While our analysis of baseline characteristics suggests that the missing data was random, we cannot completely rule out selection bias. Future studies should emphasize complete documentation of skin assessments to minimize missing data and should consider employing multiple imputation methods when appropriate.

### 4.3. Conclusions

As health systems endeavor to enhance care quality while managing costs, addressing and preventing CAPIs becomes ever more imperative [23,38]. Nurse managers play a crucial role in promoting awareness of data-intensive analysis and knowledge-based nursing management in both hospital and community settings. The shifting landscape of patient care, with a trend towards shorter hospitalizations and increased community care, emphasizes the need to integrate information seamlessly between these environments. Our study advocates for the development of proactive measures to prevent CAPIs and encourages routine PI assessments in the community. The identification of new characteristics associated with CAPIs provides a foundation for targeted interventions. Nurse managers are encouraged to prioritize the integration of these characteristics into routine assessments, leveraging continuous data quantification for timely identification and prediction of PIs.

Our findings align with those of other studies on PIs in hospitals, thereby emphasizing the value of routinely collecting and assessing data [21]. This approach tasks community nurses with identifying patients at high risk of PIs and provides information for performance improvement. As the healthcare landscape evolves, the insights from this study underscore the pivotal role of data-driven strategies in preventing CAPIs, with the ultimate aim of enhancing patient care, minimizing complications, and optimizing resource utilization in both hospitals and the community [22,39].

**Author Contributions:** Conceptualization, S.S.-T., G.G. and I.K.; methodology, S.S.-T.; software, Data scientist; validation, S.S.-T., G.G. and I.K.; formal analysis, S.S.-T.; investigation, S.S.-T.; data curation, S.S.-T.; writing—original draft preparation, G.G.; writing—review and editing, S.S.-T., G.G. and I.K.; visualization, S.S.-T.; supervision, S.S.-T.; project administration, S.S.-T. All authors have read and agreed to the published version of the manuscript.

**Funding:** This research received no external funding.

**Institutional Review Board Statement:** The study was conducted in accordance with the Declaration of Helsinki, and approved by the Institutional Review Board Hadassah University Medical Center (HMO—0582-17). 10 February 2019.

**Informed Consent Statement:** Patient consent was waived due to Big data study.

**Data Availability Statement:** Restrictions apply to the availability of these data. Data were obtained from Hadassah University Medical Center and are available from the authors with the permission of Hadassah University Medical Center.

**Acknowledgments:** The authors would like to extend their heartfelt gratitude to the Ministry of Health for their invaluable support and collaboration in conducting this study. This research was made possible through the national platform for Big Data research, TIMNA designed to serve the health system, academia, and industry by facilitating groundbreaking research in the field of health. We are especially grateful to the following individuals for their significant contributions: Meytal Avgil Tsadok, Barak Shukrun, Dror Ben Moshe, Shahar Soudry and Eli Melul. Their expertise, dedication, and unwavering support were instrumental in the successful completion of this study.

**Conflicts of Interest:** The authors declare no conflict of interests.

## References

1. Peltonen, L.M.; Pruinelli, L.; Ronquillo, C.; Nibber, R.; Peresmitre, E.L.; Block, L.; Deforest, H.; Lewis, A.; Alhuwail, D.; Ali, S.; et al. The current state of Nursing Informatics—An international cross-sectional survey. *Finn. J. ehealth eWelfare* **2019**, *11*, 220–231. [CrossRef]
2. Flaks-Manov, N.; Topaz, M.; Hoshen, M.; Balicer, R.D.; Shadmi, E. Identifying patients at highest-risk: The best timing to apply a readmission predictive model. *BMC Med. Inform. Decis. Mak.* **2019**, *19*, 118. [CrossRef] [PubMed]
3. Martin-Loeches, I.; Rose, L.; Afonso, E.; Benbenishty, J.; Blackwood, B.; Boulanger, C.; Calvino-Gunther, S.; Chaboyer, W.; Coyer, F.; Llaurado-Serra, M.; et al. Epidemiology and outcome of pressure injuries in critically ill patients with chronic obstructive pulmonary disease: A propensity score adjusted analysis. *Int. J. Nurs. Stud.* **2022**, *129*, 104222. [CrossRef] [PubMed]
4. Corbett, L.Q.; Funk, M.; Fortunato, G.; O'Sullivan, D.M. Pressure injury in a community population: A descriptive study. *J. Wound Ostomy Cont. Nurs.* **2017**, *44*, 221–227. [CrossRef]
5. Haesler, E.; Swanson, T.; Ousey, K.; Carville, K. Clinical indicators of wound infection and biofilm: Reaching international consensus. *J. Wound Care* **2019**, *28*, s4–s12. [CrossRef]
6. Coyer, F.; Labeau, S.; Blot, S. Preventing pressure injuries among patients in the intensive care unit: Insights gained. *Intensive Care Med.* **2022**, *48*, 1787–1789. [CrossRef]
7. Fernando-Canavan, L.; Gust, A.; Hsueh, A.; Tran-Duy, A.; Kirk, M.; Brooks, P.; Knight, J. Measuring the economic impact of hospital-acquired complications on an acute health service. *Aust. Health Rev.* **2020**, *45*, 135–142. [CrossRef]
8. Nghiem, S.; Campbell, J.; Walker, R.M.; Byrnes, J.; Chaboyer, W. Pressure injuries in Australian public hospitals: A cost of illness study. *Int. J. Nurs. Stud.* **2022**, *130*, 104191. [CrossRef]
9. Hauck, K.D.; Wang, S.; Vincent, C.; Smith, P.C. Healthy life-years lost and excess bed-days due to 6 patient safety incidents: Empirical evidence from English hospitals. *Med. Care* **2017**, *55*, 125–130. [CrossRef]
10. Kim, J.; Lee, J.Y.; Lee, E. Risk factors for newly acquired pressure ulcer and the impact of nurse staffing on pressure ulcer incidence. *J. Nurs. Manag.* **2022**, *30*, O1–O9. [CrossRef]
11. Yon, Y.; Mikton, C.R.; Gassoumis, Z.D.; Wilber, K.H. Elder abuse prevalence in community settings: A systematic review and meta-analysis. *Lancet Glob. Health* **2017**, *5*, e147–e156. [CrossRef] [PubMed]
12. Haesler, E. Skin care to reduce the risk of pressure injuries. *Wound Pract. Res. J. Aust. Wound Manag. Assoc.* **2018**, *26*, 111–113.
13. Jackson, D.; Durrant, L.; Bishop, E.; Walthall, H.; Betteridge, R.; Gardner, S.; Coulton, W.; Hutchinson, M.; Neville, S.; Davidson, P.M.; et al. Pain associated with pressure injury: A qualitative study of community-based, home-dwelling individuals. *J. Adv. Nurs.* **2017**, *73*, 3061–3069. [CrossRef] [PubMed]
14. Rodgers, K.; Sim, J.; Clifton, R. Systematic review of pressure injury prevalence in Australian and New Zealand hospitals. *Collegian* **2021**, *28*, 310–323. [CrossRef]
15. Haesler, E. Evidence Summary: Pressure Injuries: Preventing medical device related pressure injuries. *Wound Pract. Res. J. Aust. Wound Manag. Assoc.* **2017**, *25*, 214–216.
16. Kirkland-Khyn, H.; Teleten, O.; Joseph, R.; Maguina, P. A Descriptive Study of Hospital-and Community-acquired Pressure Ulcers/Injuries. *Wound Manag. Prev.* **2019**, *65*, 14–19. [CrossRef]
17. Khor, H.M.; Tan, J.; Saedon, N.I.; Kamaruzzaman, S.B.; Chin, A.V.; Poi, P.J.; Tan, M.P. Determinants of mortality among older adults with pressure ulcers. *Arch. Gerontol. Geriatr.* **2014**, *59*, 536–541. [CrossRef]
18. Kayser, S.A.; VanGilder, C.A.; Ayello, E.A.; Lachenbruch, C. Prevalence and analysis of medical device-related pressure injuries: Results from the international pressure ulcer prevalence survey. *Adv. Ski. Wound Care* **2018**, *31*, 276–285. [CrossRef]
19. Walker, R.M.; Gillespie, B.M.; McInnes, E.; Moore, Z.; Eskes, A.M.; Patton, D.; Harbeck, E.L.; White, C.; Scott, I.A.; Chaboyer, W. Prevention and treatment of pressure injuries: A meta-synthesis of Cochrane Reviews. *J. Tissue Viabil.* **2020**, *29*, 227–243. [CrossRef]

20. Burkhart, L.; Skemp, L.; Siddiqui, S.; Bates-Jensen, B. Developing a decision support tool to prevent community-acquired pressure injuries in spinal cord injury in ambulatory care: A nurse-led protocol for mix methods research. *Nurs. Outlook* **2021**, *69*, 127–135. [CrossRef]
21. Elli, C.; Novella, A.; Nobili, A.; Ianes, A.; Pasina, L. Factors associated with a high-risk profile for developing pressure injuries in long-term residents of nursing homes. *Med. Princ. Pract.* **2022**, *31*, 433–438. [CrossRef] [PubMed]
22. Nakagami, G.; Yokota, S.; Kitamura, A.; Takahashi, T.; Morita, K.; Noguchi, H.; Ohe, K.; Sanada, H. Supervised machine learning-based prediction for in-hospital pressure injury development using electronic health records: A retrospective observational cohort study in a university hospital in Japan. *Int. J. Nurs. Stud.* **2021**, *119*, 103932. [CrossRef] [PubMed]
23. Padula, W.V.; Armstrong, D.G.; Pronovost, P.J.; Saria, S. Predicting pressure injury risk in hospitalised patients using machine learning with electronic health records: A US multilevel cohort study. *BMJ Open* **2024**, *14*, e08254024. [CrossRef] [PubMed]
24. Tayyib, N.; Asiri, M.Y.; Danic, S.; Sahi, S.L.; Lasafin, J.; Generale, L.F.; Malubay, A.; Viloria, P.; Palmere, M.G.; Parbo, A.R.; et al. The effectiveness of the SKINCARE bundle in preventing medical-device related pressure injuries in critical care units: A clinical trial. *Adv. Ski. Wound Care* **2021**, *34*, 75–80. [CrossRef] [PubMed]
25. Aloweni, F.; Gunasegaran, N.; Lim, S.H.; Leow, B.W.; Agus, N.; Goh, I.H.; Ang, S.Y. Socio-economic and environmental factors associated with community-acquired pressure injuries: A mixed method study. *J. Tissue Viabil.* **2024**, *33*, 27–42. [CrossRef]
26. Howe, I.I.I.E.G.; Elenberg, F. Ethical challenges posed by big data. *Innov. Clin. Neurosci.* **2020**, *17*, 24.
27. Hamdan, A.; Hamdan-Mansour, A.M. Community versus Hospital Acquired Pressure Injuries: An Assessment of Predisposing Risk Factors. *Malays. J. Med. Health Sci.* **2020**, *16*, 170–176.
28. Masnoon, N.; Shakib, S.; Kalisch-Ellett, L.; Caughey, G.E. What is polypharmacy? A systematic review of definitions. *BMC Geriatr.* **2017**, *17*, 230. [CrossRef]
29. Moda Vitoriano Budri, A.; Moore, Z.; Patton, D.; O'Connor, T.; Nugent, L.; Mc Cann, A.; Avsar, P. Impaired mobility and pressure ulcer development in older adults: Excess movement and too little movement—Two sides of the one coin? *J. Clin. Nurs.* **2020**, *29*, 2927–2944. [CrossRef]
30. Galvão, E.C.; Püschel, V.A. Multimedia application in mobile platform for teaching the measurement of central venous pressure. *Rev. Esc. Enferm. USP* **2012**, *46*, 107–115. [CrossRef]
31. Friedman, L.; Avila, S.; Friedman, D.; Meltzer, W. Association between type of residence and clinical signs of neglect in older adults. *Gerontology* **2019**, *65*, 30–39. [CrossRef] [PubMed]
32. Güler, E.K.; Eşer, İ.; Khorshid, L.; Yücel, Ş.Ç. Nursing diagnoses in elderly residents of a nursing home: A case in Turkey. *Nurs. Outlook* **2012**, *60*, 21–28. [CrossRef] [PubMed]
33. Burton, R.J.; Albur, M.; Eberl, M.; Cuff, S.M. Using artificial intelligence to reduce diagnostic workload without compromising detection of urinary tract infections. *BMC Med. Inform. Decis. Mak.* **2019**, *19*, 171. [CrossRef] [PubMed]
34. Doyle, O.M.; Leavitt, N.; Rigg, J.A. Finding undiagnosed patients with hepatitis C infection: An application of artificial intelligence to patient claims data. *Sci. Rep.* **2020**, *10*, 10521. [CrossRef]
35. Shortliffe, E.H.; Sepúlveda, M.J. Clinical decision support in the era of artificial intelligence. *JAMA* **2018**, *320*, 2199–2200. [CrossRef]
36. Salomé, G.M.; Ferreira, L.M. Developing a mobile app for prevention and treatment of pressure injuries. *Adv. Ski. Wound Care* **2018**, *31*, 1–6. [CrossRef]
37. Benevides, J.L.; Coutinho, J.F.; Pascoal, L.C.; Joventino, E.S.; Martins, M.C.; Gubert, F.D.; Alves, A.M. Development and validation of educational technology for venous ulcer care. *Rev. Esc. Enferm. USP* **2016**, *50*, 0309–0316. [CrossRef]
38. Deckro, J.; Phillips, T.; Davis, A.; Hehr, A.T.; Ochylski, S. Big data in the veterans health administration: A nursing informatics perspective. *J. Nurs. Scholarsh.* **2021**, *53*, 288–295. [CrossRef]
39. Jull, A.; McCall, E.; Chappell, M.; Tobin, S. Measuring hospital-acquired pressure injuries: A surveillance program for monitoring performance improvement and estimating annual prevalence. *Int. J. Nurs. Stud.* **2016**, *58*, 71–79. [CrossRef]

healthcare

MDPI

Article

# Effectiveness of Virtual Reality in Reducing Pain and Stress During Office Hysteroscopy: A Randomized Controlled Trial

**Josep Estadella Tarriel [1,2,*], Josep Perelló Capó [1,2], Marta Simó González [3], Marta Bailón Queiruga [4], Jordi Real Gatius [5,6], Mar Gomis-Pastor [5,6], Diana Marre [7] and Elisa Llurba Olivé [1,2]**

1 Obstetrics & Gynecology Department, Hospital Universitari de la Santa Creu i Sant Pau, 08025 Barcelona, Spain
2 Pediatrics, Obstetrics and Gynecology, and Preventive Medicine and Public Health Department, Universitat Autònoma de Barcelona, 08193 Barcelona, Spain
3 Obstetrics & Gynecology Department, Hospital Universitari Arnau de Vilanova, 25198 Lleida, Spain
4 Obstetrics & Gynecology Department, Hospital Universitari Josep Trueta, 17007 Girona, Spain
5 Digital Health Validation Center, Hospital de la Santa Creu i Sant Pau, Sant Pau Campus Salut Barcelona, 08041 Barcelona, Spain
6 Institut de Recerca Sant Pau (IR SANT PAU), Sant Quintí 77 79, 08041 Barcelona, Spain
7 Department of Social and Cultural Anthropology, Universitat Autònoma de Barcelona, Bellaterra, 08193 Barcelona, Spain
* Correspondence: jestadella@santpau.cat; Tel.: +34-652-455-257

**Abstract: Introduction:** Office hysteroscopy (OH) offers a "see and treat" strategy, enabling most gynecological conditions to be addressed outside the operating room without anesthesia. Despite its convenience, the associated pain and stress remain significant barriers to its widespread success among women. Both pharmacological and non-pharmacological interventions have been explored to mitigate these challenges, albeit with mixed outcomes. **Methods:** This study aimed to evaluate the effectiveness of virtual reality (VR) in reducing pain and stress associated with OH using objective measurements. **Results:** Our findings indicate that VR significantly reduced pain during OH compared to the control group (−1.08, 95%CI; −1.93–0.23, on the Visual Analogue Scale (VAS), $p = 0.013$) and 10 min post-procedure (−1.24, 95%CI; −1.99–0.48, $p = 0.001$), without significant effects on stress-related variables. Stratified analyses further revealed that the efficacy of VR in pain reduction is influenced by individual patient characteristics, with greater effectiveness observed in women with lower baseline stress, premenopausal status and a history of childbirth, regardless of vaginal delivery. **Conclusions:** VR represents a promising strategy for managing OH-associated pain, with its effectiveness largely depending on patient-specific variables.

**Keywords:** office hysteroscopy; virtual reality; pain; anxiety; stress; gynecology; analgesia; trial

## 1. Introduction

Hysteroscopy is a minimally invasive endoscopic technique that enables direct visualization of the uterine cavity and constitutes the gold standard for the diagnosis and treatment of most intrauterine pathologies, such as endometrial polyps, submucosal fibroids or uterine malformations [1]. Improvements in instrumentation and techniques have enabled these procedures to be performed in an office setting without anesthesia [2]. Office hysteroscopy (OH) marked a significant paradigm shift in gynecological interventions [3], notably reducing the costs associated with traditional operating-room procedures [4] and allowing for a "see and treat" approach, enabling therapeutic intervention immediately after observing any pathological condition in the same session [5]. Additionally, OH without anesthesia provides a quick recovery and a faster reincorporation of the patient into normal daily activities. OH has proven highly effective in addressing most gynecological conditions [1,6] with a 90% success rate [7]. Despite its benefits, the primary limitation of OH remains the pain associated with the procedure, reported in many cases as moderate and severe [8]. This significantly affects patient's tolerance and occasionally leads to discontinuation of the technique [9,10].

Several factors may affect patients' tolerance of the OH procedure, such as vaginal delivery history, menopausal status or chronic pain [11–13]. In addition to these factors, anxiety plays a crucial role in influencing the perception of pain and, therefore, in the acceptance of the procedure [14,15]. Several studies have shown that longer waiting times before the procedure [16] and the low expertise of the specialist performing OH [9] can increase patient anxiety and pain perception. Therefore, addressing both factors is essential for improving the overall acceptance and success of the procedure and highlights the need for effective strategies applicable to all patients.

Efforts to alleviate pain and anxiety associated with OH have led to the exploration of several pharmacological strategies, including nonsteroidal anti-inflammatory drugs (NSAIDs), local analgesics, opioids and paracervical blocks [17]. However, given the subjective nature of pain perception [17], there is extensive heterogeneity in the results obtained for each therapeutic approach [5,18–21].

Relatively recent efforts have focused on non-pharmacological strategies for pain reduction. A particularly promising innovation is the use of virtual reality (VR) devices that can recreate three-dimensional (3D) immersive environments. This technology is becoming increasingly accessible in medical settings, demonstrating success in reducing pain and anxiety for patients undergoing treatments like burn wound care, dental procedures, labour, and minor gynecological procedures [22–27]. However, when applied to OH, there are few studies published on this topic, with a low number of patients and inconsistent results. Some studies have highlighted its effectiveness in alleviating discomfort [8,28], while others reported no significant improvements in pain and anxiety levels [29–31]. The overall conclusion of these studies indicates the necessity for further research involving a larger sample size to enhance the generalizability of the findings.

For this reason, in this study, we aimed to assess the efficacy of VR in OH patients, focusing on pain and stress levels and using objective measures to overcome the limitations of previous research. In the following sections, we will describe the materials and methods used in the study, followed by the presentation of the results. Finally, a comprehensive review and comparison of the relevant studies has been conducted and will be presented in detail in the Section 4, providing the necessary context for the interpretation of the results.

## 2. Materials and Methods

### *2.1. Study Design*

An unblinded, randomized, parallel-group and open clinical trial was conducted at two tertiary hospitals (Santa Creu i Sant Pau Hospital. Barcelona, Spain; and Arnau de Vilanova Hospital. Lleida, Spain) between February 2020 and June 2023 (Figure 1). The study was approved by and regulated by the ethics committees of both centres and registered on ClinicalTrials (code NCT04721587).

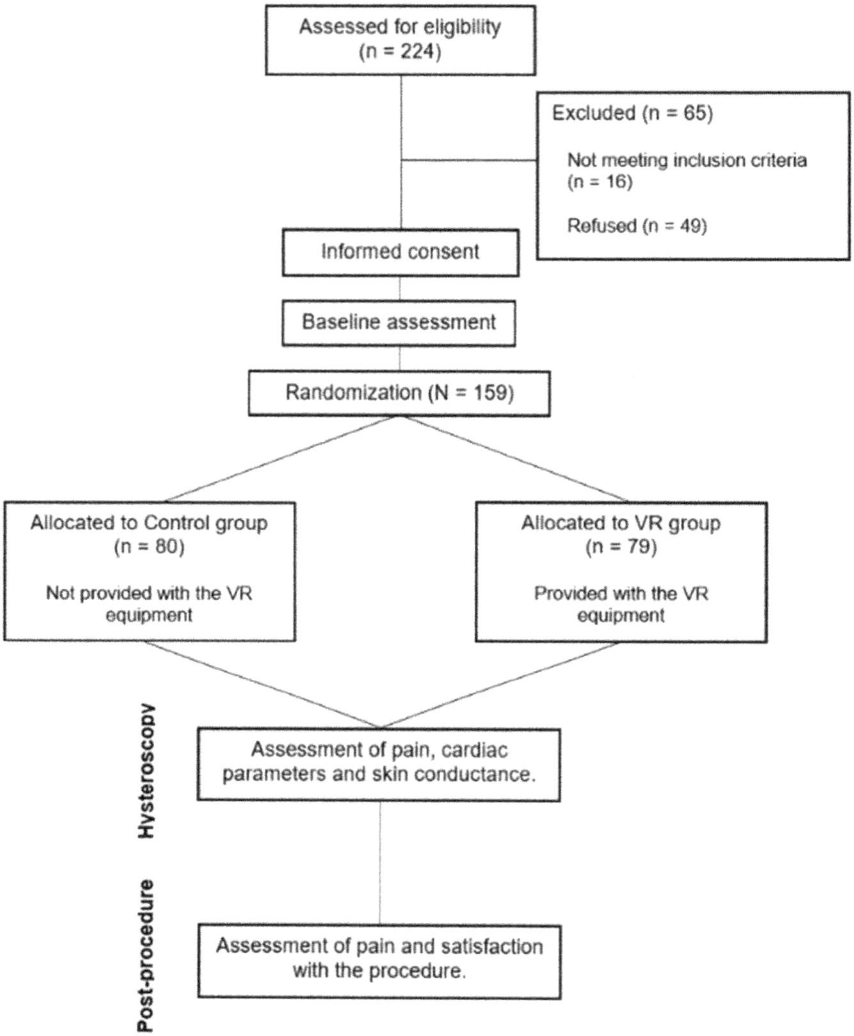


**Figure 1.** CONSORT diagram of the study.

### 2.2. Study Participants and Eligibility Criteria

Patients scheduled for an office hysteroscopy were invited to participate in the study and were selected based on the eligibility criteria: over 18 years of age, able to understand and accept the study procedures (hysteroscopy, 3D VR protocol pre- and during the procedure, physiological measurements of stress- and pain-related parameters, anxiety, pain and satisfaction reports regarding the procedure), and not taking anxiolytic treatment. All participants signed the informed consent and were excluded from the clinical trial if they met one or more of the following exclusion criteria: inability to understand the study's characteristics and procedures; under 18 years of age; pregnant; and having a prior diagnosis of an anxiety disorder (or being under anxiolytic treatment), psychosis, or other severe mental disorders due to the close relationship between anxiety and the perceived level of pain, as well as the modulation of these levels by anxiolytic drug,; additionally, as recommended by VR device manufacturers, we excluded women suffering from vertigo, epilepsy, or an active ear infection or with a diagnosis of arterial hypertension or the presence of cardiovascular diseases as they should not use this technology due to the potential risk of exacerbating their underlying condition.

### 2.3. Recruitment and Randomization Process

After accepting participation in the study and signing the informed consent, participants were randomly allocated a group through a secure computer online system with a randomization scheme based on a permuted block of random block sizes (Clinapsis software v.1 [32], which was applied to assist in the design and management of epidemiological and clinical studies and designed by the Statistics and Methodological support unit of the Research Institute of Santa Creu i Sant Pau Hospital); this ensured equal probability for both interventions. Due to the nature of the study, blinding of patients or healthcare professionals was not feasible; however, the allocation was concealed until randomization. Those patients in the intervention group were equipped with a portable, standalone VR headset PICO G2 (Pico XR, Mountain View, CA). Women allocated to the control group did not receive the VR headsets, and the OH was performed as a routine procedure. The required sample size for this study was determined based on a minimum detectable difference of 1.5 points on the VAS for pain perception, with an assumed standard deviation (SD) of 3 points. A potential rate of non-assessable cases below 10% was considered, alongside a probability of a type I error set at the usual value of 5% (alpha of 0.05), with a minimum required power of 80% (type II error, beta of 0.20). The sample size was calculated as 160 participants; however, due to recruitment constraints related to the COVID-19 pandemic, the final enrollment included 80 patients in the CTL group and 79 in the VR group.

### 2.4. Hysteroscopy Procedure

All procedures were performed in an office setting according to the centres' standard clinical practice. The procedures were performed by four experienced consultant gynecologists (JE, MB, MS, JP). Hysteroscopic instrumentation (scissors and graspers, tissue removal devices, bioplar electrodes) was selected by the facultative based on patient's pathology and the specific procedure required, following clinical criteria. The different hysteroscopes available were 5.0 mm (Truclear 5C) or 4.3 mm (Bettochi) rigid hysteroscopes. Hysteroscopy was performed using a vaginoscopic approach (without speculum or cervical tenaculum), with 0.9% saline solution used as a distension medium with pressures ranging 80–100 mmHg. Thirty minutes before the hysteroscopy, all the participants were administered a single 600 mg dose of Ibuprofen and a single 2.5 mg dose of Diazepam, as per routine clinical practice. No additional local anesthesia or recovery analgesia was administered beyond the standard protocol.

### 2.5. VR Intervention

Patients allocated to the intervention group underwent OH as stated above, with the addition of a VR experience. VR environments were provided by a portable, standalone VR headset PICO G2 (Pico XR, Mountain View, CA, USA), with a head-mounted display with built-in audio speakers. Prior to the hysteroscopy procedure, patients in the VR group viewed a 7 min conscious and guided relaxation "body-scan" procedure, a recognized relaxation technique in mindfulness and meditation supported by scientific evidence [33] (environment developed by XRHealth (R)). Once the OH procedure began, a different scenario was displayed with patients immersed in a distracting 3D environment called "Under the Sea", representing a videogame-like environment where patients were asked to look for specific sea life (environment developed by XRHealth (R)). Participants were required to keep the VR device in place but could remove it if they experienced discomfort or any adverse effects. All equipment underwent proper cleaning with wipes before and after each procedure.

### 2.6. Outcomes and Measurements

The primary outcome measures were patient-reported pain scores during the procedure and 10 min after completion, measured using a Visual Analogue Scale (VAS) ranging from 0 to 10, where 0 represented "Absence of pain" and 10 "The worst pain conceivable", which is a validated scale that is easy to use and able to detect significant changes [34]. The baseline characteristics of the participants were compiled and included the following: age, pre or postmenopausal stage, pregnancy history, pre-hysteroscopy State-Trait Anxiety Inventory (STAI) state (STAI-S) and trait (STAIT-T) scores, cervical and endometrial preparation for the procedure, diagnosis and the protocol carried out in the patient.

Secondary outcomes included objective parameters related to pain and anxiety (heart rate, blood pressure, sweating) before, during, and after the hysteroscopic procedure. To collect these data, all participants underwent cardiac parameter monitoring before and after the procedure using a validated blood pressure monitor (OMRON M2 Plus, OMRON, Kyoto, Japan). Additionally, they were equipped with a Fitbit Charge 3 device (Fitbit Inc., San Francisco, CA, USA) to measure average heart rate and an Esense Skin Response device (Mindfield Biosystems, Gronau, Germany) to evaluate sweating through increases in skin conductance, since changes in these parameters have been defined as stress indicators [35–38].

Before the procedure, the participants' anxiety status was evaluated using the validated STAI, a psychological tool divided into two questionnaires [39]. The STAI-S questionnaire defines the patient's anxiety at a specific moment, describing the current emotional state. On the other hand, the STAIT-T questionnaire defines anxiety as a personality trait, describing the patient's tendency to experience anxiety in diverse situations over time. Each questionnaire includes 20 statements, with participants indicating their level of agreement on a scale from 0 to 3, where 0 represents "Total disagreement" and 3 indicates "Total agreement". The total sum of the items was calculated and ranged between 0 and 60, with relaxation-related items scoring in reverse. A threshold STAI score of 24 was established to classify patients with normal or high anxiety status/trait. This threshold corresponds to the average of Spanish women and also p50 of the STAI-T distribution [40].

After the process, all participants completed a final questionnaire assessing their experience with the hysteroscopic procedure and a separate questionnaire specifically related to using the VR device and the environments displayed to evaluate patient satisfaction, with this strategy as a potential alternative for reducing gynecological pain and discomfort associated with OH.

### 2.7. Statistical Analysis

Quantitative measures were summarized using the mean and standard deviation (SD), while qualitative measures were described using frequencies and percentages. The main analysis focused on comparing quantitative outcomes between study groups using an unpaired Student's *t*-test. The *t*-test was applied under the assumption of independence of observations and heteroscedasticity; therefore, the variance was estimated using the Welch (or Satterthwaite) approximation. The analyses were performed using the compareGroups R package (v.4.8.0) [41]. The effect size was computed using Cohen's d approach.

The same approach was performed by stratifying the data based on the individual characteristics of the participants to assess the impact of VR intervention in specific profiles. Stratification factors included baseline STAI-T score (under or over 24 points), menopausal status (premenopausal or postmenopausal), pregnancy history (parous or non-parous) and vaginal or non-vaginal delivery in childbirth. A complete case analysis was conducted, excluding missing values from each analysis by removing data from participants with incomplete information. A $p$-value of <0.05 was considered statistically significant, and 95% confidence intervals were applied without accounting for multiple testing corrections. Data management and statistical analyses were performed using the R software package (v.4.3.0) [42].

## 3. Results

### *3.1. Baseline Characteristics of the Study Groups*

No baseline differences were observed between groups regarding clinical variables, anxiety or stress levels of the participants. Both groups also presented similar distributions in the diagnosis of the participants and the procedures performed (Table 1).

**Table 1.** Baseline characteristics of the study population.

| Variable | CTL ($n$ = 80) | VR ($n$ = 79) |
|---|---|---|
| Age, mean years (SD) | 45.6 (9.9) | 43.3 (10) |
| Menopause, $n$ (%): | | |
| Premenopause | 57 (71.20) | 63 (79.70) |
| Postmenopause | 23 (28.70) | 16 (20.30) |
| Pregnancy history, $n$ (%): | | |
| Nulliparous | 32 (40) | 27 (34.20) |
| Parous | 48 (60) | 52 (65.80) |
| Initial STAI-T Score, mean (SD) | 16.50 (8.65) | 18.10 (7.34) |
| Initial STAI-S Score, mean (SD) | 18.30 (9.69) | 19.20 (9.85) |
| Cervical preparation, $n$ (%): | | |
| No | 72 (90) | 72 (91.10) |
| Yes | 8 (10) | 7 (8.86) |
| Endometrial preparation, $n$ (%): | | |
| No | 73 (91.20) | 66 (83.50) |
| Yes | 7 (8.75) | 13 (16.50) |
| Diagnosis, $n$ (%): | | |
| Normality | 10 (12.50) | 13 (16.50) |
| Endometrial Polyp | 44 (55) | 39 (49.40) |
| Fibroid | 9 (11.20) | 8 (10.10) |
| Retention of IUD | 7 (8.75) | 9 (11.40) |
| RPOC | 3 (3.75) | 4 (5.06) |
| Intrauterine adhesions | 2 (2.50) | 2 (2.53) |
| Others | 5 (6.25) | 4 (5.06) |
| Procedure, $n$ (%): | | |
| None | 10 (12.50) | 14 (17.70) |
| Targeted Biopsy | 14 (17.50) | 12 (15.20) |
| Polypectomy | 45 (56.20) | 39 (49.40) |
| RPOC removal | 3 (3.75) | 4 (5.06) |
| IUD removal | 7 (8.75) | 8 (10.10) |
| Oppium technique | 1 (1.25) | 2 (2.53) |

Note: CTL, control; VR, virtual reality; STAI, State-Trait Anxiety Inventory; IUD, Intrauterine Device; RPOC, Retained products of conception; SD, standard deviation.

### *3.2. Effects of VR on Pain Perception and Stress*

Reported pain during and after the procedure is shown in Table 2 and Figure 2 (effect sizes described in Table S1). Patients in the VR group reported significantly lower pain levels compared to the control group during hysteroscopy (4.51 vs. 5.59 on the VAS, $p$-value = 0.013). These differences became even more pronounced 10 min post-procedure, with the VR group reporting significantly lower pain levels (2.09 vs. 3.33, $p$-value = 0.001).

**Table 2.** Comparison of pain- and stress-related variables.

| Variable | Control ($n$ = 80) | VR ($n$ = 79) | $p$-Value | Mean Diff (CI) |
|---|---|---|---|---|
| Pain intra, mean VAS (SD) | 5.59 (2.50) | 4.51 (2.90) | 0.013 | −1.08 (−1.93–−0.23) |
| Pain post, mean VAS (SD) | 3.33 (2.57) | 2.09 (2.24) | 0.001 | −1.24 (−1.99–−0.48) |
| Basal Heart Rate, mean bpm (SD) | 74.70 (8.17) | 76.60 (9.69) | 0.170 | 1.97 (−0.86–4.81) |
| Final Heart Rate, mean bpm (SD) | 70.10 (9.41) | 73.60 (10.50) | 0.027 | −3.56 (0.41–6.71) |
| Basal Systolic Blood Pressure, mean mmHg (SD) | 125 (17.90) | 124 (16.20) | 0.641 | −1.27 (−6.65–4.10) |
| Final Systolic Blood Pressure, mean mmHg (SD) | 119 (17.90) | 120 (15.60) | 0.759 | 0.82 (−4.47–6.12) |
| Basal Diastolic Blood Pressure, mean mmHg (SD) | 79.10 (12.40) | 78 (11.10) | 0.572 | −1.06 (−4.77–2.64) |
| Final Diastolic Blood Pressure, mean mmHg (SD) | 79.20 (10.70) | 79.40 (12.30) | 0.951 | 0.11 (−3.52–3.75) |
| Maximum Skin Conductance, mean µS (SD) | 2485 (2667) | 2264 (1866) | 0.562 | −221.24 (−973.44–530.966) |
| Increase in Skin Conductance, mean µS (SD) | 1367 (1921) | 1070 (1139) | 0.257 | −297.16 (−813.79–219.48) |

Note: CTL, control; CI, confidence interval; bpm, beats per minute; Mean diff, mean difference; VR, virtual reality; VAS, Visual Analogue Scale; SD, standard deviation.

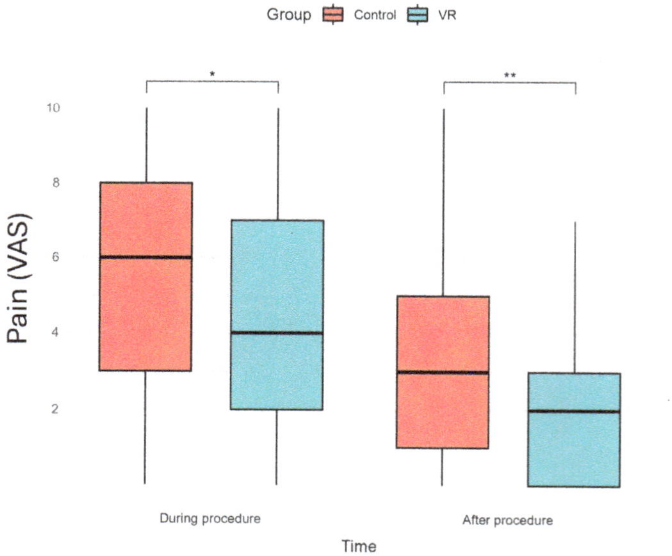


**Figure 2.** Boxplot of VR effects on perceived pain by patients in the control (orange) and VR group (green) during and after office hysteroscopy ($n$ = 179). (* $p < 0.05$ ** $p < 0.001$). Note: VR, virtual reality; VAS, Visual Analogue Scale. The box represents the range in which the middle 50% of all values lie, with the lower end indicating the 1st quartile and the upper end the 3rd quartile.

Both groups exhibited comparable basal systolic and diastolic arterial pressure before hysteroscopy, which remained unaltered after the procedure without significant differences between the control and the VR groups (Table 2). Skin conductance measurements in the control group were comparable to those in the VR group, with VR not influencing this parameter. However, while the baseline heart rate (HR) was identical in both groups, a significant increase was observed in the VR group following the hysteroscopy (70.1 vs. 73.6, $p$-value = 0.027) (Table 2).

### 3.3. STAI-T Stratification

In total, 120 patients (63 from the control group and 57 from the VR group) scored below 24 points, while the remaining 38 (17 from the control and 21 from the VR groups) scored equal to or higher than 24. One patient did not complete the questionnaire properly and was excluded from this analysis. In the low-anxiety group, pain perception during the procedure was significantly lower in the VR group compared to the control group (5.56 vs. 4.56, $p$-value = 0.052), and these differences persisted 10 min post-intervention (3.29 vs. 1.95, $p$-value = 0.002) (Figure 3A, Table S2). Additionally, the final HR was higher in the VR group than in the control group (69.9 vs. 73.8, $p$-value = 0.047). No significant differences were observed between groups in arterial pressure or skin conductance. In contrast, participants with high anxiety scores showed no significant differences in pain perception or objective parameters between the control and VR groups, either during the procedure or 10 min after its completion.

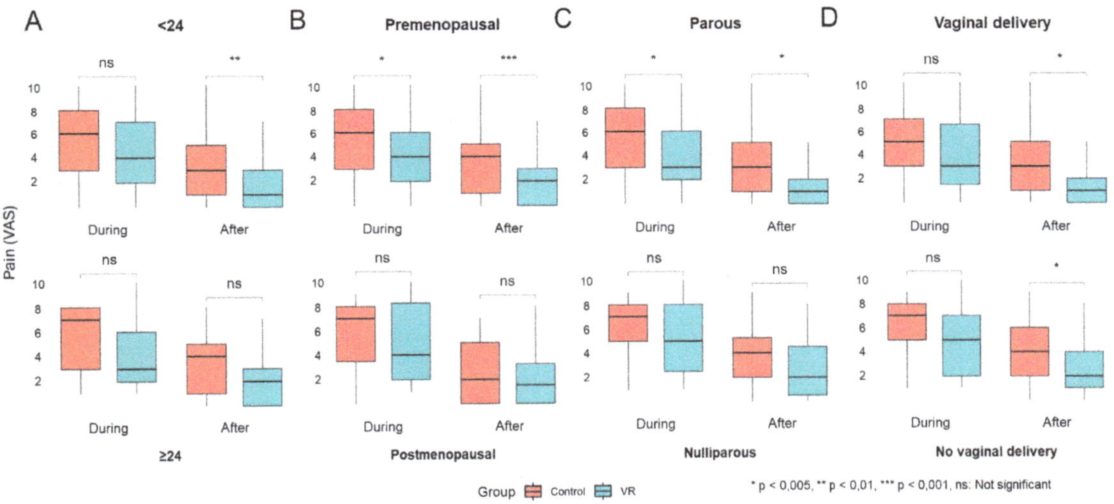


**Figure 3.** Boxplot of VR effects on perceived pain by patients in the control (orange) and VR group (green) during and after office hysteroscopy across stratified subgroups. (**A**) According to STAI-T score < 24 (up) or ≥24 (down). (**B**) According to the menopausal stage, premenopausal (up) or postmenopausal (down). (**C**) According to pregnancy history, parous (up) or nulliparous (down). (**D**) According to vaginal delivery, yes (up) or no (down). (* $p < 0.05$ ** $p < 0.01$ *** $p < 0.001$ ns: not significant.) Note: VR, virtual reality.

### 3.4. Menopausal Stage Stratification

VR significantly reduced pain perception in premenopausal women (5.58 vs. 4.37, $p$-value = 0.012) but did not affect postmenopausal patients (Figure 3B, Table S3). These differences persisted in pain perceived after the procedure (3.63 vs. 2.05, $p$-value < 0.001), while these changes were not statistically significant in postmenopausal women. According to menopausal stratification, cardiac and skin conductance parameters remained unaffected.

### 3.5. Pregnancy History Stratification

A total of 100 patients had a history of pregnancy (parous), while 59 were non-parous (Figure 3C, Table S4). In parous women, VR significantly reduced pain during the procedure (5.29 vs. 4.08, $p$-value = 0.028). This effect was not observed in non-parous women. The differences persisted post-procedure, with parous women continuing to report lower pain perception levels when submitted to VR (3.04 vs. 1.79, *p*-value = 0.01), while no significant changes were observed in non-parous women. Additionally, VR significantly increased HR in parous women (70.2 vs. 74.8, *p*-value = 0.019). No differences were observed in other parameters of pregnancy history stratification.

### 3.6. Vaginal Delivery Stratification

Eighty-three women had a history of vaginal delivery, and seventy-six women had no pregnancy history or the delivery route was through cesarian section (no vaginal delivery). Unlike previous stratifications, no significant differences were observed in pain perception during the hysteroscopy between the control and VR groups, regardless of vaginal delivery history. However, a non-significant trend was observed in the no vaginal delivery subpopulation (6.08 vs. 4.94, *p*-value = 0.059) (Figure 3D, Table S5). Nevertheless, VR significantly reduced pain perception post-procedure in both groups (2.83 vs. 1.65, *p*-value = 0.027 for vaginal delivery and 3.83 vs. 2.61, *p*-value = 0.031 for non-vaginal delivery). The HR averages were comparable across both groups, and no significant differences were identified in other cardiac parameters or in skin conductance.

### 3.7. Patient Satisfaction Regarding the Hysteroscopic Procedure and the Use of VR

No difference regarding overall procedure satisfaction, intimacy level, quality of the information about the procedure or satisfaction with the duration of intervention was observed between groups (Table 3). Although not statistically significant, 27 patients in the control group (38.8%) and 16 in the intervention group (20,3%) experienced nausea or dizziness at some point during the procedure.

**Table 3.** Patient's satisfaction with the procedure.

| Variable | CTL (*n* = 80) | VR (*n* = 79) |
|---|---|---|
| Overall satisfaction with the procedure, *n* (%) | | |
| Very satisfied | 71 (88.80) | 73 (92.40) |
| Somewhat satisfied | 7 (8.80) | 5 (6.30) |
| Little satisfied | 0 (0) | 0 (0) |
| Somewhat dissatisfied | 1 (1.30) | 0 (0) |
| Very dissatisfied | 1 (1.30) | 1 (1.30) |
| Assessment of nurse's attendance, *n* (%) | | |
| Very kind | 77 (96.30) | 77 (97.50) |
| Relatively kind | 3 (3.80) | 2 (2.50) |
| Neutral | 0 (0) | 0 (0) |
| Relatively unkind | 0 (0) | 0 (0) |
| Very unkind | 0 (0) | 0 (0) |
| Assessment of gynecologist's attendance, *n* (%) | | |
| Very kind | 79 (98.80) | 76 (96.20) |
| Relatively kind | 1 (1.30) | 3 (3.80) |
| Neutral | 0 (0) | 0 (0) |
| Relatively unkind | 0 (0) | 0 (0) |
| Very unkind | 0 (0) | 0 (0) |
| Level of intimacy during the procedure, *n* (%) | | |
| High | 67 (83.80) | 62 (78.50) |
| Good | 12 (15) | 16 (20.3) |
| Moderate | 1 (1.30) | 1 (1.30) |
| Scarce | 0 (0) | 0 (0) |
| Bad | 0 (0) | 0 (0) |

**Table 3.** *Cont.*

| Variable | CTL (*n* = 80) | VR (*n* = 79) |
|---|---|---|
| Quality level of the information received, *n* (%) | | |
| High | 73 (91.30) | 75 (94.90) |
| Good | 5 (6.30) | 4 (5.10) |
| Moderate | 1 (1.30) | 0 (0) |
| Scarce | 1 (1.30) | 0 (0) |
| Bad | 0 (0) | 0 (0) |
| Duration of the procedure, *n* (%) | | |
| Very acceptable | 68 (85) | 62 (78.50) |
| Slightly acceptable | 3 (3.80) | 6 (7.60) |
| Correct | 6 (7.50) | 11 (13.90) |
| Slightly prolonged | 2 (2.50) | 0 (0) |
| Very prolonged | 1 (1.30) | 0 (0) |
| Presence of nausea or dizziness, *n* (%) | | |
| No | 53 (66.30) | 63 (79.90) |
| In certain moments | 15 (18.80) | 10 (12.70) |
| Slightly | 8 (10) | 6 (7.60) |
| Quite a few | 4 (5) | 0 (0) |
| During all the procedure | 0 (0) | 0 (0) |

Note: CTL, control; VR, virtual reality.

Patient feedback regarding satisfaction with the VR device and the generated 3D environment is listed in Table 4. Among VR users, most participants (72.2%) found the headset very comfortable, while 21.5% described it as relatively comfortable. Only four patients reported medium comfort, and one patient experienced relative uncomfortableness.

**Table 4.** Patients' satisfaction regarding the use of VR devices and environments.

| Variable | Overall (*n* = 79) |
|---|---|
| VR headset comfort, *n* (%) | |
| Very comfortable | 57 (72.20) |
| Relatively comfortable | 17 (21.50) |
| Somewhat comfortable | 4 (5.10) |
| Relatively uncomfortable | 1 (1.30) |
| Very uncomfortable | 0 (0) |
| Quality of the mindfulness 3D environment, *n* (%) | |
| Very good | 46 (58.20) |
| Good | 30 (38) |
| Regular | 2 (2.50) |
| Bad | 1 (1.30) |
| Very bad | 0 (0) |
| Quality of the 3D environment during the procedure, *n* (%) | |
| Very good | 44 (55.70) |
| Good | 27 (34.20) |
| Regular | 7 (8.90) |
| Bad | 1 (1.30) |
| Very bad | 0 (0) |

**Table 4.** *Cont.*

| Variable | Overall (*n* = 79) |
|---|---|
| To what extent would use VR again in other treatments, *n* (%) | |
| Not for sure | 3 (3.80) |
| Probably not | 0 (0) |
| Maybe | 8 (10.10) |
| Probably yes | 24 (30.40) |
| Yes for sure | 44 (55.70) |
| Overall satisfaction with VR experience, *n* (%) | |
| Very satisfied | 55 (69.60) |
| Somewhat satisfied | 20 (25.30) |
| Little satisfied | 2 (2.50) |
| Somewhat dissatisfied | 1 (1.30) |
| Very dissatisfied | 1 (1.30) |
| Overall satisfaction with VR procedure, *n* (%) | |
| Very nice | 55 (69.60) |
| Quite nice | 20 (25.30) |
| Poor | 3 (3.80) |
| Unpleasant | 1 (1.30) |
| Very bad | 0 (0) |

Note: CTL, control; VR, virtual reality; 3D, three-dimensional.

In evaluating the quality of the mindfulness 3D environment, 58.2% of patients rated it as very good and 38% as good, with two reports of regular quality and one case of bad quality. The assessment of the quality of the 3D environments followed a similar trend: 55.7% rated it as very good and 34.2% as good, with seven participants describing it as regular and one as bad.

Overall, the VR experience was highly satisfactory, with 55.7% of users indicating they would definitively use it again and 30.4% considering it likely for future use. Eight participants were undecided, while only three would not consider using it again.

Finally, 69.6% of the patients reported being very satisfied with the overall VR experience, while 25.3% were somewhat satisfied. Only two patients were slightly satisfied; one was somewhat dissatisfied, and another was very dissatisfied.

## 4. Discussion

The present study demonstrates that VR significantly reduces pain associated with OH, both during the procedure and 10 min post-procedure. Furthermore, our findings underscore the importance of individual patient factors. Baseline anxiety and clinical variables such as the menopausal state, the pregnancy history or vaginal delivery birth can significantly influence the effectiveness of this therapeutic approach.

Non-pharmacological interventions like music or hypnosis have recently been used in clinical settings to reduce perceived pain, though with mixed results [43–45]. Nevertheless, VR has emerged as an effective option for alleviating perceived pain during invasive medical procedures. The results of our study demonstrate that VR significantly reduces the pain perceived during and after OH, aligning with previous studies [28]. In a comparable work, Pelazas et al. also reported a decrease in pain levels in patients using VR, although anxiety was not assessed [8]. However, some other contradictory results have been published. Fouks et al. found no benefit of VR on pain during OH, though they emphasized that their procedures were more prolonged, which may account for elevated pain perception [29]. Furthermore, patients were asked about analgesic use, which may have introduced a selection bias. Another study by Sewel et al. reported contradictory outcomes, reporting no benefits of VR on pain perception [39]. This study also involved the operator's discretionary use of extra local anesthetics and analgesics, which may have influenced the observed results. Fouks and Sewel's studies also had fewer participants than ours, a limitation frequently described as crucial in this type of research.

In our work, we observed that the final HR significantly changed with the use of VR. While strategies like music have been shown to decrease HR due to their calming effects [44], VR has exhibited the opposite outcome [29]. This likely stems from the immersive nature of the 3D scenarios, which are often unfamiliar to patients and have a stimulating and excitatory impact that increases their HR [18]. This is consistent with previous findings that report that VR can provoke solid psychophysiological sensations [46,47].

Our findings indicate that the efficacy of VR in reducing pain is associated with some patients' clinical characteristics, specifically their STAI-T score. The results showed that VR significantly reduced pain in patients with an STAI-T score below the cut-off of 24 points (the median for the female Spanish population of the STAI-T score) [40]. This result, although unexpected, supports the idea of VR functioning as a distraction tool. According to the control gate theory [48], pain perception is multimodal and influenced by additional stimuli; thus, high anxiety levels can impair an individual's ability to focus on a distraction, influencing pain perception. Therefore, patients with higher anxiety scores may have more difficulty engaging with or paying attention to the 3D virtual environment, diminishing VR's analgesic effect. High-anxiety individuals often experience intrusive thoughts and attentional interferences, which reduce their capacity to focus on VR as a pain management tool [49]. This suggests that while VR can be effective in patients with lower anxiety, its benefit might be reduced in those with high anxiety.

Secondly, our results showed that VR was associated with a significant decrease in pain reported by premenopausal women, but this significance was not reached in the postmenopausal group. Research indicates that postmenopausal women tend to report higher pain levels during hysteroscopy due to physiological changes associated with menopause, such as increased vaginal dryness and cervical stenosis, restricting hysteroscope access through the cervical canal and increasing pain levels [50]. Given this, it is unsurprising that postmenopausal women often require more anesthetics [51] and also respond better to local analgesics [17]. These physiological factors likely contribute to the moderate but effective pain relief observed with VR in premenopausal women, as this population may not fully benefit from anesthetics but remains susceptible to non-pharmacological interventions like VR due to their relatively lower overall pain. This makes VR a viable alternative for managing pain in premenopausal women, offering an analgesic effect when standard treatments may be insufficient.

A similar conclusion can be drawn from the pregnancy history stratification of our study. The results showed that the use of VR significantly reduced OH-associated pain in women with a pregnancy history. Nulliparous women are less likely to have cervical canal expansion, making the hysteroscopy process more painful [12,52–54]. Their pain levels may interfere with the efficacy of other approaches, but VR has proven effective in reducing pain in this group. Our findings, in line with the existing literature, highlight that women with a history of vaginal delivery generally experience less pain during hysteroscopy due to a naturally more dilated cervical canal. This postulates the pregnancy history of the patients as a crucial factor in determining VR effectiveness [50]. The results strengthen the hypothesis that VR is more effective in populations experiencing lower baseline hysteroscopy pain. In such cases, the subtle but noticeable analgesic effects of VR can be better observed. Nevertheless, additional studies should clarify the clinical relevance of the observed findings.

Our study incorporated skin conductance evaluations during the procedure to measure anxiety and stress in real time. This approach has been validated as a reliable marker of anxiety across different settings [35–37]. However, our results showed no significant differences in skin conductance or the other cardiac parameters measured throughout the procedure. These findings support the hypothesis that pain perception is more closely related to trait anxiety than to state anxiety, as suggested by Kokanali [16]. Previous research has indicated that technologies like VR may help reduce OH-associated anxiety [28,31,55]. However, our analysis is the first to demonstrate with objective parameters that anxiety levels do not fluctuate significantly during the procedure. Instead, it appears that baseline anxiety levels influence how pain is perceived both during and after the procedure, which might explain the conflicting outcomes in the literature regarding anxiety reduction.

This study represents the most comprehensive trial to date evaluating the efficacy of VR in reducing OH-associated pain. Previous research on the topic had smaller sample sizes [8,28–31], leading to inconsistent results and a call for larger trials involving more participants to obtain robust evidence for VR effectiveness [55–57].

Our research also addressed critical points raised by previous works. For instance, it has been proposed that different 3D environments could increase variability [55]. In our study, participants were exposed to the same 3D environment, reducing heterogeneity in the outcomes; however, Pelazas et al. suggested that more significant results could be obtained by selecting a specific 3D reality by the patient. It is hypothesized that adapted 3D experiences, where patients can choose a 3D immersion based on their preferences, can have more significant results. [8]. A comparable strategy was applied in music-based interventions, where different styles were tailored to individual tastes [44]. Our study groups also represented the general population, including patients undergoing a broad spectrum of gynecological procedures instead of focusing on one intervention, a key factor as exposed previously [31].

By stratifying the data according to clinical characteristics, we examined subpopulations more likely to benefit from VR and/or to confirm the consistency of the overall findings. Finally, analyzing anxiety during hysteroscopy remains a complex challenge due to the characteristics of the study. Nevertheless, we have evaluated anxiety levels in real-time for the first time during OH. Our study also adhered to recommendations by Malaris et al., which encouraged the authors to gather patient feedback on the 3D environment used in VR interventions [22]. The results from the final satisfaction questionnaires highlighted that the technique was widely regarded as comfortable and of high quality. Most participants expressed a willingness to use the technology again and showed a high likelihood of recommending it to others, reinforcing VR's feasibility and patient approval for future application in medical settings.

### *Limitations and Strengths of This Study*

This study has certain limitations that should be considered when interpreting the findings. First, the characteristics of the study impede the conduct of a blind trial, which might result in the underreporting of pain by the VR group and overreporting by the control group. Secondly, while we aimed to recruit more participants, the COVID-19 pandemic severely restricted the recruitment. Additionally, this protocol did not incorporate headphones for sound stimulation, which some authors suggest enhances the immersive and distracting qualities of the 3D environment. However, other authors consider that complete isolation can have detrimental effects on pain perception and anxiety levels [31]. Another limitation was the variability in the hysteroscopic equipment used, as different instruments were adapted to patients' needs. Moreover, including various gynecological procedures could contribute to the heterogeneity of results. Another concern is the possible recall bias from patients completing the VAS questionnaire post-procedure. Fouks et al. also highlighted the potential placebo effect of VR on post-procedure pain, suggesting that further analysis is needed to clarify the full impact of VR [29]. Finally, the results obtained from the stratification should be cautiously considered since the separation into unbalanced groups of patients might affect the statistical power of the study.

Despite these limitations, the study has several strengths that contribute to its validity and relevance in clinical settings. First, the use of real-time anxiety measurement through skin conductance represents a novel and objective method for evaluating anxiety during medical procedures. These objective data enhance the reliability of our findings compared to studies relying solely on subjective self-report measures.

Additionally, our large and diverse sample, including patients with a range of gynecological conditions, provides a more comprehensive view of VR's effectiveness in different clinical scenarios. By stratifying the data based on key clinical factors, such as anxiety levels, menopausal status, and pregnancy history, our study offers valuable insights into how individual patient characteristics could influence the effectiveness of VR interventions. These data may help identify specific patient subgroups that may benefit most from VR and individualize the analgesic strategy for OH procedures.

Furthermore, the high patient satisfaction with the VR experience, as indicated by the post-procedure surveys, supports the feasibility and acceptability of VR as a non-pharmacological pain management tool in medical procedures.

## 5. Conclusions

Virtual reality effectively reduces pain associated with OH, and its effectiveness depends on patient-specific variables. The anxiety trait and the gynecological clinical history, as well as the menopausal state, condition the efficacy of VR to decrease the pain associated with hysteroscopy. Further development of VR devices and the environments displayed may be an effective strategy for pain management that is affordable for medical settings.

**Supplementary Materials:** The following supporting material can be downloaded at: https://www.mdpi.com/article/10.3390/healthcare13020131/s1, Table S1. Effect sizes (Cohen's d) for each outcome measure of pain- and stress-related variables; Table S2. Comparative of pain and stress variables according to stratification based on STAI-T results; Table S3. Comparative of pain and stress variables according to stratification based on menopausal stage, Table S4. Comparative of pain and stress variables according to stratification based on pregnancy history; Table S5. Comparative of pain and stress variables according to stratification based on history of vaginal delivery.

**Author Contributions:** Conceptualization, J.E.T., J.P.C., M.S.G. and M.B.Q.; Methodology, J.E.T., J.P.C., M.S.G. and M.B.Q.; Software, J.R.G.; Validation, J.R.G.; Formal Analysis, J.R.G.; Investigation, J.E.T., J.P.C., M.S.G. and M.B.Q.; Resources, J.E.T.; Data Curation, J.E.T.; Writing—Original Draft Preparation, J.E.T. and J.P.C.; Writing—Review and Editing, J.E.T., J.P.C., M.S.G., M.B.Q., J.R.G., M.G.-P., D.M. and E.L.O.; Supervision, J.E.T.; Project Administration, J.E.T.; Funding Acquisition, M.G.-P. All authors have read and agreed to the published version of the manuscript.

**Funding:** Hospital de Sant Pau's Digital Health Validation Center provided funding to assist in the preparation and writing of this manuscript.

**Institutional Review Board Statement:** The study was conducted according to the guidelines of the Declaration of Helsinki and approved by the Ethics Committee of the Institut de Recerca de Hospital de la santa Creu i Sant Pau (Code IIBSP-VIR-2019-75) on 9 October 2019.

**Informed Consent Statement:** Informed consent was obtained from all subjects involved in the study.

**Data Availability Statement:** The datasets presented in this article are not readily available because they belong to medical records.

**Acknowledgments:** We would like to express our sincere gratitude to all those who made this study possible. Special thanks go to Judit Guix, Sara Marín and Elisabet San Agustin for their dedication and invaluable assistance during the research process. But, above all, we would like to thank all the patients who generously participated in the study. We also extend our appreciation to Hospital de Sant Pau's Digital Health Validation Center for their support with the statistical analysis and assistance in the preparation and writing of this manuscript. This work has been carried out as part of the author's doctoral thesis, JET, at the Autonomous University of Barcelona (Spain).

**Conflicts of Interest:** The authors declare no conflicts of interest.

## Abbreviations

The following abbreviations are used in this manuscript:

| | |
|---|---|
| OH | office hysteroscopy |
| STAI | State-Trait Anxiety Inventory |
| RPOC | retained products of conception |
| IUD | Intrauterine Device |
| NSAIDs | nonsteroidal anti-inflammatory drugs |
| VAS | Visual Analogue Scale |
| HR | heart rate |
| VR | virtual reality |
| 3D | three-dimensional |

## References


1. Bosteels, J.; van Wessel, S.; Weyers, S.; Broekmans, F.J.; D'Hooghe, T.M.; Bongers, M.Y.; Mol, B.W.J. Hysteroscopy for treating subfertility associated with suspected major uterine cavity abnormalities. *Cochrane Database Syst. Rev.* **2018**, *12*, CD009461. [CrossRef] [PubMed]
2. Wright, K.N.; Hamilton, K.; Kosturakis, A. An Overview of Office Hysteroscopy. *Curr. Obstet. Gynecol. Rep.* **2024**, *13*, 88–96. [CrossRef]
3. Gimpelson, R.J.; Rappold, H.O. A comparative study between panoramic hysteroscopy with directed biopsies and dilatation and curettage: A review of 276 cases. *Am. J. Obstet. Gynecol.* **1988**, *158*, 489–492. [CrossRef] [PubMed]
4. Bennett, A.; Lepage, C.; Thavorn, K.; Fergusson, D.; Murnaghan, O.; Coyle, D.; Singh, S.S. Effectiveness of Outpatient Versus Operating Room Hysteroscopy for the Diagnosis and Treatment of Uterine Conditions: A Systematic Review and Meta-Analysis. *J. Obstet. Gynaecol. Can.* **2019**, *41*, 930–941. [CrossRef] [PubMed]
5. Salazar, C.A.; Isaacson, K.B. Office Operative Hysteroscopy: An Update. *J. Minim. Invasive Gynecol.* **2018**, *25*, 199–208. [CrossRef] [PubMed]
6. van Dongen, H.; de Kroon, C.D.; Jacobi, C.E.; Trimbos, J.B.; Jansen, F.W. Diagnostic hysteroscopy in abnormal uterine bleeding: A systematic review and meta-analysis. *BJOG* **2007**, *114*, 664–675. [CrossRef]
7. Sardo, A.D.S.; Calagna, G.; Scognamiglio, M.; O'Donovan, P.; Campo, R.; De Wilde, R.L. Prevention of intrauterine post-surgical adhesions in hysteroscopy. A systematic review. *Eur. J. Obstet. Gynecol. Reprod. Biol.* **2016**, *203*, 182–192. [CrossRef] [PubMed]
8. Pelazas-Hernández, J.A.; Varillas-Delgado, D.; González-Casado, T.; Cristóbal-Quevedo, I.; Alonso-Bermejo, A.; Ronchas-Martínez, M.; Cristóbal-García, I. The Effect of Virtual Reality on the Reduction of Pain in Women with an Indication for Outpatient Diagnostic Hysteroscopy: A Randomized Controlled Trial. *J. Clin. Med.* **2023**, *12*, 3645. [CrossRef]
9. Pegoraro, A.; Santos, M.E.; Takamori, J.T.; Carvalho, W.A.P.; Oliveira, R.; Barbosa, C.P.; van Nimwegen, Â. Prevalence and intensity of pain during diagnostic hysteroscopy in women attending an infertility clinic: Analysis of 489 cases. *Einstein* **2020**, *18*, eAO4916. [CrossRef] [PubMed]
10. Paulo, A.A.S.; Solheiro, M.H.R.; Paulo, C.O.S.; Afreixo, V.M.A. What proportion of women refers moderate to severe pain during office hysteroscopy with a mini-hysteroscope? A systematic review and meta-analysis. *Arch. Gynecol. Obstet.* **2016**, *293*, 37–46. [CrossRef]
11. Vitale, S.G.; Caruso, S.; Ciebiera, M.; Török, P.; Tesarik, J.; Vilos, G.A.; Cholkeri-Singh, A.; Gulino, F.A.; Kamath, M.S.; Cianci, A. Management of anxiety and pain perception in women undergoing office hysteroscopy: A systematic review. *Arch. Gynecol. Obstet.* **2020**, *301*, 885–894. [CrossRef] [PubMed]
12. Bettocchi, S.; Nappi, L.; Ceci, O.; Selvaggi, L. What does 'diagnostic hysteroscopy' mean today? The role of the new techniques. *Curr. Opin. Obstet. Gynecol.* **2003**, *15*, 303–308. [CrossRef] [PubMed]
13. Cicinelli, E.; Rossi, A.C.; Marinaccio, M.; Matteo, M.; Saliani, N.; Tinelli, R. Predictive factors for pain experienced at office fluid minihysteroscopy. *J. Minim. Invasive Gynecol.* **2007**, *14*, 485–488. [CrossRef] [PubMed]

14. Gambadauro, P.; Navaratnarajah, R.; Carli, V. Anxiety at outpatient hysteroscopy. *Gynecol. Surg.* **2015**, *12*, 189–196. [CrossRef] [PubMed]
15. Gupta, J.K.; Clark, T.J.; More, S.; Pattison, H. Patient anxiety and experiences associated with an outpatient "one-stop" "see and treat" hysteroscopy clinic. *Surg. Endosc.* **2004**, *18*, 1099–1104. [CrossRef]
16. Kokanali, M.K.; Cavkaytar, S.; Guzel, A.; Topçu, H.O.; Eroğlu, E.; Aksakal, O.; Doğanay, M. Impact of preprocedural anxiety levels on pain perception in patients undergoing office hysteroscopy. *J. Chin. Med. Assoc.* **2014**, *77*, 477–481. [CrossRef] [PubMed]
17. Ahmad, G.; Attarbashi, S.; O'Flynn, H.; Watson, A.J. Pain relief in office gynaecology: A systematic review and meta-analysis. *Eur. J. Obstet. Gynecol. Reprod. Biol.* **2011**, *155*, 3–13. [CrossRef] [PubMed]
18. Ahmad, G.; Saluja, S.; O'Flynn, H.; Sorrentino, A.; Leach, D.; Watson, A. Pain relief for outpatient hysteroscopy. *Cochrane Database Syst. Rev.* **2017**, *10*, Cd007710. [CrossRef]
19. De Silva, P.M.; Mahmud, A.; Smith, P.P.; Clark, T.J. Analgesia for Office Hysteroscopy: A Systematic Review and Meta-analysis. *J. Minim. Invasive Gynecol.* **2020**, *27*, 1034–1047. [CrossRef] [PubMed]
20. Allen, R.H.; Micks, E.; Edelman, A. Pain relief for obstetric and gynecologic ambulatory procedures. *Obstet. Gynecol. Clin. North Am.* **2013**, *40*, 625–645. [CrossRef] [PubMed]
21. Wong, A.Y.; Wong, K.; Tang, L.C. Stepwise pain score analysis of the effect of local lignocaine on outpatient hysteroscopy: A randomized, double-blind, placebo-controlled trial. *Fertil. Steril.* **2000**, *73*, 1234–1237. [CrossRef]
22. Mallari, B.; Spaeth, E.K.; Goh, H.; Boyd, B.S. Virtual reality as an analgesic for acute and chronic pain in adults: A systematic review and meta-analysis. *J. Pain. Res.* **2019**, *12*, 2053–2085. [CrossRef] [PubMed]
23. Malloy, K.M.; Milling, L.S. The effectiveness of virtual reality distraction for pain reduction: A systematic review. *Clin. Psychol. Rev.* **2010**, *30*, 1011–1018. [CrossRef] [PubMed]
24. Li, A.; Montaño, Z.; Chen, V.J.; Gold, J.I. Virtual reality and pain management: Current trends and future directions. *Pain. Manag.* **2011**, *1*, 147–157. [CrossRef] [PubMed]
25. Smith, V.; Warty, R.R.; Sursas, J.A.; Payne, O.; Nair, A.; Krishnan, S.; da Silva Costa, F.; Wallace, E.M.; Vollenhoven, B. The Effectiveness of Virtual Reality in Managing Acute Pain and Anxiety for Medical Inpatients: Systematic Review. *J. Med. Internet Res.* **2020**, *22*, e17980. [CrossRef] [PubMed]
26. Frey, D.P.; Bauer, M.E.; Bell, C.L.; Low, L.K.; Hassett, A.L.; Cassidy, R.B.; Boyer, K.D.; Sharar, S.R. Virtual Reality Analgesia in Labor: The VRAIL Pilot Study-A Preliminary Randomized Controlled Trial Suggesting Benefit of Immersive Virtual Reality Analgesia in Unmedicated Laboring Women. *Anesth. Analg.* **2019**, *128*, e93–e96. [CrossRef] [PubMed]
27. Chan, J.J.I.; Yeam, C.T.; Kee, H.M.; Tan, C.W.; Sultana, R.; Sia, A.T.H.; Sng, B.L. The use of pre-operative virtual reality to reduce anxiety in women undergoing gynecological surgeries: A prospective cohort study. *BMC Anesthesiol.* **2020**, *20*, 261. [CrossRef]
28. Deo, N.; Saeed Khan, K.; Mak, J.; Allotey, J.; Jose Gonzalez Carreras, F.; Fusari, G.; Benn, J. Authors' reply re: Virtual reality for acute pain in outpatient hysteroscopy: A randomised controlled trial. *BJOG* **2021**, *128*, 770. [CrossRef] [PubMed]
29. Fouks, Y.; Kern, G.; Cohen, A.; Reicher, L.; Shapira, Z.; Many, A.; Yogev, Y.; Rattan, G. A virtual reality system for pain and anxiety management during outpatient hysteroscopy—A randomized control trial. *Eur. J. Pain* **2022**, *26*, 600–609. [CrossRef]
30. Brunn, E.; Cheney, M.; Hazen, N.; Morozov, V.; Robinson, J.K. Virtual-Reality Effects on Acute Pain During Office Hysteroscopy: A Randomized Controlled Trial. *J. Gynecol. Surg.* **2022**, *38*, 214–220. [CrossRef]
31. Sewell, T.; Fung, Y.; Al-Kufaishi, A.; Clifford, K.; Quinn, S. Does virtual reality technology reduce pain and anxiety during outpatient hysteroscopy? A randomised controlled trial. *BJOG* **2023**, *130*, 1466–1472. [CrossRef] [PubMed]
32. Clinapsis: Para Compartir Información Clínica. Available online: https://www.clinapsis.com/index.php/auth/login (accessed on 1 December 2024).
33. Ussher, M.; Spatz, A.; Copland, C.; Nicolaou, A.; Cargill, A.; Amini-Tabrizi, N.; McCracken, L.M. Immediate effects of a brief mindfulness-based body scan on patients with chronic pain. *J. Behav. Med.* **2014**, *37*, 127–134. [CrossRef]
34. Delgado, D.A.; Lambert, B.S.; Boutris, N.; McCulloch, P.C.; Robbins, A.B.; Moreno, M.R.; Harris, J.D. Validation of Digital Visual Analog Scale Pain Scoring With a Traditional Paper-based Visual Analog Scale in Adults. *J. Am. Acad. Orthop. Surg. Glob. Res. Rev.* **2018**, *2*, e088. [CrossRef] [PubMed]
35. Memar, M.; Mokaribolhassan, A. Stress level classification using statistical analysis of skin conductance signal while driving. *SN Appl. Sci.* **2021**, *3*, 64. [CrossRef]
36. Bari, D.S.; Aldosky, H.Y.Y.; Tronstad, C.; Martinsen, Ø.G. The correlations among the skin conductance features responding to physiological stress stimuli. *Skin. Res. Technol.* **2021**, *27*, 582–588. [CrossRef] [PubMed]
37. Kyriakou, K.; Resch, B.; Sagl, G.; Petutschnig, A.; Werner, C.; Niederseer, D.; Liedlgruber, M.; Wilhelm, F.H.; Osborne, T.; Pykett, J. Detecting Moments of Stress from Measurements of Wearable Physiological Sensors. *Sensors* **2019**, *19*, 3805. [CrossRef]
38. Sugimine, S.; Saito, S.; Takazawa, T. Normalized skin conductance level could differentiate physical pain stimuli from other sympathetic stimuli. *Sci. Rep.* **2020**, *10*, 10950. [CrossRef]
39. Buela-Casal, G.; Guillén-Riquelme, A. Short form of the Spanish adaptation of the State-Trait Anxiety Inventory. *Int. J. Clin. Health Psychol.* **2017**, *17*, 261–268. [CrossRef]

40. Spielberger, C.D.; Gorsuch, R.L.; Lushene, R.E. Cuestionario de ansiedad estado-rasgo. *Madr. Tea* **1982**, *1*. Available online: https://web.teaediciones.com/Ejemplos/STAI-Manual-Extracto.pdf (accessed on 1 December 2024).
41. Subirana, I.; Sanz, H.; Vila, J. Building Bivariate Tables: The compareGroups Package for R. *J. Stat. Softw.* **2014**, *57*, 1–16. [CrossRef]
42. R Core Team. *A Language and Environment for Statistical Computing*, v.4.8.0.; R Foundation for Statistical Computing: Vienna, Austria, 2022.
43. Deffieux, X.; Gauthier, T.; Menager, N.; Legendre, G.; Agostini, A.; Pierre, F. Hysteroscopy: Guidelines for clinical practice from the French College of Gynaecologists and Obstetricians. *Eur. J. Obstet. Gynecol. Reprod. Biol.* **2014**, *178*, 114–122. [CrossRef] [PubMed]
44. Angioli, R.; Nardone, C.D.C.; Plotti, F.; Cafà, E.V.; Dugo, N.; Damiani, P.; Ricciardi, R.; Linciano, F.; Terranova, C. Use of music to reduce anxiety during office hysteroscopy: Prospective randomized trial. *J. Minim. Invasive Gynecol.* **2014**, *21*, 454–459. [CrossRef] [PubMed]
45. Mak, N.; Reinders, I.M.A.; Slockers, S.A.; Westen, E.; Maas, J.W.M.; Bongers, M.Y. The effect of music in gynaecological office procedures on pain, anxiety and satisfaction: A randomized controlled trial. *Gynecol. Surg.* **2017**, *14*, 14. [CrossRef] [PubMed]
46. Chirico, A.; Ferrise, F.; Cordella, L.; Gaggioli, A. Designing Awe in Virtual Reality: An Experimental Study. *Front. Psychol.* **2017**, *8*, 2351. [CrossRef] [PubMed]
47. Joye, Y.; Bolderdijk, J.W. An exploratory study into the effects of extraordinary nature on emotions, mood, and prosociality. *Front. Psychol.* **2014**, *5*, 1577. [CrossRef] [PubMed]
48. Melzack, R.; Wall, P.D. Pain mechanisms: A new theory. *Science* **1965**, *150*, 971–979. [CrossRef] [PubMed]
49. Areces, D.; Rodríguez, C.; García, T.; Cueli, M.; González-Castro, P. The Influence of State and Trait Anxiety on the Achievement of a Virtual Reality Continuous Performance Test in Children and Adolescents with ADHD Symptoms. *J. Clin. Med.* **2021**, *10*, 2534. [CrossRef] [PubMed]
50. de Carvalho, J.A.; de Amorim, M.M.R.; Costa, A.A.R.; Neto, L.C.A. Pain evaluation in outpatients undergoing diagnostic anesthesia-free hysteroscopy in a teaching hospital: A cohort study. *J. Minim. Invasive Gynecol.* **2007**, *14*, 729–735. [CrossRef]
51. Nagele, F.; O'Connor, H.; Davies, A.; Badawy, A.; Mohamed, H.; Magos, A. 2500 Outpatient diagnostic hysteroscopies. *Obs. Gynecol.* **1996**, *88*, 87–92. [CrossRef]
52. Malu, A.; Patvekar, M.; Kolate, D.; Laxmi, K.D. Ambulatory Hysteroscopy: Evaluating Pain and Determining Factors. *J. Obstet. Gynecol. India* **2023**, *73*, 434–439. [CrossRef] [PubMed]
53. Coimbra, A.C.; Falcão, V.; Pinto, P.; Cavaco-Gomes, J.; Fernandes, A.S.; Martinho, M. Predictive Factors of Tolerance in Office Hysteroscopy—A 3-Year Analysis from a Tertiary Center. *Rev. Bras. De Ginecol. E Obs.* **2023**, *45*, 38–42. [CrossRef] [PubMed]
54. Zayed, S.M.; Elsetohy, K.A.; Zayed, M.; Fouda, U.M. Factors affecting pain experienced during office hysteroscopy. *Middle East Fertil. Soc. J.* **2015**, *20*, 154–158. [CrossRef]
55. Cohen, N.; Nasra, L.A.; Paz, M.; Kaufman, Y.; Lavie, O.; Zilberlicht, A. Pain and anxiety management with virtual reality for office hysteroscopy: Systemic review and meta-analysis. *Arch. Gynecol. Obstet.* **2024**, *309*, 1127–1134. [CrossRef] [PubMed]
56. Baradwan, S.; Alshahrani, M.S.; AlSghan, R.; Alyafi, M.; Elsayed, R.E.; Abdel-Hakam, F.A.; Moustafa, A.A.; Hussien, A.E.; Yahia, O.S.; Shama, A.A.; et al. The effect of virtual reality on pain and anxiety management during outpatient hysteroscopy: A systematic review and meta-analysis of randomized controlled trials. *Arch. Gynecol. Obstet.* **2024**, *309*, 1267–1280. [CrossRef] [PubMed]
57. Vitagliano, A.; Dellino, M.; Favilli, A.; D'Amato, A.; Nicolì, P.; Laganà, A.S.; Noventa, M.; Bochicchio, M.A.; Cicinelli, E.; Damiani, G.R. Patients' Use of Virtual Reality Technology for Pain Reduction during Outpatient Hysteroscopy: A Meta-analysis of Randomized Controlled Trials. *J. Minim. Invasive Gynecol.* **2023**, *30*, 866–876. [CrossRef] [PubMed]

healthcare

MDPI

Article

# Exploring the Impact of Positive Psychology-Based Virtual Music Therapy on Mental Health in Stressed College Students during COVID-19: A Pilot Investigation

Jinwoo Han [1,2], Hyejin Lee [1], Teri Kim [3] and Sangyeol Lee [1,4,*]

1 Department of Public Health, Graduate School, Wonkwang University, Iksan 54538, Republic of Korea; hanjw.stress@gmail.com (J.H.); stcaecil@hanmail.net (H.L.)
2 Department of Arts Therapy, Daegu Catholic University, Gyeongsan 38430, Republic of Korea
3 Division of Health and Sport Science, Dongguk University-WISE, Gyeongju 38066, Republic of Korea; terikim@dongguk.ac.kr
4 Department of Psychiatry, School of Medicine, Wonkwang University, Iksan 54538, Republic of Korea
* Correspondence: psysangyeol@hanmail.net

**Abstract:** This study explored the effectiveness of a virtual music therapy program, based on positive psychotherapy principles, in college students during the COVID-19 pandemic. Twenty-four undergraduate students with partial PTSD were initially assigned to either an experimental group or a control group, with 11 participants in each group by the study's end. The experimental group underwent 15 video sessions of the therapy program, completing one session per weekday over 3 weeks. The program involved worksheets targeting goals aligned with positive psychology, such as positive affect, life meaning, personal strengths, gratitude, hope, and happiness. The activities included writing music autobiographies, creating and analyzing song lyrics, and exploring various music pieces. The effectiveness of the intervention was measured using the 21-item Depression Anxiety Stress Scale and the Korean Version of Positive Psychological Capital (K-PPC) before, immediately after, and 3 weeks post-program. The experimental group showed significant improvements in stress ($F = 5.759$, $p < 0.05$), anxiety ($F = 4.790$, $p < 0.01$), depression ($F = 5.740$, $p < 0.01$), self-efficacy ($F = 3.723$, $p < 0.05$), resilience ($F = 4.739$, $p < 0.05$), and the K-PPC total score ($F = 3.740$, $p < 0.05$) compared with the control group. These improvements were maintained at the 3-week follow-up. The findings suggest that positive psychology-based virtual music therapy can significantly enhance the mental health of highly stressed college students, especially during challenging times such as the COVID-19 pandemic.

**Keywords:** virtual music therapy; positive psychotherapy; mental health; stress reduction; anxiety; depression; self-efficacy; resilience; COVID-19

## 1. Introduction

The global crisis of coronavirus disease 2019 (COVID-19) has had a profound impact on human lives, causing numerous infections and deaths [1]. The uncertainty surrounding the situation and the experience of quarantine have adversely affected people's mental health. During the COVID-19 pandemic, the prevalence rates of various mental health issues, including depression, anxiety, stress, sleep problems, and overall psychological distress, were observed to be higher in the general population [2,3]. Resulting from the COVID-19 situation, individuals were required to develop coping skills to respond to the sudden changes, such as isolation, infection anxiety, employment restrictions, telecommuting, reduced working hours, and economic impacts [4]. Studies have shown that the pandemic has exacerbated existing mental health conditions and triggered new ones across diverse populations. A systematic review reported increased rates of anxiety, depression, and stress-related symptoms, with healthcare workers, young adults, and individuals with pre-existing mental health conditions being particularly vulnerable [5]. The prevalence of insomnia and sleep disturbances surged during the pandemic, further contributing to the overall psychological distress [6]. The economic consequences, including job losses and financial instability, have been identified as key stressors amplifying mental health problems. Frontline healthcare workers experienced significant psychological distress, including burnout and PTSD symptoms, due to prolonged exposure to high-risk environments and the moral dilemmas posed by resource limitations [7]. Furthermore, research suggests that infectious disease outbreaks can induce stress and contribute to post-traumatic stress disorder (PTSD) symptoms not only in directly infected individuals but also in uninfected populations. For example, a study by Brooks et al. explored the psychological impact of quarantine and isolation measures during infectious disease outbreaks, including COVID-19 [8]. They found elevated levels of stress, anxiety, and PTSD symptoms among individuals regardless of their direct infection status. This underscores the broad-reaching psychological effects of infectious disease outbreaks on mental health.

While the COVID-19 pandemic negatively affected mental health across genders, ages, and races, this study specifically targeted college students undergoing a crucial transition from adolescence to young adulthood, marked by a newfound independence. During this phase, they cultivate diverse relationships, pursue academic goals, and reflect on their identities and career paths. However, this period also correlates with an increased prevalence of mental disorders, such as emotional distress, anxiety, and substance use [9]. Changes in educational and employment landscapes have exacerbated challenges related to identity formation, emotional turmoil, and financial strain [10]. Consequently, stress, anxiety, depression, alcohol consumption, and drug use have escalated among college students during the pandemic, underscoring the urgent need for support and intervention [10–12].

To address the mental health challenges among college students, promoting positive factors such as self-efficacy, optimism, hope, and resilience is crucial. Positive psychotherapy, a method rooted in character strengths, emphasizes positive affect [13]. Positive affect, which is a positive factor in personal development and achievement, encompasses inner joy, physical and mental well-being, satisfaction, life balance, and practical aspects that influence human thoughts, emotions, and behavior [14]. Studies have suggested that a higher positive affect is associated with reduced stress, anxiety, and depression, as well as a higher quality of life in college students during the COVID-19 pandemic [15,16]. Positive affect is linked to positive thinking processes, which involve looking at difficult situations in a favorable light and thinking positively about one's own characteristics and current emotional states [17]. Increased positive affect and positive rumination contribute to a clearer emotional awareness, while employing positive affect as a coping strategy leads to a decreased experience of negative affect in daily life events [17]. This suggests that the principles of positive psychotherapy can serve as effective coping strategies for improving mental health.

To foster resilience and well-being amidst the profound mental health challenges wrought by the COVID-19 pandemic, there arises a pressing need for interventions grounded in positive psychotherapy. In particular, positive psychology-based music therapy is an intervention based on the principles of positive psychotherapy developed by Martin Seligman, aiming to improve an individual's positive affect, such as strengths, gratitude, and hope, while fostering a deeper sense of meaning in life and the pursuit of overall happiness [18]. In addition, positive psychology-based therapy recognizes the significance of social connections, where individuals can obtain intellectual and emotional satisfaction in their relationships with others as an essential element for a happy life along with personal growth [19]. Recently, there has been a steady increase in research on positive psychology-based music therapy in various populations, such as infants, children, adolescents, patients, and the older adults [20–22]. By incorporating activities such as singing, playing instruments, listening to music, and writing lyrics, this approach enables clients to comfortably and authentically engage in therapeutic experiences [23]. Through this process, they can cognitively identify their problems, deal with related emotions, and develop new perspectives for applying and solving psychological problems.

Virtual music therapy emerges as a promising avenue for intervention, harnessing the therapeutic potential of music to cultivate positive emotions, enhance coping mechanisms, and facilitate psychological growth [24]. Furthermore, given the pandemic's constraints on face-to-face services and the limited mental health personnel, addressing individual psychological difficulties consistently poses significant challenges [25]. In this context, the digital realm affords unprecedented opportunities for the remote delivery of music therapy interventions, enabling individuals to access therapeutic resources from the confines of their homes.

Recently, the effectiveness of virtual music therapy as a coping strategy for mental health during the COVID-19 pandemic has been reported. For example, clinical staff working with patients with COVID-19 participated in a remote receptive music therapy intervention over a 5-week period and indicated a significant decrease in the intensity of tiredness, sadness, fear, and worry [26]. A study that conducted a 12-day program of home-based music therapy in children with developmental delay reported a significant improvement in children's sleep quality and a reduction in parental distress [26]. However, existing studies on music therapy during the COVID-19 pandemic have certain limitations. These studies typically offered one-on-one personalized therapy sessions, limited experiences to passive listening to music, and primarily focused on clinical populations [26,27]. Consequently, there remains a gap in research regarding the impact of virtual music therapy on addressing the psychological challenges faced by healthy young adults during the pandemic. Furthermore, in the previous studies of music therapy, the main activity has been listening to specific music, which limited participants' cognitive efforts to actively identify and overcome their situation or problem.

Therefore, this study endeavored to address this gap by developing a self-administered virtual music therapy program grounded in positive psychology principles. The aim of the present study was to investigate the program's effects on stress, anxiety, depression, and positive affect in college students during the COVID-19 pandemic. By integrating the principles of positive psychology and music therapy into a digital platform, the study aimed to assess its effectiveness in providing collegiate participants with a comprehensive approach to mental health, empowering individuals to navigate the challenges of the pandemic with resilience and optimism.

## 2. Materials and Methods

### 2.1. Participants

Participants were recruited from four universities located in the J province and one university located in the D metropolitan area in South Korea. To achieve the desired power of the study, calculated using the software G*Power 3.1.9.7, the sample size was determined based on an effect size of 0.50, a significance level of 0.05, and a power of 0.75. The minimum number of participants required was found to be 11 for the experimental group and 11 for the control group, totaling 22 participants. The inclusion criteria for this study included college students aged 20 to 29 years enrolled in a regular undergraduate program during the study period. Participants were required to score higher than 18 points on the Impact of Event Scale-Revised Korean version (IES-R-K), indicating partial post-traumatic stress disorder (PTSD) [28]. Additionally, participants needed to demonstrate the ability to commit to the entire duration of the study, attending all the therapy sessions and completing all the assessments. Applicants were excluded if they had undergone psychiatric treatment in the past, were currently receiving psychiatric treatment, or were undergoing any type of psychological counseling, including music therapy. A total of 45 individuals applied to participate in this study, and after screening with the IES-R-K, 24 participants were confirmed. All of these participants met the remaining inclusion and exclusion criteria for the study and were non-randomly assigned to either the experimental group ($n$ = 13), participating in the positive psychology-based virtual music therapy program, or the control group ($n$ = 11), receiving no treatment. Two participants dropped out of the experimental group during the study, resulting in a final count of 11 participants in both the experimental and control groups (Figure 1). All the participants received a prior explanation of the research, including its purpose, procedures, the positive psychology-based virtual music therapy program, and the expected benefits, and provided written consent. Approval for this study was obtained from the Institutional Review Board for Ethics in Human Research at Wonkwang University (approval no. WKIRB-202102-HR-005). This study's clinical trial has been registered with the Clinical Research Information Service (CRIS) associated with the WHO International Clinical Trials Registry Platform (ICTRP) (registration number: KCT0009532).

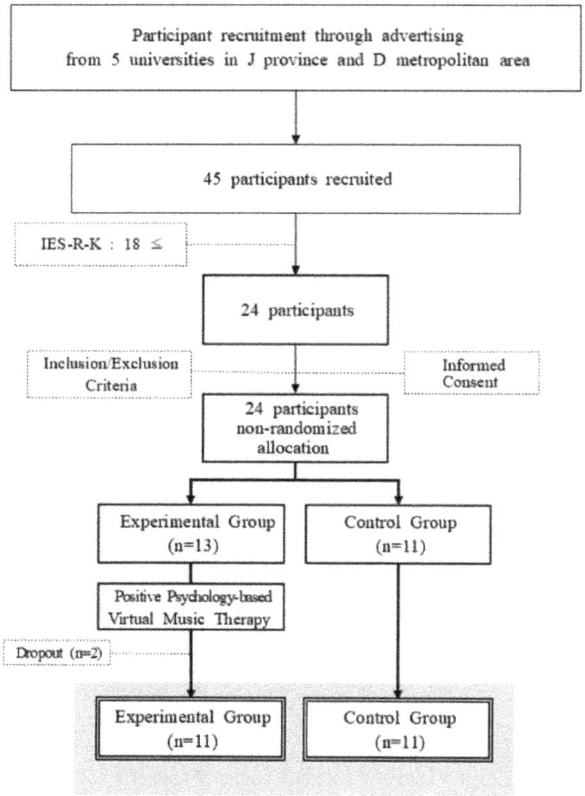


**Figure 1.** CONSORT flow diagram of participant allocation and progression.

### 2.2. *Measures*

#### 2.2.1. Impact of Event Scale-Revised Korean Version (IES-R-K)

The Korean Version of the Impact of Event Scale-Revised (IES-R-K) [24], which was adapted from the original version, was employed as an inclusion criterion [29,30]. This scale consists of 22 items that are restructured into six items for intrusion (e.g., intrusive thoughts, nightmares), six for avoidance (e.g., avoidance of reminders of the traumatic event), five for hyperarousal (e.g., heightened startle response), and five for sleep disturbance and emotional numbing symptoms. This scale uses a 5-point Likert scale ranging from 0 (not at all) to 4 (extremely high). The cutoff points for screening for full PTSD and partial PTSD were 24/25 and 17/18, respectively. The overall Cronbach's $\alpha$ for the items was 0.89.

2.2.2. 21-Item Version of the Depression Anxiety Stress Scale (DASS 21)

To assess changes in depression, anxiety, and stress resulting from participation in the positive psychology-based virtual music therapy program, we used the 21-Item Version of the Depression Anxiety Stress Scale (DASS-21), which was adapted from the original 42-item version [31–33]. The scale consists of three subscales: depression, anxiety, and stress, each with seven items. It utilizes a 4-point Likert scale (0 to 3), with subscale scores obtained by doubling the raw scores. For depression, scores of 0–9 were considered normal and 10–13, 14–20, 21–27, and ≥28 were considered as mild, moderate, severe, and extremely severe depression, respectively. For anxiety, scores of 0–7 were considered normal and 8–9, 10–14, 15–19, and ≥20 were as considered mild, moderate, severe, and extremely severe anxiety. For stress, scores of 0–14 were considered normal and 15–18, 19–25, 26–33, and ≥34 were considered as mild, moderate, severe, and >extremely severe stress. The Cronbach's alpha for the entire scale was 0.926, and for the depression, anxiety, and stress subscales, the Cronbach's alpha values were 0.81, 0.84, and 0.85, respectively.

2.2.3. Korean Version of the Positive Psychological Capital (K-PPC)

We evaluated the changes in positive psychological resources among participants using the Korean Version of Positive Psychological Capital (K-PPC), adapted from the Positive Psychological Capital (PsyCap) [34,35]. Consisting of 18 items and four sub-factors, the scale assesses an individual's positive psychological state, characterized by belief in their ability to pursue goals (hope), confidence in their skills (self-efficacy), capacity to rebound from setbacks (resilience), and an optimistic outlook on future outcomes (optimism), based on a 5-point Likert scale. Overall, Cronbach's $\alpha$ of the scale was 0.93, with the Cronbach's $\alpha$ of each sub-factor as follows: self-efficacy 0.879, optimism 0.822, hope 0.837, and resilience 0.723.

### 2.3. Procedure

Prior to the first session of the positive psychology-based virtual music therapy program, the purpose of the study was explained to the participants in both the experimental and control groups, and informed consent was obtained. Sociodemographic characteristics, IES-R-K, DASS 21, and K-PPC scores were obtained from both groups. The experimental group participants received 15 sessions' worth of video clips of the positive psychology-based virtual music therapy program along with accompanying worksheets at the outset of the research, which they could download onto their personal electronic devices. They were instructed to complete one session per weekday over a 3-week period, granting them autonomy to engage in the program without the constraints of time and space. The DASS 21 and K-PPC scores were reassessed in both groups immediately after the 3-week program concluded, as well as at a 3-week follow-up. This study was conducted in two phases. The first phase took place from 17 February to 20 April 2021, during which the pre, post, and follow-up tests were administered. The second phase occurred from 27 May to 8 July 2021, and followed the same procedure as the first phase, with the pre, post, and follow-up tests conducted during this period.

### 2.4. Intervention: Positive Psychology-Based Virtual Music Therapy

Based on the Positive Psychotherapy Clinical Manual and the items of the DASS 21 and K-PPC, we developed a virtual music therapy program incorporating elements of positive psychology, such as positive affect, meaning of life, personal strengths, gratitude, hope, and happiness [13,18–21]. The validity of the program was confirmed through consultations with a psychiatrist and two music therapists. The program duration was 3 weeks, with sessions held five times per week, totaling 15 sessions. Each session lasted for 20 min, and all sessions were delivered to participants in a pre-recorded video format. Throughout the program, participants were instructed to engage in tasks aligned with the session theme, such as writing down thoughts, emotions, relationships, and reflections, as directed by the therapist in the video.

The structure of each session was as follows: sessions 1–4 focused on the cognitive perspective of self-awareness, sessions 5–8 on the emotional perspective of self-awareness, and sessions 9–15 on exploring the meaning of life and relationships with others. In each session, the consistent elements included the relaxation and presence phase to bring attention to the here and now through breathing and muscle relaxation, the practice and reflection phase to achieve session-specific goals, and finally, the stage of acceptance where the content recognized during the practice and reflection stages is accepted without judgment.

Music served three purposes in this program. First, music was used to facilitate the exploration of cognition, emotion, and relationships, enhancing the overall experience. Second, it was used as a means for the participants to actively express and reflect on their experiences, fostering insight and self-awareness. Finally, music provided enjoyment, aiding in coping with anxiety or depression, and induced mood changes through aesthetic experiences [13].

This program strategically incorporated musical elements including tempo, tonality, melody, musical texture, timbre, and orchestration. Throughout the sessions, a piano melody in a major key with a BPM of 65 and the sound of ocean waves were consistently provided to the participants as part of the theme-related working process. The therapist also provided piano and guitar accompaniments with a steady beat and a root note to create a safe and predictable musical environment. In addition, depending on the theme of each session, third and fourth chords were added during the music appreciation to provide a richer musical experience. In addition to appreciating the music, the program included activities such as music autobiography, creating new lyrics, analyzing song lyrics, and comparing different pieces of music to help participants achieve session-specific goals. The specific structure of the program, including session goals and content based on positive psychotherapy, is detailed in Table 1.

**Table 1.** Structure of the positive psychology-based virtual music therapy program.

| Elements of Positive Psychotherapy | | Positive Psychology-Based Virtual Music Therapy | | |
|---|---|---|---|---|
| **Session** | **Element** | **Theme** | **Focus** | **Contents** |
| 1 | Positive Introduction and Gratitude Journal | Self-awareness and introduction | Cognitive understanding of myself | Write a music autobiography. |
| 2 | Character and Signature Strengths | Finding my strengths | | Select strength keywords and match them with my music autobiography. |
| 3 | Practical Wisdom | Using my strengths | | Write advice for a given story using my strengths. |
| 4 | A Better Version of Me | The future of me who has grown up | | Write a message (lyrics) to my future self to a rap beat. |
| 5 | Open and Closed Memories | Encounter with emotions | Affective understanding of myself | After listening to a song in two different versions (major and minor), discuss the feelings they evoke. |
| 6 | Forgiveness | A tolerant attitude | | Reflect on others' mistakes towards me and my emotions, considering forgiveness. |
| 7 | Maximizing vs. Satisficing | A fulfilling life | | Talk about music that brings me satisfaction and the elements of a fulfilling life. |
| 8 | Gratitude | Expressing gratitude | | Write a letter expressing gratitude to someone I am grateful for. |

**Table 1.** *Cont.*

| Elements of Positive Psychotherapy | | Positive Psychology-Based Virtual Music Therapy | | |
|---|---|---|---|---|
| **Session** | **Element** | **Theme** | **Focus** | **Contents** |
| 9 | Hope and Optimism | Door of Hope | The meaning of life and relationship with others | Discuss experiences of finding hope in despair and my expectations for the future. |
| 10 | Post-traumatic Growth | To grow beyond pain | | Listen to songs about overcoming pain and growth, and reflect on their meanings. |
| 11 | Slowness and Savoring | Speed control and mindfulness | | Listen to music with a slow tempo to discover thoughts and reflect on slowness in life. |
| 12 | Positive Relationships | Positively connected you and me | | Find the strengths of the people around me and write instruments and lyrics for the music. |
| 13 | Positive Communication | Communication with positivity | | Write a positive letter to someone with concerns. |
| 14 | Altruism | Compassion | | Recall misunderstandings with others, past gifts, and associated emotions. |
| 15 | Meaning and Purpose | The meaning and purpose of life | | Write a letter to myself reflecting on aspirations, desired legacy, and how I want to be remembered. |

The elements of positive psychotherapy correspond to the session-based program components outlined in the Positive Psychotherapy Clinician Manual by Tayyab Rashid and Martin Seligman [13]. Based on this framework, the themes, focus, and contents of Positive Psychology-based Virtual Music Therapy were developed through consultation with a psychiatrist and two professional music therapists.

### *2.5. Data Analysis*

A homogeneity test between the experimental and control groups was conducted prior to the study using an independent *t*-test. To analyze the differences in stress, anxiety, depression, and positive psychological capital across the groups (experimental and control) and time points (pre-test, post-test, and follow-up), separate repeated-measures analyses of variance (ANOVAs) were conducted on the DASS 21 subfactors (stress, anxiety, and depression) and the K-PPC subfactors (self-efficacy, optimism, hope, resilience, and total score). All the statistical analyses were performed using SPSS 22.0, and an alpha value of 0.05 was set as the significance level.

## 3. Results

### *3.1. Homogeneity Test of Participant Characteristics*

The homogeneity test results for the sociodemographic characteristics, IES-R-K, DASS 21, and K-PPC variables between each group are presented in Table 2. There were no statistically significant differences between the two groups in terms of the sociodemographic characteristics for any of the items.

**Table 2.** Homogeneity test results for the sociodemographic characteristics and pre-tested outcome measures.

| Variables | | Experimental Group (N = 11) | Control Group (N = 11) | $t/X^2$ | $p$ |
|---|---|---|---|---|---|
| Age (years) | M ± SD | 21.18 ± 1.47 | 21.36 ± 2.25 | −0.224 | 0.825 |
| Sex (N, %) | Male<br>Female | 1 (9.1)<br>10 (90.9) | 1 (9.1)<br>10 (90.9) | 0.000 | 1.000 |
| Academic Year (N, %) | First<br>Second<br>Third<br>Fourth | 0 (0)<br>2 (18.2)<br>4 (36.4)<br>5 (45.4) | 2 (18.2)<br>1 (9.1)<br>1 (9.1)<br>7 (63.6) | 4.467 | 0.215 |
| Religion (N, %) | Christianity<br>Buddhism<br>None | 9 (81.8)<br>0 (0)<br>2 (18.2) | 5 (45.5)<br>1 (9)<br>5 (45.5) | 03.429 | 0.180 |
| Sleeping Time (hour) | M ± SD | 5.96 ± 1.46 | 6.36 ± 1.34 | −0.685 | 0.501 |
| IES-R-K | | 36.55 ± 13.02 | 32.18 ± 6.21 | 1.003 | 0.332 |
| DASS 21 | Stress | 14.00 ± 8.94 | 9.45 ± 6.07 | 1.394 | 0.181 |
| | Anxiety | 8.36 ± 8.66 | 3.64 ± 2.94 | 1.714 | 0.102 |
| | Depression | 9.45 ± 6.46 | 5.09 ± 4.13 | 1.888 | 0.076 |
| K-PPC | Total | 60.73 ± 9.34 | 61.09 ± 9.09 | −0.093 | 0.927 |
| | Self-Efficacy | 16.27 ± 2.97 | 16.64 ± 2.84 | −0.294 | 0.772 |
| | Optimism | 17.73 ± 2.90 | 16.55 ± 3.14 | 0.916 | 0.370 |
| | Hope | 17.55 ± 2.54 | 17.00 ± 3.41 | 0.426 | 0.675 |
| | Resilience | 9.18 ± 3.06 | 10.91 ± 2.47 | −1.457 | 0.161 |

To verify the homogeneity between the two groups, independent sample *t*-tests were conducted for age, sleeping time, IES-R-K, DASS 21, and K-PPC. Chi-square tests were used for sex, academic year, and religion. N, number of participants; M, Mean; SD, standard deviation; IES-R-K, the Impact of Event Scale-Revised Korean Version; DASS 21, the 21-item version of the Depression Anxiety Stress Scale; K-PPC, the Korean version of positive psychological capital.

### 3.2. Outcome Measures

#### 3.2.1. DASS 21

In the analyses of the DASS 21 as a function of group and time, the statistically significant main effects of time emerged in the stress (F = 19.907, $p < 0.001$), anxiety (F = 9.487, $p < 0.01$), and depression (F = 10.472, $p < 0.01$) variables. In addition, significant group-by-time interaction effects were observed in the stress (F = 5.759, $p < 0.05$), anxiety (F = 4.790, $p < 0.01$), and depression (F = 5.740, $p < 0.01$) variables. The results revealed a significant decrease in stress, anxiety, and depression within the experimental group following the positive psychology-based virtual music therapy, with these improvements sustained at the 3-week follow-up. However, no such changes were observed within the control group (Table 3, Figure 2).

**Table 3.** Comparisons of the DASS 21 and K-PPC as a function of group and time using repeated measures ANOVAs.

| Variables | | | Experimental Group (N = 11) | Control Group (N = 11) | Group | Time | Group by Time |
|---|---|---|---|---|---|---|---|
| | | | M ± SD | M ± SD | F | F | |
| DASS 21 | Stress | pre | 14.00 ± 8.94 | 9.45 ± 6.07 | 0.018 | 19.907 *** | 5.759 * |
| | | post | 4.73 ± 3.26 | 7.09 ± 6.28 | | | |
| | | follow-up | 2.73 ± 3.50 | 5.82 ± 7.67 | | | |
| | Anxiety | pre | 8.36 ± 8.66 | 3.64 ± 2.94 | 0.460 | 9.487 ** | 4.790 * |
| | | post | 2.18 ± 1.89 | 2.18 ± 3.28 | | | |
| | | follow-up | 0.73 ± 1.35 | 2.55 ± 4.48 | | | |
| | Depression | pre | 9.45 ± 6.46 | 5.09 ± 4.13 | 0.005 | 10.472 ** | 5.740 * |
| | | post | 1.82 ± 3.63 | 3.27 ± 4.13 | | | |
| | | follow-up | 2.18 ± 3.40 | 4.73 ± 7.00 | | | |
| K-PPC | Total | pre | 60.73 ± 9.34 | 61.09 ± 9.09 | 0.920 | 17.235 *** | 3.740 * |
| | | post | 70.00 ± 8.80 | 64.64 ± 9.12 | | | |
| | | follow-up | 69.91 ± 8.25 | 64.27 ± 10.95 | | | |
| | Self-efficacy | pre | 16.27 ± 2.97 | 16.64 ± 2.84 | 0.643 | 14.381 *** | 3.723 * |
| | | post | 19.82 ± 3.34 | 17.64 ± 2.50 | | | |
| | | follow-up | 19.00 ± 2.49 | 18.00 ± 3.80 | | | |
| | Optimism | pre | 17.73 ± 2.90 | 16.55 ± 3.14 | 2.200 | 3.914 * | 0.688 |
| | | post | 19.64 ± 2.54 | 17.91 ± 3.75 | | | |
| | | follow-up | 19.18 ± 2.75 | 16.64 ± 4.27 | | | |
| | Hope | pre | 17.55 ± 2.54 | 17.00 ± 3.41 | 1.420 | 7.317 ** | 0.714 |
| | | post | 19.55 ± 3.30 | 17.73 ± 2.20 | | | |
| | | follow-up | 19.91 ± 1.92 | 18.64 ± 3.04 | | | |
| | Resilience | pre | 9.18 ± 3.06 | 10.91 ± 2.47 | 0.192 | 6.235 ** | 4.739 * |
| | | post | 11.00 ± 2.68 | 11.36 ± 2.01 | | | |
| | | follow-up | 11.82 ± 2.48 | 11.00 ± 2.37 | | | |

N, number of participants; M, Mean; SD, standard deviation; DASS 21, the 21-item version of the Depression Anxiety Stress Scale; K-PPC, the Korean version of positive psychological capital. * $p < 0.05$, ** $p < 0.01$, *** $p < 0.001$.

### 3.2.2. K-PPC

The analyses of the K-PPC as a function of group and time revealed statistically significant main effects of time emerged in self-efficacy ($F = 14.381$, $p < 0.001$), optimism ($F = 3.914$, $p < 0.05$), hope ($F = 7.317$, $p < 0.01$), resilience ($F = 6.235$, $p < 0.01$), and total score ($F = 17.235$, $p < 0.001$). Additionally, significant group-by-time interaction effects were found in self-efficacy ($F = 3.723$, $p < 0.05$), resilience ($F = 4.739$, $p < 0.05$), and total score ($F = 3.740$, $p < 0.05$). These results suggest that the positive psychology-based virtual music therapy program effectively enhanced the positive psychological capital of the participants, particularly in terms of self-efficacy and resilience, with these improvements maintained at the 3-week follow-up. However, significant changes were not observed in the control group (see Figure 2 and Table 3).

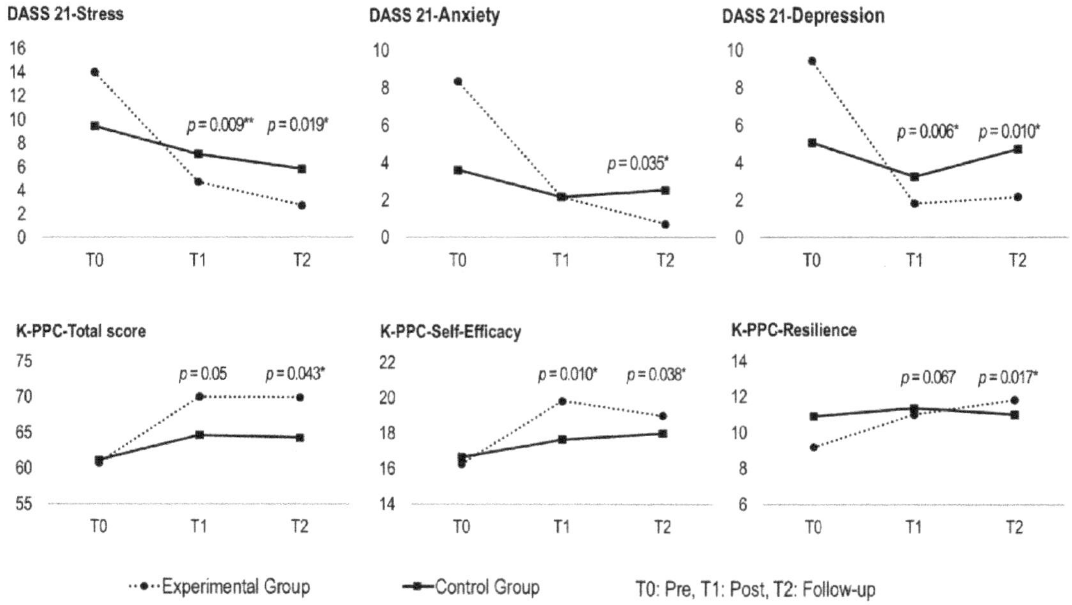


**Figure 2.** Differences in stress, anxiety, depression, self-efficacy, optimism, hope, and resilience as a result of two (groups: experimental and control) by three (time points: pre-test, post-test, and follow-up) repeated measures ANOVAs. * $p < 0.05$, ** $p < 0.01$.

## 4. Discussion

This study investigated the effects of positive psychology-based virtual music therapy on stress, anxiety, depression, and positive psychological capital (self-efficacy, optimism, hope, and resilience) among college students experiencing high levels of stress during the COVID-19 pandemic. Notably, participants enrolled in the 3-week program experienced significant reductions in stress, anxiety, and depression, coupled with notable enhancements in positive psychological capital, with a particular emphasis on self-efficacy and resilience.

The participants in this study were undergraduate students who showed a tendency for post-traumatic stress disorder on the IES-R-K, indicating their vulnerability to stress. High stress levels in a restricted environment can lead to negative thoughts and emotions and can limit the perspective of looking at current problems in a positive light and thinking about a hopeful future. The students in this study also highlighted the challenges they encountered while adjusting to the educational and technological changes brought about by the COVID-19 pandemic. They expressed feelings of stress and fatigue from coping with the increased volumes of online information and assignments, as well as the considerable time spent in front of computer screens on a daily basis. Consequently, reports of impaired mental health among college students during the COVID-19 era have been consistently documented on a global scale [10–12]. Primarily, the observed reductions in stress, anxiety, and depression in the experimental group align with previous research highlighting the therapeutic benefits of music therapy in promoting emotional well-being and reducing psychological distress [36–39]. In this study, listening to music and participating in diverse musical activities designed to offer enjoyable and meaningful experiences throughout the 15 sessions proved to be effective strategies for coping with negative emotions. In each session, the participants were encouraged to write down their honest feelings and thoughts about the given theme on a worksheet and apply them to their daily lives as actions. Previous research has reported the positive impact of expressive writing on reducing symptoms of depression, anxiety, and stress, thus supporting the effectiveness of the intervention in this study [40].

For college students, heightened depressive symptoms and decreased well-being during the COVID-19 pandemic have been linked to feelings of social isolation and loneliness [41]. In this context, engaging in virtual music therapy sessions may have offered opportunities for participants to connect with the therapist and perceive themselves as part of a collective endeavor with others, even if not physically present. This sense of social connection and belongingness cultivated during the sessions could have served as a protective factor against the negative psychological impacts of social isolation and loneliness. Studies have suggested that practices such as meditation, mindfulness sessions, engaging in phone or online counseling, and participating in digital mental health programs can serve as effective alternatives for alleviating psychological distress and feelings of isolation [42,43].

This study also demonstrated the effectiveness of the positive psychology-based virtual music therapy program in enhancing positive psychological capital, particularly resilience and self-efficacy. Previous studies on the impact of music-based interventions on resilience and self-efficacy have not been abundant. In addition, existing studies present inconsistent findings regarding whether music therapy significantly enhances resilience and self-efficacy, with study participants primarily comprised of clinical populations, particularly children or adolescents [44–50]. However, it appears that the elements of positive psychology blended into the music therapy program in this study resulted in significant improvements in resilience and efficacy in the undergraduate participants. As presented in Table 1, the program was designed not only to provide relaxation and enjoyment through music but also to enable participants to reflect on past, present, and future events, emotions, and hopes, as well as their personal strengths and relationships through various activities. Such an approach, combining elements of positive psychotherapy with the therapeutic use of music to actively engage participants in activities, might be more conducive to enhancing the overall positive psychological capital, including resilience and self-efficacy, compared with the traditional receptive music therapy approach, which focuses on the passive experience of listening to or experiencing music. This interpretation can be supported by previous studies that have reported the effects of positive psychotherapy on establishing a psychologically safe environment, increasing social connectedness, raising internal hope, and modifying perceptions of coping strategies, ultimately leading to behavioral changes [18–31].

The experimental group participants in this study received 15 sessions' worth of video clips and worksheets at the outset of the research. They were instructed to complete one session per weekday over a 3-week period, granting them autonomy to choose their preferred time and location to perform specific tasks. This emphasis on self-regulation aligns with the research suggesting that autonomy-supportive environments can bolster resilience and self-efficacy through enhanced motivation and perceived competence [51,52]. According to Deci and Ryan's self-determination theory, when individuals feel autonomous and self-directed in their actions, they experience higher intrinsic motivation, which fosters greater engagement, persistence, and overall psychological well-being [51]. Furthermore, adhering to a daily routine has a positive impact on psychological resilience [53]. Engaging in any regular activity voluntarily can provide a sense of routine and structure, helping individuals to cope with negative emotions more effectively. Therefore, participating in the virtual music therapy program as a structured daily routine might have promoted feelings of control and predictability, thereby increasing resilience and self-efficacy.

The present study has several limitations. There may be selection bias along with the limitation of a small sample size. Excluding individuals who have a history of psychiatric treatment or are currently undergoing psychiatric or psychological counseling introduces potential selection bias in this study. By excluding these participants, the study may inadvertently sample individuals who are generally healthier or less prone to severe mental health issues compared with the broader college student population. Moreover, participants who voluntarily chose to be in the experimental group may have a heightened interest in music therapy or mental health concerns. This self-selection could influence their responses and outcomes, as their motivation and engagement with the therapy may differ from those who did not choose to participate in the intervention. Furthermore, since the intervention delivered music therapy content to participants through pre-recorded video files, it may have been somewhat limited in terms of its therapeutic effectiveness due to communication constraints, such as the therapist's inability to directly interact with and offer immediate feedback to the client. Therefore, future research should examine how the impacts of positive psychology-based music therapy on mental health differ from the outcomes of this study when delivered in a virtual environment where therapists and clients can interact in real time. In this study, participants were given the autonomy to engage in the program at their preferred time and location. However, despite significant improvement, it is unclear whether this autonomy played a role in enhancing (or diminishing) the effectiveness of the intervention itself. Future research could provide stronger evidence by comparing outcomes when participants have autonomy versus when they adhere to a researcher-determined schedule. Additionally, while worksheets were utilized in the program, their contents were not analyzed or provided with feedback in this study. Incorporating a qualitative analysis of the worksheet data in future research would yield valuable insights.

In summary, this study delved into the effects of positive psychology-based virtual music therapy on stress, anxiety, depression, and positive psychological capital among college students amidst the backdrop of the COVID-19 pandemic. The results illuminated significant reductions in stress, anxiety, and depression alongside notable enhancements in positive psychological capital, particularly in terms of self-efficacy and resilience among participants. These findings are significant given the documented challenges faced by college students during the pandemic, including increased stress levels and mental health issues. This study underscores the potential of positive psychology-based virtual music therapy as a scalable intervention for addressing mental health challenges among college students, particularly in the context of the COVID-19 pandemic, by leveraging technology and evidence-based therapeutic approaches.

## 5. Conclusions

The findings of the present study suggest the potential of positive psychology-based virtual music therapy as a promising and scalable intervention for addressing stress, anxiety, and depression, and enhancing positive psychological resources among college students. By leveraging technology and evidence-based therapeutic approaches, such interventions have the potential to empower individuals to cultivate resilience and well-being, particularly in challenging circumstances such as the ongoing COVID-19 pandemic. The scalability of this approach is further facilitated by the nature of the program, which allows participants to choose their preferred time and place of participation in a virtual setting. This flexibility may enhance accessibility and effectiveness, making it a valuable tool for promoting mental health in diverse populations. The observed positive outcomes align with previous research highlighting the therapeutic benefits of music therapy in promoting emotional well-being. Moreover, the integration of expressive writing and virtual social connection within the therapy sessions contributed to the effectiveness of the intervention. The emphasis on positive psychology principles, combined with the therapeutic use of music, proved instrumental in fostering resilience and self-efficacy among participants, a notable contribution given the limited research in this area.

**Author Contributions:** Conceptualization, J.H. and H.L.; methodology, J.H. and S.L.; software, J.H. and T.K.; validation, J.H. and S.L.; formal analysis, J.H. and T.K.; investigation, J.H. and H.L; resources, J.H. and S.L.; data curation, J.H. and S.L.; writing—original draft preparation, J.H. and T.K.; writing—review and editing, H.L. and S.L.; visualization, J.H. and T.K.; supervision, H.L. and S.L. All authors have read and agreed to the published version of the manuscript.

**Funding:** This research received no specific grant from any funding agency in the public, commercial, or not-for-profit sectors.

**Institutional Review Board Statement:** The study was conducted in accordance with the Declaration of Helsinki and approved by the Institutional Review Board for Ethics in Human Research at Wonkwang University (approval no. WKIRB-202102-HR-005).

**Informed Consent Statement:** Informed consent was obtained from all subjects involved in the study.

**Data Availability Statement:** The data presented in this study are openly available in Google Docs at [https://docs.google.com/spreadsheets/d/1pixJV6lNkXIDnvRabgnCMF1pxW1wU9z1/edit?usp=sharing&ouid=115163458442950089664&rtpof=true&sd=true], accessed on 20 July 2024.

**Conflicts of Interest:** The authors declare no conflicts of interest.

## References

1. Baud, D.; Qi, X.; Nielsen-Saines, K.; Musso, D.; Pomar, L.; Favre, G. Real estimates of mortality following COVID-19 infection. *Lancet Infect. Dis.* **2020**, *20*, 773. [CrossRef] [PubMed]
2. Wasim, A.; Truong, J.; Bakshi, S.; Majid, U. A systematic review of fear, stigma, and mental health outcomes of pandemics. *J. Ment. Health* **2023**, *32*, 920–934. [CrossRef] [PubMed]
3. Lakhan, R.; Agrawal, A.; Sharma, M. Prevalence of depression, anxiety, and stress during COVID-19 pandemic. *J. Neurosci. Rural Pract.* **2020**, *11*, 519–525. [CrossRef] [PubMed]
4. Smit, A.N.; Juda, M.; Livingstone, A.; Stephanie, R.U.; Mistlberger, R.E. Impact of COVID-19 social-distancing on sleep timing and duration during a university semester. *PLoS ONE* **2021**, *16*, e0250793. [CrossRef] [PubMed]
5. Xiong, J.; Lipsitz, O.; Nasri, F.; Lui, L.M.; Gill, H.; Phan, L.; Chen-Li, D.; Iacobucci, M.; Ho, R.; Majeed, A.; et al. Impact of COVID-19 pandemic on mental health in the general population: A systematic review. *J. Affect. Disord.* **2020**, *277*, 55–64. [CrossRef] [PubMed]
6. Rajkumar, R.P. COVID-19 and mental health: A review of the existing literature. *Asian J. Psychiatry* **2020**, *52*, 102066. [CrossRef] [PubMed]
7. Vindegaard, N.; Benros, M.E. COVID-19 pandemic and mental health consequences: Systematic review of the current evidence. *Brain Behav. Immun.* **2020**, *89*, 531–542. [CrossRef] [PubMed]
8. Brooks, S.K.; Webster, R.K.; Smith, L.E.; Woodland, L.; Wessely, S.; Greenberg, N.; Rubin, G.J. The psychological impact of quarantine and how to reduce it: Rapid review of the evidence. *Lancet* **2020**, *395*, 912–920. [CrossRef]
9. Auerbach, R.P.; Mortier, P.; Bruffaerts, R.; Alonso, J.; Benjet, C.; Cuijpers, P.; Demyttenaere, K.; Ebert, D.D.; Green, J.G.; Hasking, P.; et al. WHO world mental health surveys international college student project: Prevalence and distribution of mental disorders. *J. Abnorm. Psychol.* **2018**, *127*, 623. [CrossRef]
10. Husky, M.M.; Kovess-Masfety, V.; Swendsen, J.D. Stress and anxiety among university students in France during COVID-19 mandatory confinement. *Compr. Psychiatry* **2020**, *102*, 152191. [CrossRef]
11. Gritsenko, V.; Skugarevsky, O.; Konstantinov, V.; Khamenka, N.; Marinova, T.; Reznik, A.; Isralowitz, R. COVID 19 fear, stress, anxiety, and substance use among Russian and Belarusian university students. *Int. J. Ment. Health Addict.* **2021**, *19*, 2362–2368. [CrossRef] [PubMed]
12. Konstantopoulou, G.; Pantazopoulou, S.; Iliou, T.; Raikou, N. Stress and depression in the exclusion of the COVID-19 pandemic in Greek university students. *Eur. J. Public Health Stud.* **2020**, *3*, 91–99. [CrossRef]
13. Rashid, T.; Seligman, M.P. *Positive Psychotherapy: Clinician Manual*; Oxford University Press: Oxford, UK, 2018.
14. McDowell, I. Measures of self-perceived well-being. *J. Psychosom. Res.* **2010**, *69*, 69–79. [CrossRef] [PubMed]
15. Kim, S.Y. A convergence study of stress caused by the epidemic of COVID-19, quality of life and positive psychological capital. *J. Korea Converg. Soc.* **2020**, *11*, 423–431. [CrossRef]
16. Lee, Y.J. An Analysis of Positive Psychological Capital Influencing Emotional Reactions of College Students under COVID-19. *J. Humanit. Soc. Sci. 21* **2020**, *11*, 2885–2899. [CrossRef]
17. Li, Y.I.; Starr, L.R.; Hershenberg, R. Responses to positive affect in daily life: Positive rumination and dampening moderate the association between daily events and depressive symptoms. *J. Psychopathol. Behav. Assess.* **2017**, *39*, 412–425. [CrossRef]
18. Lee Duckworth, A.; Steen, T.A.; Seligman, M.E. Positive psychology in clinical practice. *Annu. Rev. Clin. Psychol.* **2005**, *1*, 629–651. [CrossRef]
19. Magyar-Moe, J.L.; Owens, R.L.; Conoley, C.W. Positive psychological interventions in counseling: What every counseling psychologist should know. *Couns. Psychol.* **2015**, *43*, 508–557. [CrossRef]
20. Yoon, H.Y.; Seo, S.B.; Park, J.Y. Effects of Positive Psychology-Based Music Therapy on Family Members' Attitudes towards Gambling Addicts. *J. Korea Converg. Soc.* **2019**, *10*, 269–279. [CrossRef]
21. Kwok, S.Y. Integrating positive psychology and elements of music therapy to alleviate adolescent anxiety. *Res. Soc. Work Pract.* **2019**, *29*, 663–676. [CrossRef]
22. Jackson, N.A. Music therapy and chronic mental illness: Overcoming the silent symptoms. *Music Ther. Perspect.* **2015**, *33*, 90–96. [CrossRef]
23. Ziv, N.; Chaim, A.B.; Itamar, O. The effect of positive music and dispositional hope on state hope and affect. *Psychol. Music* **2011**, *39*, 3–17. [CrossRef]

24. Croom, A.M. Music practice and participation for psychological well-being: A review of how music influences positive emotion, engagement, relationships, meaning, and accomplishment. *Music. Sci.* **2015**, *19*, 44–64. [CrossRef]
25. Chirico, A.; Maiorano, P.; Indovina, P.; Milanese, C.; Giordano, G.G.; Alivernini, F.; Iodice, G.; Gallo, L.; De Pietro, G.; Lucidi, F.; et al. Virtual reality and music therapy as distraction interventions to alleviate anxiety and improve mood states in breast cancer patients during chemotherapy. *J. Cell. Physiol.* **2020**, *235*, 5353–5362. [CrossRef] [PubMed]
26. Giordano, F.; Scarlata, E.; Baroni, M.; Gentile, E.; Puntillo, F.; Brienza, N.; Gesualdo, L. Receptive music therapy to reduce stress and improve wellbeing in Italian clinical staff involved in COVID-19 pandemic: A preliminary study. *Arts Psychother.* **2020**, *70*, 101688. [CrossRef] [PubMed]
27. Bompard, S.; Liuzzi, T.; Staccioli, S.; D'Arienzo, F.; Khosravi, S.; Giuliani, R.; Castelli, E. Home-based music therapy for children with developmental disorders during the COVID-19 pandemic. *J. Telemed. Telecare* **2023**, *29*, 211–216. [CrossRef] [PubMed]
28. Eun, H.J.; Kwon, T.W.; Lee, S.M.; Kim, T.H.; Choi, M.R.; Cho, S.J. A study on reliability and validity of the Korean Version of Impact of Event Scale-Revised. *J. Korean Neuropsychiatr. Assoc.* **2005**, *44*, 303–310.
29. Horowitz, M.; Wilner, N.; Alvarez, W. Impact of event scale: A measure of subjective stress. *Psychosom. Med.* **1979**, *41*, 209–218. [CrossRef]
30. Weiss, D.S.; Marmar, C.R. The Impact of Event Scale-Revised. In *Assessing Psychological Trauma and PTSD*; Wilson, J.P., Keane, T.M., Eds.; Guilford Press: New York, NY, USA, 1997; pp. 399–411.
31. Lee, E.H.; Moon, S.H.; Cho, M.S.; Park, E.S.; Kim, S.Y.; Han, J.S.; Cheio, J.H. The 21-item and 12-item versions of the depression anxiety stress scales: Psychometric evaluation in a Korean population. *Asian Nurs. Res.* **2019**, *13*, 30–37. [CrossRef]
32. Lovibond, P.F.; Lovibond, S.H. The structure of negative emotional states: Comparison of the Depression Anxiety Stress Scales (DASS) with the Beck Depression and Anxiety Inventories. *Behav. Res. Ther.* **1995**, *33*, 335–343. [CrossRef]
33. Henry, J.D.; Crawford, J.R. The short-form version of the Depression Anxiety Stress Scales (DASS-21): Construct validity and normative data in a large non-clinical sample. *Br. J. Clin. Psychol.* **2005**, *44*, 227–239. [CrossRef] [PubMed]
34. Lim, T.H. Validation of the Korean version of positive psychological capital (K-PPC). *J. Coach. Dev.* **2014**, *16*, 157–166.
35. Luthans, F.; Youssef-Morgan, C.M. Psychological capital: An evidence-based positive approach. *Annu. Rev. Organ. Psychol. Organ. Behav.* **2017**, *4*, 339–366. [CrossRef]
36. Umbrello, M.; Sorrenti, T.; Mistraletti, G.; Formenti, P.; Chiumello, D.; Terzoni, S. Music therapy reduces stress and anxiety in critically ill patients: A systematic review of randomized clinical trials. *Minerva Anestesiol.* **2019**, *85*, 886–898. [CrossRef] [PubMed]
37. de la Rubia Ortí, J.E.; García-Pardo, M.P.; Iranzo, C.C.; Madrigal, J.J.C.; Castillo, S.S.; Rochina, M.J.; Gascó, V.J.P. Does music therapy improve anxiety and depression in alzheimer's patients? *J. Altern. Complement. Med.* **2018**, *24*, 33–36. [CrossRef] [PubMed]
38. Mohammadi, A.Z.; Shahabi, T.; Panah, F.M. An evaluation of the effect of group music therapy on stress, anxiety and depression levels in nursing home residents. *Can. J. Music Ther.* **2011**, *17*, 55–68.
39. Hwang, E.Y.; Oh, S.H. A comparison of the effects of music therapy interventions on depression, anxiety, anger, and stress on alcohol-dependent clients: A pilot study. *Music Med.* **2013**, *5*, 136–144. [CrossRef]
40. Guo, L. The delayed, durable effect of expressive writing on depression, anxiety and stress: A meta-analytic review of studies with long-term follow-ups. *Br. J. Clin. Psychol.* **2023**, *62*, 272–297. [CrossRef]
41. Holm-Hadulla, R.M.; Wendler, H.; Baracsi, G.; Storck, T.; Herpertz, S.C. Depression and social isolation during the COVID-19 pandemic in a student population: The effects of establishing and relaxing social restrictions. *Front. Psychiatry* **2023**, *14*, 1200643. [CrossRef]
42. Pizzoli, S.M.F.; Marzorati, C.; Mazzoni, D.; Pravettoni, G. An internet-based intervention to alleviate stress during social isolation with guided relaxation and meditation: Protocol for a randomized controlled trial. *JMIR Res. Protoc.* **2020**, *9*, e19236. [CrossRef]
43. Farris, S.R.; Grazzi, L.; Holley, M.; Dorsett, A.; Xing, K.; Pierce, C.R.; Estave, P.M.; O'Connell, N.; Wells, R.E. Online mindfulness may target psychological distress and mental health during COVID-19. *Glob. Adv. Health Med.* **2021**, *10*, 21649561211002461. [CrossRef]
44. Blauth, L.; Oldfield, A. Research into increasing resilience in children with autism through music therapy: Statistical analysis of video data. *Nord. J. Music Ther.* **2022**, *31*, 454–480. [CrossRef]
45. Burns, D.S.; Robb, S.L.; Haase, J.E. Exploring the feasibility of a therapeutic music video intervention in adolescents and young adults during stem-cell transplantation. *Cancer Nurs.* **2009**, *32*, E8–E16. [CrossRef] [PubMed]
46. Choi, A.N.; Cha, E.S. The Effect of Group Music Therapy on the Emotional Stabilisation and the Self-Efficacy of Juvenile Delinquents. *J. Fam. Better Life* **2007**, *25*, 1–14.
47. Letwin, L.; Silverman, M.J. No between-group difference but tendencies for patient support: A pilot study of a resilience-focused music therapy protocol for adults on a medical oncology/hematology unit. *Arts Psychother.* **2017**, *55*, 116–125. [CrossRef]
48. Lim, H.A.; Befi, C.M. Music therapy career aptitude and generalized self-efficacy in music therapy students. *J. Music Ther.* **2014**, *51*, 382–395. [CrossRef]
49. Silverman, M.J. Effects of music therapy on drug avoidance self-efficacy in patients on a detoxification unit: A three-group randomized effectiveness study. *J. Addict. Nurs.* **2014**, *25*, 172–181. [CrossRef] [PubMed]
50. Silverman, M.J. Music therapy for coping self-efficacy in an acute mental health setting: A randomized pilot study. *Community Ment. Health J.* **2019**, *55*, 615–623. [CrossRef]

51. Deci, E.L.; Ryan, R.M. The "what" and "why" of goal pursuits: Human needs and the self-determination of behavior. *Psychol. Inq.* **2000**, *11*, 227–268. [CrossRef]
52. Ataii, M.; Saleh-Sedghpour, B.; Asadzadeh-Dahraei, H.; Sadatee-Shamir, A. Effect of Self-regulation on Academic Resilience Mediated by Perceived Competence. *Int. J. Behav. Sci.* **2021**, *15*, 156–161. [CrossRef]
53. Suckow, E.J.; Henderson-Arredondo, K.; Hildebrand, L.; Jankowski, S.R.; Killgore, W.D. 70 Daily Routine and Psychological Resilience. *J. Int. Neuropsychol. Soc.* **2023**, *29*, 579–580. [CrossRef]

*healthcare*

MDPI

*Article*

# Artificial Intelligence in Postoperative Care: Assessing Large Language Models for Patient Recommendations in Plastic Surgery

**Cesar A. Gomez-Cabello [1], Sahar Borna [1], Sophia M. Pressman [1], Syed Ali Haider [1], Ajai Sehgal [2], Bradley C. Leibovich [2,3] and Antonio J. Forte [1,2,*]**

[1] Division of Plastic Surgery, Mayo Clinic, Jacksonville, FL 32224, USA
[2] Center for Digital Health, Mayo Clinic, Rochester, MN 55905, USA
[3] Department of Urology, Mayo Clinic, Rochester, MN 55905, USA
* Correspondence: forte.antonio@mayo.edu

**Abstract:** Since their release, the medical community has been actively exploring large language models' (LLMs) capabilities, which show promise in providing accurate medical knowledge. One potential application is as a patient resource. This study analyzes and compares the ability of the currently available LLMs, ChatGPT-3.5, GPT-4, and Gemini, to provide postoperative care recommendations to plastic surgery patients. We presented each model with 32 questions addressing common patient concerns after surgical cosmetic procedures and evaluated the medical accuracy, readability, understandability, and actionability of the models' responses. The three LLMs provided equally accurate information, with GPT-3.5 averaging the highest on the Likert scale (LS) ($4.18 \pm 0.93$) ($p = 0.849$), while Gemini provided significantly more readable ($p = 0.001$) and understandable responses ($p = 0.014$; $p = 0.001$). There was no difference in the actionability of the models' responses ($p = 0.830$). Although LLMs have shown their potential as adjunctive tools in postoperative patient care, further refinement and research are imperative to enable their evolution into comprehensive standalone resources.

**Keywords:** large language models; artificial intelligence; plastic surgery; postoperative care; patient resource; patient-centered outcomes; patient satisfaction

## 1. Introduction

The advancement of artificial intelligence (AI) offers new opportunities for healthcare improvements and individualized patient care. Large language models (LLMs) represent a breakthrough in applied AI and medical practice. They learn and understand the complex patterns and structures in typical language by leveraging natural language processing (NLP) and deep learning (DL) techniques, in particular, transformer architectures [1]. LLMs can process, interpret, and summarize vast amounts of internet data in real time and generate human-like text responses [2,3]. Since their release, LLMs have shown promise in providing accurate medical knowledge throughout distinct medical fields, encouraging the medical community to actively explore their potential applications and determine how to best leverage their capabilities.

Plastic surgery is a constantly innovating field that relies on updated, accurate tools to provide patient-centered outcomes [4]. In particular, cosmetic surgery is a major ever-evolving field with a rising demand due to its growing social acceptance. In 2022, there were 26.2 million surgical and minimally invasive cosmetic and reconstructive procedures in the United States, with a 19% increase in cosmetic surgery since 2019 [5]. Plastic surgeons are challenged to provide comprehensive information and support to an increasing number of patients [3]. LLMs, in particular, Open AI's ChatGPT, have proved to be helpful throughout the specialty, with the ability to generate and detect areas for improvement and potential research [4]. ChatGPT has even proved to have a comparable level of knowledge to 50% of first-year integrated plastic surgery residents, as shown by in-service exam scores [6].

While most LLM research focuses on their clinical decision capabilities, such as diagnosis and treatment, one very promising application is as a patient resource. Given its accessibility, patients already rely on the Internet as their primary source of information and make decisions based on the information they find, risking themselves being misinformed [2,7]. Previous studies have shown that despite some inherent limitations, LLMs can provide accurate information for patients seeking insights into cosmetic procedure details, outcomes, risks, and benefits [2,3,8]. Additionally, they offer immediate, multilingual, round-the-clock access to information, which is crucial for addressing concerns and questions outside of regular office hours and ensuring equity.

In plastic surgery, the postoperative period is as important as the surgical procedure itself, and in some cases even more so, as the patient's final outcome and the procedure's long-term success depend on it [9]. Although surgeons offer clear verbal and printed postoperative care recommendations, patients may struggle to retain or implement them due to their postoperative emotional state. This forces them to keep looking for their surgeons and their staff's help outside of office hours, sometimes overburdening the surgical staff. Approaches to decrease these burdens may include limiting notifications or delegating responses to less-trained support staff [10]. These limit access to high-quality care and lead to the common patient misconception that they are forgotten once their surgery has finished. The immediate and accurate responses provided by LLMs can reduce anxiety and improve patient satisfaction [11–13].

Building on previous work assessing LLMs' use in the perioperative period [2,3,8,14,15], we aimed to evaluate and compare the ability of the currently readily available LLMs, ChatGPT-3.5, ChatGPT-4, and Google's Gemini, formerly Bard, to provide postoperative care recommendations to patients who underwent any one of the five most common cosmetic plastic surgery procedures according to the American Society of Plastic Surgeons (ASPS) in 2022 [5] in the absence of utilizing a retrieval-augmented generation (RAG) approach. As accessibility is fundamental to achieving equal health distribution, we decided to include the publicly available version of ChatGPT in our comparison.

## 2. Methods

### 2.1. Study Design

We created a set of 32 questions addressing the most common concerns patients have at our clinic after liposuction (n = 7), breast augmentation (n = 6), abdominoplasty (n = 6), mastopexy (n = 6), and blepharoplasty (n = 7). Each question was presented to each LLM using a combination of specialized medical terminology and common language to reflect the various ways in which a typical plastic surgery patient might phrase their questions. Moreover, we did not employ any specialized prompting engineering techniques, such as contextualization or role play, to ensure that the responses obtained were not a result of these methods, as a typical patient may not be aware of them or be comfortably familiarized with them. We only asked each question once and in different chats. After every question was asked to one model, another was tested. Figure 1 portrays an example of the questions. In addition, we have included the full set of questions provided to the LLMs and the responses retrieved in Supplementary File S1 and in a Supplementary File S2, respectively.

| Question | GPT-3.5 | GPT-4 | Gemini |
|---|---|---|---|
| I had a breast lift some years ago and I feel that my breast are starting to sag, is that something normal or should I go with my surgeon? | "It's not uncommon for the results of a breast lift surgery (mastopexy) to change over time. Factors such as aging, gravity, pregnancy, weight fluctuations, and genetics can all influence breast shape and position. It's essential to understand that breast tissue can naturally sag or droop over the years, even after a successful breast lift procedure. However, whether or not you should consult with your surgeon depends on your specific concerns and goals.<br>Here are some considerations:<br>Normal Aging Process: Over time, the effects of gravity, loss of skin elasticity, and changes in breast tissue can lead to a gradual return of some degree of sagging. This is a normal part of the aging process.<br>Post-Surgery Changes: While a breast lift can provide long-lasting results, it does not stop the aging process. Your breasts may continue to change in appearance over the years, which could include some degree of sagging.<br>Consultation with Your Surgeon: If you are concerned about changes in the appearance of your breasts or feel that they are sagging more than you are comfortable with, it's a good idea to consult with your original surgeon or a board-certified plastic surgeon. They can evaluate your current breast condition and discuss potential options for improvement.<br>Breast Lift Revision: In some cases, a breast lift revision surgery may be recommended if you are dissatisfied with the degree of sagging. A revision procedure can help restore breast shape and position. Your surgeon will assess your specific needs and discuss the best approach for achieving your desired outcome.<br>Lifestyle Factors: Lifestyle factors such as maintaining a stable weight, wearing supportive bras, and protecting your skin from excessive sun exposure can help minimize the progression of breast sagging over time.<br>Realistic Expectations: It's important to have realistic expectations about the results of cosmetic surgery. While a breast lift can provide significant improvement, it may not completely halt the natural aging process.<br>Consulting with your surgeon is the first step in addressing your concerns and exploring potential solutions. They can provide personalized advice and recommendations based on your individual situation and goals." | "It's not uncommon for some degree of breast sagging to occur after a breast lift, especially as the years pass. This can be due to several factors, including aging, gravity, changes in weight, hormonal fluctuations, and the natural loss of skin elasticity over time. Even after surgical lifting, these factors can contribute to changes in breast shape and position.<br>However, if you notice significant changes or if you're concerned about the appearance of your breasts, it's a good idea to consult with your surgeon. They can assess whether what you're experiencing is within the normal range of changes following a breast lift or if there might be a need for a revision surgery or other interventions. Your surgeon can provide personalized advice based on your specific situation, including your initial surgical outcome, your current concerns, and your overall health and goals.<br>Maintaining a stable weight, wearing supportive bras, especially during exercise, and taking care of your skin can help maintain your results for as long as possible. But, it's important to have realistic expectations and understand that some changes over time are inevitable.<br>If you're feeling unsure or worried, scheduling a consultation with your surgeon is the best way to get peace of mind and make informed decisions about your care." | "It's important to understand that the results of any cosmetic procedure, including breast lifts, are not permanent. While they can offer significant improvements in appearance and satisfaction for many years, various factors can contribute to a return of sagging over time. These can include:<br>Natural aging: As we age, our skin loses elasticity and collagen, which can lead to drooping of tissues throughout the body, including the breasts.<br>Gravity: Gravity continuously exerts a downward pull on the breasts, and while a lift addresses this to some extent, it can't completely counteract its effects over time.<br>Weight fluctuations: Significant weight gain and loss can stretch the skin and underlying supporting tissues, contributing to sagging.<br>Pregnancy: Subsequent pregnancies after a lift can stretch the skin and affect the results.<br>Given that it's been several years since your procedure and you're experiencing renewed sagging, it's not necessarily unusual but consulting with your original surgeon is highly recommended.<br>They are best equipped to:<br>Evaluate your specific situation: They can assess the degree of sagging, the condition of your skin, and any other contributing factors.<br>Discuss your options: Based on their evaluation, they can discuss whether additional surgery might be appropriate, or if alternative methods like supportive bras or specific exercises might be beneficial.<br>Address your concerns: They can answer your questions, address any anxieties you might have, and provide you with realistic expectations for potential next steps.<br>Remember, maintaining open communication with your original surgeon throughout the process is crucial for achieving the best possible outcome and addressing any concerns you may have." |
| What can I do to avoid or decrease edema after eyelid surgery? | "Edema, or swelling, is a common occurrence after eyelid surgery (blepharoplasty). While some degree of swelling is normal during the initial stages of recovery, there are steps you can take to minimize and manage it. Here are some tips to help avoid or decrease edema after eyelid surgery:<br>Follow Your Surgeon's Instructions: Adhere to all post-operative instructions provided by your plastic surgeon. These instructions are tailored to your specific case and are essential for a smooth recovery.<br>Elevate Your Head: Sleeping with your head elevated at a 30-45 degree angle can help reduce swelling. Use extra pillows to prop yourself up, or consider sleeping in a reclining chair for the first few days.<br>Cool Compresses: Applying cold compresses to the eyelids can help reduce swelling and discomfort. Use clean, cold, damp washcloths or gel packs, and follow your surgeon's recommendations for timing and duration.<br>Avoid Heat: Avoid hot showers, hot tubs, saunas, or anything that increases blood flow to the face during the early stages of recovery, as heat can exacerbate swelling.<br>Limit Physical Activity: Rest and avoid strenuous physical activities in the first few days to minimize swelling. Gradually increase your activity level as advised by your surgeon.<br>Hydrate: Drink plenty of water to stay hydrated, as proper hydration can help reduce swelling and promote healing.<br>Eye Drops: If prescribed or recommended by your surgeon, use lubricating eye drops or artificial tears to keep your eyes moist and comfortable. Dry eyes can contribute to discomfort and swelling.<br>Avoid Salt: Reduce your salt intake, as excess sodium can lead to fluid retention and increased swelling.<br>Protect Your Eyes: Use any protective measures, such as eye shields or glasses, as instructed by your surgeon to prevent accidental rubbing or pressure on the eyes.<br>Avoid Allergens: Minimize exposure to allergens, such as dust and pollen, that can irritate the eyes and worsen swelling.<br>Avoid Alcohol and Caffeine: Alcohol and caffeine can dehydrate the body, so it's best to limit or avoid them during the early recovery period.<br>Proper Nutrition: Follow a well-balanced diet rich in fruits and vegetables, which can support healing and reduce inflammation.<br>Stay Relaxed: Stress and anxiety can contribute to swelling, so try to stay relaxed and avoid situations that may cause unnecessary stress.<br>Follow-Up Appointments: Attend all follow-up appointments with your surgeon so they can monitor your progress and make any necessary adjustments to your post-operative care plan.<br>It's important to be patient during the recovery process, as swelling can take time to subside completely. In most cases, the majority of swelling should resolve within a few weeks, with gradual improvement over the following months. If you have concerns about the extent of swelling or any other post-operative issues, contact your surgeon for guidance and reassurance" | "Post-operative edema (swelling) is a common occurrence after eyelid surgery (blepharoplasty) and typically resolves over time. However, there are several strategies you can employ to minimize swelling and promote a smoother recovery. Here are some tips:<br>Cold Compresses: Applying cold compresses or ice packs to the eye area can significantly reduce swelling, especially during the first 48 hours after surgery. Be sure to wrap the ice pack in a clean cloth to avoid direct contact with your skin.<br>Elevation: Keep your head elevated higher than your chest when lying down. This can be achieved by using extra pillows under your head while sleeping or resting. Elevation helps reduce swelling by improving venous return and decreasing fluid accumulation.<br>Avoid Strenuous Activities: Limit activities that can increase blood pressure to your head, such as bending over, lifting heavy objects, or performing strenuous exercises, as they can exacerbate swelling.<br>Follow Your Surgeon's Instructions: Your surgeon will provide specific aftercare instructions, including how to care for your incisions, when to return for follow-up visits, and the use of any prescribed medications or ointments. Adhering to these instructions is crucial for minimizing swelling and preventing complications.<br>Stay Hydrated: Drinking plenty of water can help reduce swelling by flushing excess fluids out of your body.<br>Limit Salt Intake: Excessive salt can contribute to fluid retention. Reducing your salt intake can help minimize swelling.<br>Avoid Smoking and Alcohol: Smoking can delay healing, and alcohol can lead to fluid retention. Both should be avoided during the recovery period.<br>Use Prescribed Medications: If your surgeon prescribes medications to help reduce swelling, such as anti-inflammatory drugs, be sure to take them as directed.<br>Protect Your Skin: Follow any recommendations for sun protection, as sun exposure can contribute to swelling and affect healing.<br>Healthy Diet: Eating a balanced diet rich in vitamins and minerals can support your body's healing process.<br>Remember, recovery times and experiences vary from person to person. If you have concerns about swelling or any aspect of your recovery, it's important to contact your surgeon. They can provide advice tailored to your specific situation and intervene if necessary to address any complications." | "While completely avoiding edema (swelling) after eyelid surgery is not possible, there are several steps you can take to minimize its severity and duration:<br>Cold compresses: Apply cold compresses to your eyelids for 10-15 minutes at a time, several times a day, especially during the first 24-48 hours after surgery. Wrap a gel ice pack or a clean washcloth soaked in cold water in a thin towel to prevent direct contact with the skin.<br>Head elevation: Keep your head elevated at night by using extra pillows or sleeping in a reclining chair. This helps reduce fluid accumulation around the eyes.<br>Avoid straining: Avoid strenuous activities, bending over, or lifting heavy objects for at least 2 weeks after surgery. These activities can increase blood pressure in your head and worsen swelling.<br>Limit salt intake: Reducing your salt intake can help minimize fluid retention throughout your body, including around your eyes.<br>Quit smoking: Smoking can impair healing and increase the risk of complications, including swelling. If you smoke, quitting at least 4 weeks before surgery is recommended.<br>Gentle cleansing: Avoid rubbing your eyes or using harsh soaps or cosmetics around the eyes. Gently cleanse the area with a mild cleanser as instructed by your doctor.<br>Sleep: Getting enough sleep is crucial for healing. Aim for 7-8 hours of sleep each night.<br>Medications: Your doctor may prescribe pain medication or anti-inflammatory medication to help manage swelling and discomfort. Take these medications exactly as directed.<br>Remember, these are general recommendations, and it's crucial to follow your doctor's specific instructions for post-operative care after eyelid surgery. They will provide you with detailed guidance on how to care for your eyes and minimize swelling." |

**Figure 1.** *Cont.*

| Question | GPT-3.5 | GPT-4 | Gemini |
| --- | --- | --- | --- |
| I just had a liposuction and I feel like I am gaining weight, is this normal? | "I'm not a doctor, but I can try to provide you with some general information about liposuction and weight fluctuations.<br><br>Liposuction is a surgical procedure designed to remove fat cells from specific areas of the body. While it can result in immediate reductions in localized fat, it's important to understand that liposuction doesn't prevent future weight gain. If you're experiencing weight fluctuations after liposuction, several factors could be contributing to this:<br><br>Swelling: Swelling is a common side effect after liposuction, and it can take several weeks to months for the swelling to subside completely. During this period, you may feel like you've gained weight due to the increased fluid retention and inflammation.<br>Lifestyle and Diet: Your post-liposuction weight can be influenced by your lifestyle and dietary choices. If you're consuming more calories than you're burning, you can still gain weight, even after the procedure.<br>Redistribution of Fat: Liposuction removes fat from specific areas, but it doesn't affect fat distribution in the rest of your body. This means that if you consume excess calories, your body may store fat in other areas, potentially leading to weight gain.<br>Muscle Changes: After liposuction, it's important to maintain or build muscle tone in the treated areas to prevent sagging and maintain a balanced appearance. If you're not engaging in regular exercise, muscle loss can contribute to changes in your body's shape.<br>Psychological Factors: Sometimes, people may experience changes in their body image or perception after cosmetic procedures, which can lead to concerns about weight gain even if there's no significant physical change.<br>If you have concerns about weight gain or changes in your body after liposuction, it's crucial to consult with your plastic surgeon or a medical professional who can provide personalized advice and address your specific situation. They can help you understand the causes of any changes you're experiencing and provide guidance on maintaining a healthy lifestyle to achieve your desired results." | "After liposuction, experiencing fluctuations in weight is not uncommon. Here are a few points to consider that might explain why you feel like you're gaining weight:<br><br>Swelling: The most common reason for feeling like you've gained weight shortly after liposuction is swelling. The body's response to the surgery involves retaining fluid in the treated areas, which can make you feel heavier or look puffier than before. This swelling can last for several weeks to months.<br>Fluid Retention: In addition to swelling in the surgical area, your body might retain fluids more generally as part of the healing process. This can also contribute to a sensation of weight gain.<br>Diet and Activity Levels: Your diet and activity levels post-surgery can also impact your weight. If you're consuming more calories than you're expending, especially during your recovery period when your physical activity might be limited, you might notice weight gain.<br>Temporary Weight Gain: It's also worth noting that liposuction removes fat cells from the body, but if you don't maintain a stable weight by balancing caloric intake with physical activity, the remaining fat cells in your body can grow, leading to weight gain.<br>Healing Process: The body is in a state of healing and recovery after liposuction, and it can take time for the final results to be visible. The initial weight gain or bloated feeling usually resolves as the body heals.<br>Lymphatic System Response: The lymphatic system plays a crucial role in removing fluids and waste from your body. Liposuction can temporarily disrupt the normal function of the lymphatic system, leading to fluid accumulation.<br>It's important to follow your surgeon's post-operative instructions closely, including wearing compression garments if recommended, maintaining a healthy diet, staying hydrated, and gradually returning to exercise under guidance. These steps can help minimize swelling and support your recovery.<br><br>If you're concerned about your weight gain after liposuction, it's best to discuss this with your surgeon. They can assess your situation to determine whether what you're experiencing is a normal part of the healing process or if there's another underlying issue that needs to be addressed." | "While it's understandable to feel concerned about weight gain after liposuction, it's important to remember that experiencing a perceived increase in weight after the procedure can be normal. Here's a breakdown of the points to consider:<br><br>1. Liposuction is not a weight loss solution: Liposuction aims to reshape specific areas by removing fat cells. It's not intended for overall weight loss.<br><br>2. Initial weight fluctuations:<br>• Fluid retention: During healing, your body might retain fluids, leading to a temporary increase on the scale.<br>• Inflammation: The surgical process itself can cause inflammation, which can contribute to a feeling of puffiness or weight gain.<br><br>3. Fat cells vs. remaining fat:<br>• The treated areas have fewer fat cells, so even with weight gain, they won't expand as much as untreated areas.<br>• However, the remaining fat cells throughout your body can still grow if you gain weight overall.<br><br>Here's what you can do:<br><br>Consult your doctor: They can assess your individual situation, provide reassurance, and address any specific concerns you have.<br>Maintain a healthy lifestyle: Continue a balanced diet and regular exercise routine to promote overall health and maintain your results.<br>Be patient: Allow your body time to heal fully, which can take several weeks or even months. The final results of liposuction might not be fully visible until several months after the procedure.<br>If you have any significant concerns or questions about your recovery process, always consult your doctor for personalized guidance." |
| It's been 2 weeks since my breast augmentation surgery, can I start doing yoga? | "After breast augmentation surgery, it's crucial to follow your surgeon's specific post-operative instructions, including guidelines for physical activity and exercise. While I can provide some general information, it's essential to consult with your plastic surgeon before resuming any exercise routine, including yoga.<br><br>Here are some general considerations for resuming yoga or other forms of physical activity after breast augmentation:<br><br>Consult Your Surgeon: Your surgeon is the best source of guidance for when it's safe to resume exercise. They will consider your individual healing progress and recommend an appropriate timeline.<br>Early Post-Operative Period (First Few Weeks): During the first few weeks after breast augmentation, you will likely be advised to avoid strenuous activities, including yoga, that involve chest expansion, stretching, or intense movements. Your body needs time to heal, and strenuous exercise can increase the risk of complications.<br>Gradual Return to Exercise: As you progress through your recovery, your surgeon may gradually allow you to reintroduce gentle physical activities. This timeline can vary based on individual factors and the extent of your surgery.<br>Listen to Your Body: Pay close attention to how your body feels during and after yoga or any physical activity. If you experience pain, discomfort, or unusual sensations, stop immediately and consult with your surgeon.<br>Modify Your Practice: When you are cleared to resume yoga, consider modifying your practice to avoid putting excess strain on your chest muscles and incisions. Use props, avoid deep stretches, and choose gentle yoga poses that don't involve significant chest or arm movement.<br>Supportive Bra: Ensure that you are wearing a supportive sports bra or the recommended post-surgical bra during any physical activity to provide adequate support and minimize breast movement.<br>Remember that everyone's recovery timeline is unique, and it's essential to prioritize your healing during this period. Rushing back into strenuous exercise too soon can lead to complications and affect your surgical results. Always consult with your plastic surgeon to ensure that your exercise plan aligns with your recovery and healing process." | "It's important to follow the guidance of your surgeon or healthcare provider when resuming physical activities after breast augmentation surgery. The timeline for when you can start doing yoga varies depending on the individual, the specifics of the surgery, and the type of yoga you plan to practice.<br><br>Generally, light activities can be resumed within a few days to a week after surgery, but it's crucial to avoid any exercises that involve heavy lifting, strenuous activities, or significant stretching of the chest muscles for at least 4-6 weeks. Some gentle yoga poses that do not put pressure on the chest or involve stretching the arms overhead might be permissible earlier, but poses that strain the chest, back, or shoulders should be avoided until your surgeon gives you the green light.<br><br>Here are a few guidelines for resuming yoga after breast augmentation:<br><br>Wait for Clearance: Get explicit clearance from your surgeon before starting yoga or any form of exercise. They might provide specific guidelines based on your recovery progress.<br>Start Slow: Begin with gentle, low-impact poses and avoid any asanas that put pressure on your chest or involve stretching or compressing the surgical area.<br>Listen to Your Body: Pay close attention to your body's signals. If you feel any pain or discomfort, stop immediately and consult your healthcare provider.<br>Modify Poses: Consider modifying poses to reduce strain on your chest and incisions. A yoga instructor familiar with post-surgery recovery can offer personalized modifications.<br>It's essential to prioritize healing and allow your body enough time to recover fully before returning to your regular yoga practice or any physical activities. Recovery times can vary, and rushing the process may lead to complications or prolong the healing period. Always consult with your healthcare provider for advice tailored to your specific situation and recovery progress." | "While it's tempting to get back to your yoga routine after 2 weeks, it's generally not recommended to resume yoga practice so soon after breast augmentation surgery. Most surgeons advise waiting for 4 to 6 weeks for your body to heal adequately before engaging in any activity that puts strain on the chest area, including yoga.<br><br>Here's why waiting is important:<br><br>Healing: The initial weeks are crucial for proper healing and minimizing the risk of complications like displaced implants or delayed wound closure. Engaging in yoga poses, especially those involving upper body movements, can put undue stress on the surgical site and hinder the healing process.<br>Discomfort: You might still experience soreness and discomfort in your chest and upper body during the first few weeks. Attempting yoga poses could exacerbate this discomfort and hinder your ability to focus on proper form and alignment.<br>However, it's important to consult with your plastic surgeon for specific guidance. They are best equipped to assess your individual recovery progress and advise on when it's safe to resume specific activities like yoga. They may even suggest modified yoga poses or alternative exercises suitable for your current stage of recovery.<br><br>In the meantime, you can focus on low-impact activities like walking or gentle stretching to stay active during your recovery." |
| Is it normal to feel abdominal numbness after a tummy tuck? | "Yes, it is normal to experience abdominal numbness after a tummy tuck (abdominoplasty) procedure. Numbness in the abdominal area is a common side effect of the surgery and is typically due to the disruption of sensory nerves during the procedure. This numbness can extend to various areas of the abdominal region and may vary in intensity from person to person.<br><br>Here are some key points to keep in mind regarding abdominal numbness after a tummy tuck:<br><br>Temporary Sensation Changes: Numbness or altered sensation in the abdominal area is usually temporary. Over time, sensation gradually returns, but it can take several months to a year or more for full sensation to come back in some cases.<br>Nerve Regeneration: As your body heals, damaged nerves will begin to regenerate, leading to a gradual return of sensation. However, the process can be slow and may not result in the same level of sensation as before the surgery.<br>Patience is Key: Be patient and allow your body time to heal. Avoid any activities that could put excessive strain on the abdominal area during the initial recovery period to minimize the risk of complications or prolonged numbness.<br>Follow-Up Appointments: Attend all scheduled follow-up appointments with your plastic surgeon. They will monitor your healing progress and can provide guidance on managing any concerns related to sensation changes.<br>Scar Management: Proper scar care and management can also play a role in the overall healing process. Follow your surgeon's recommendations for scar care to optimize the appearance of your tummy tuck scar.<br>It's important to communicate any concerns or questions about sensation changes with your plastic surgeon during your post-operative follow-up visits. They can provide you with personalized advice and address any specific issues related to your recovery. In most cases, abdominal numbness is a normal part of the healing process and should gradually improve over time" | "Yes, it is normal to feel abdominal numbness after a tummy tuck (abdominoplasty). This surgical procedure involves making incisions, tightening muscles, and removing excess skin and fat from the abdomen, which can affect the nerves in the area. Nerve endings in the skin and subcutaneous tissues may be disrupted or damaged during the procedure, leading to temporary or sometimes prolonged numbness in the treated area.<br><br>The extent and duration of the numbness can vary depending on the specifics of the surgery, such as the amount of tissue removed, the technique used, and individual healing processes. For most patients, the sensation gradually returns over months as the nerves regenerate, but it can take up to a year or more for full sensation to return. In some cases, there may be areas of permanent numbness, but this is less common.<br><br>It's important to follow your surgeon's post-operative instructions carefully and attend all follow-up appointments to monitor your healing process. If you have concerns about the numbness or if it is accompanied by signs of infection or other complications, you should contact your surgeon for advice." | "Yes, experiencing abdominal numbness after a tummy tuck is completely normal. In fact, it's one of the most common side effects of the surgery.<br><br>During a tummy tuck, some nerves in the treated area are inevitably disturbed or severed. This disrupts the communication between the nerves and the brain, leading to a temporary loss of sensation in the affected area.<br><br>The numbness can range from mild to complete and can affect the entire abdomen, specific areas like the lower abdomen or around the scar, or even extend to the upper thighs. You might also experience tingling, prickling, or a feeling of tightness in the area.<br><br>The good news is that this numbness is usually temporary. In most cases, sensation gradually returns over time, with most patients regaining normal feeling within 6 to 9 months after surgery. However, it's important to note that some patients may experience a permanent slight decrease in sensation, particularly around the scar.<br><br>Here are some additional things to keep in mind:<br><br>It's important to be patient: Don't expect your feeling to return overnight. The healing process takes time, and nerve regeneration can be slow.<br>Talk to your doctor: If you are concerned about the numbness or if it seems to be worsening, be sure to speak to your doctor. They can assess your individual situation and provide guidance.<br>Gentle massage: Once your incisions are fully healed and your doctor gives the go-ahead, gentle massage of the affected area may help promote nerve healing.<br>If you are considering a tummy tuck, it is important to be aware of the potential for temporary numbness and to discuss this with your doctor beforehand." |

**Figure 1.** Examples of the questions provided to the LLMs.

### 2.2. Employment of Language Models

Our goal was to evaluate the capabilities of the currently available LLMs to the public without utilizing an RAG approach. To do this, we used the models' responses based on their current training. After learning grammar, vocabulary, and context during pre-training with a vast dataset of internet text, the models are fine-tuned on specific datasets tailored to specialized tasks such as text generation or conversation [1]. Models such as GPT and Gemini are further trained using extensive internet-sourced text data, such as books, articles, wikis, and websites, including high-level-evidence medical research [1,14,16]. This training enables the models to provide accurate medical information.

### 2.3. Evaluation Tools

We evaluated and compared each LLM response's accuracy, readability, understandability, and actionability.

For medical accuracy, we utilized a 5-point Likert scale with the following values: 1 point: completely incorrect, 2 points: partially incorrect, 3 points: partially correct and incorrect, 4 points: partially correct, and 5 points: completely correct. To score each answer, we used as ground truth the ASPS's webpage [17–21] and textbooks such as *The Art of Aesthetic Surgery* [22] and *Essentials of Plastic Surgery* [23]. Three independent authors (C.A.G.C., S.B., and S.A.H.) analyzed and graded the responses. Any discrepancies were discussed to reach a consensus, and when not possible, the most common score assigned by the authors was used.

We used the Flesch Reading Ease (FRE) score and the Flesch–Kincaid Grade Level (FKGL) to assess readability. The FRE gives a score between 1 and 100, with scores around 100 meaning that the document is extremely easy to read. Scoring between 70 and 80 is equivalent to school-grade level 8. The FKGL assesses the approximate reading grade level of a text. If a text has an FKGL of 8, the reader needs a grade 8 reading level or above to understand it. Both tests take into account the number of sentences, words, and syllables to emit a score [24]. According to the American Medical Association (AMA) [25] and the National Institute of Health (NIH) [26], readability scores should not exceed 6th and 8th-grade levels, respectively. We calculated the FRE score and the FKGL for every model's response using a free online calculator.

We employed the Patient Education Materials Assessment Tool (PEMAT) [27] to measure the understandability and actionability of the LLMs' responses. While it is recommended for the evaluation of printed or audiovisual materials, we decided to use it as it is a systematic method designed to determine whether patients will be able to understand and act on the information provided. According to the developers' website, materials are understandable when consumers can process and explain key messages regardless of their backgrounds and level of health literacy. On the other hand, materials are actionable when patients can identify what they can do based solely on the information provided, regardless of their background and health literacy level. There are two versions of the PEMAT, for printable and for audiovisual materials. We used the printable version, which consists of 17 understandability items and 7 actionability items. Each item was rated as agree (1 point), disagree (0 points), or N/A (not applicable). The sum of the total points was divided by the total possible points (excluding items with N/A), and the result was multiplied by 100. A higher score indicates that the material is more understandable or actionable. We gave an understandability and actionability score to every response given by the LLMs.

### 2.4. Statistical Analysis

We calculated and charted the mean, mode, standard deviation (SD), and range of the evaluated metrics of the models' responses using a Microsoft Excel spreadsheet (Version 2403 Build 16.0.17425.20236) 64-bit). To compare the models' performance, we employed the analyses of variance (ANOVA) and Tukey's post hoc analysis when applicable. ANOVA and Tukey's post hoc test were calculated using Microsoft Excel's statistical package. We considered a $p$-value < 0.05 as statistically significant.

## 3. Results

### 3.1. Medical Accuracy

Overall, the three LLMs provided accurate information, with no statistically significant difference ($p = 0.85$). ChatGPT-3.5 obtained the highest mean score of 4.19 ± 0.93, followed by GPT-4 with a mean of 4.16 ± 0.88 and Gemini with a mean of 4.06 ± 0.91. The three models' scores ranged between 2 and 5 points, with 81% of the answers provided by ChatGPT-4 scoring higher than 4. The same was true for 78% and 75% of ChatGPT-3.5's and Gemini's answers, respectively (Figure 2).

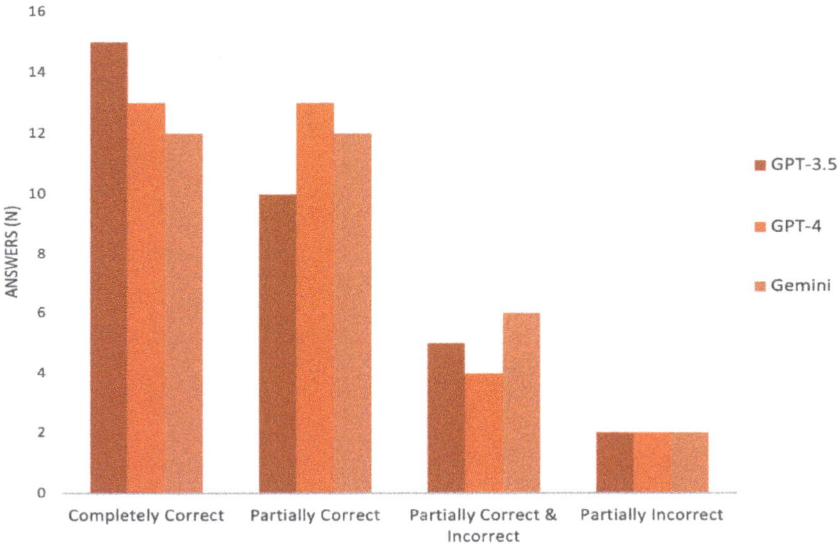


**Figure 2.** Likert scale scores per LLM.

### 3.2. Readability

Gemini's responses were significantly more readable than those of ChatGPT-3.5 and 4. The average FRE score for Gemini was 43.72 ± 10.2, which was significantly higher than ChatGPT-3.5's 33.7 ± 6.8 and ChatGPT-4's 33.7 ± 6.2 ($p = 0.001$). This translated to a significantly lower FKGL average for Gemini's responses (10.92 ± 2.0) than those of ChatGPT-3.5 (12.88 ± 1.0) and ChatGPT-4 (13.6 ± 1.3), with a $p$-value of 0.001. While 53% of the responses provided by Gemini required a college reading level, it was the only model with responses requiring a 10th to 12th-grade reading level (31%). In contrast, almost 72% of ChatGPT-4 responses required a college reading level, and 41% of those from ChatGPT-3.5 were nearly at a college graduate reading level (Figure 3).

### 3.3. Understandability and Actionability

Gemini provided more understandable responses, with an average PEMAT understandability score of 90.97 ± 3.0%. This was statistically different from ChatGPT-4, with an average score of 85.13 ± 4.9% ($p = 0.001$), and ChatGPT-3.5, which averaged at 88.31 ± 2.7% ($p = 0.014$). ChatGPT-3.5 also obtained a significantly higher average understandability score than GPT-4, with a $p$-value of 0.002. Regarding actionability, ChatGPT-4 provided the most actionable responses, with an average of 58.7 ± 8.7%. Both ChatGPT-3.5 and Gemini averaged 57.5%; however, Gemini's responses ranged among higher scores, 40–80%, as compared to ChatGPT-3.5, which scored as lower as 20% and only reached a maximum score of 60%. Nevertheless, there was no statistically significant difference in actionability among these models ($p = 0.83$) (Figure 4).

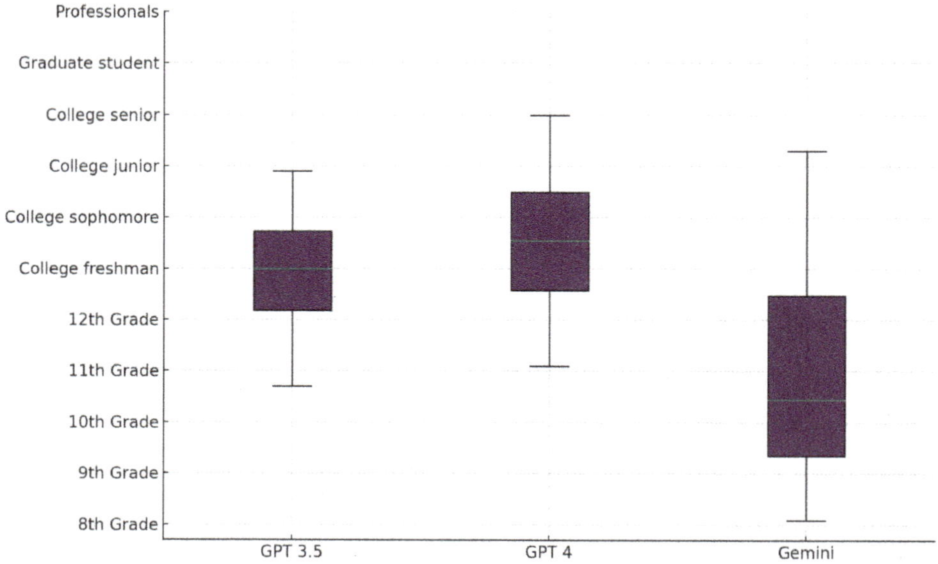


**Figure 3.** A box and whisker plot of the readability scores per LLM. Each box represents the interquartile range (25–75% of data), the line inside the box shows the median, and the whiskers extend to the smallest and largest values within 1.5 times the interquartile range from the lower and upper quartiles, respectively.

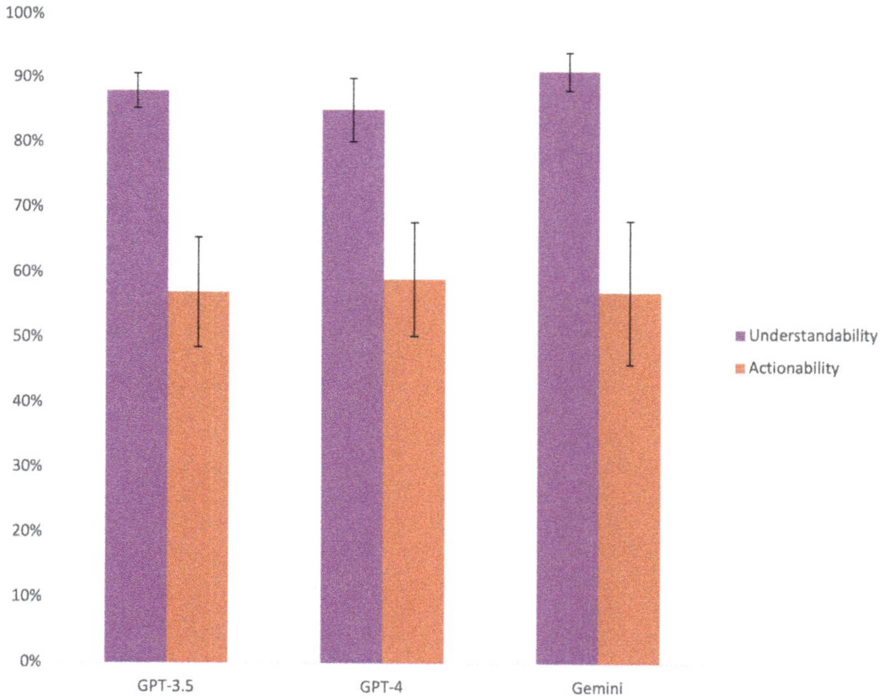


**Figure 4.** Understandability and actionability scores per LLM. Bars represent average score; error bars represent standard deviation.

## 4. Discussion

In this modern era, the vast, instantaneous access to medical information acts as a double-edged sword. While patients can easily access helpful information to guide their decisions, they can also easily be misinformed, risking making prejudicial decisions. As they are publicly available, LLMs may present as a solution by offering accurate information presented as a human-like conversation text. One study even showed that patients preferred chatbot responses over physicians' as they were perceived as more empathetic [10]. In specialties with rising demands, such as plastic surgery, these models may be pivotal as they can serve a vast number of patients simultaneously.

In plastic surgery, several studies have analyzed LLMs' capabilities for answering patient questions in the pre- and postoperative period for breast surgery [2,3,8], blepharoplasty [14], rhinoplasty [15], and oculoplastic surgery [28]. This underscores their potential as extremely helpful and valuable adjunctive tools for patient management and the importance of exploring their capabilities, with further visualization toward independent tools (Figure 5). To our knowledge, this is the first study comparing the two versions of ChatGPT and Gemini.

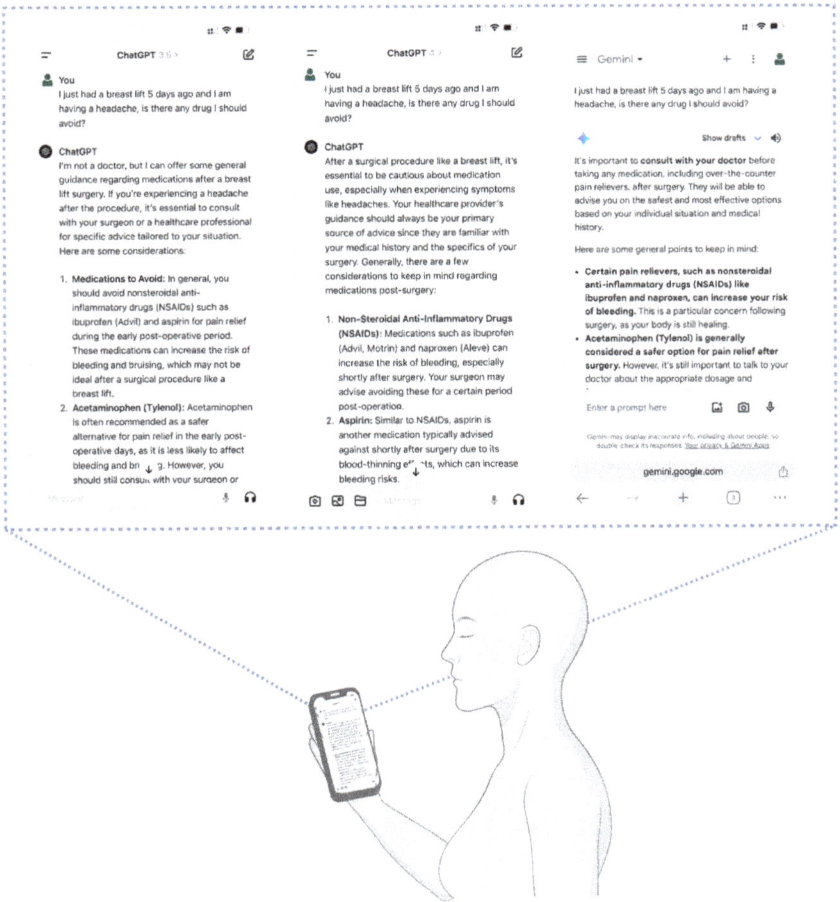


**Figure 5.** Examples of prompts given to the LLMs and an illustration of the LLMs as adjunctive tools for postoperative care. Created with BioRender [29].

Optimally, LLMs would be able to provide accurate medical information and, when not, at least provide non-harmful advice without over-alerting patients, which would further burden physicians. In our study, the three LLMs provided accurate information at least 75% of the time. Although ChatGPT-3.5 had entirely correct answers almost 47% of the time, it also responded partially incorrectly nearly 22% of the time. The latter was also true for 25% of Gemini's responses. Conversely, ChatGPT-4 was at least partially correct 81% of the time. However, there was no significant difference in the accuracy among the models. This was the opposite in Al-Sharif et al. [28] and in Abi-Rafeh et al. [2], where GPT-3.5 outperformed Bard in providing comprehensive, accurate responses.

Even though there was no statistical difference, we identified that ChatGPT-4's responses were more comprehensive and straightforward than those of ChatGPT-3.5 and Gemini, as they were usually preceded or followed by unnecessary, unuseful content. It was common for all of the models to recommend asking or visiting their surgeon, even when the questions were unrelated to life-threatening scenarios. However, Gemini stated four times that it was unable to provide any medical advice as it was just an LLM and instead encouraged patients to visit a doctor. Similarly, ChatGPT-3.5 started its response by saying it was not a doctor before providing an accurate response twice. This may be an attempt to avoid accountability or a way to express their limitations as LLMs, but it was not the case for ChatGPT-4.

Despite their impressive ability to process information, LLMs still struggle to provide completely accurate responses, which remains the most prevailing concern in their use among specialties [30]. ChatGPT-3.5's latest update was in March 2022, which hinders its ability to answer questions with updated information after that date. Although ChatGPT-4 was last updated in April 2023, the same can still be true. Both GPT-4 and Gemini can access the Internet to provide updated information; nevertheless, their responses are primarily based on their training data [4]. This risks the models being biased as they cannot only inherit but also amplify biases present in their training data [31,32], perpetuating inequalities related to factors such as race, gender, and socioeconomic status [1,11]. Moreover, LLMs may generate fabricated responses, often referred to as hallucinations, when lacking information, which can result in deviations from established practices [30]. Statistical parity ensures that the demographics used for training the models are the same as the demographics of the population where they will be implemented, which can be achieved with specialized training [31,32]. However, for now, it is crucial to analyze inaccurate responses and verify the information generated by the models [30–32].

Our study determined none of the responses as completely incorrect, only partially incorrect. This may be seen in the scenario of an acute postoperative period of a patient who underwent an abdominoplasty and wanted to know how many days she had to stay in bed. ChatGPT-4 suggested gentle walks around the house and no strenuous activities but failed to mention the number of days. On the other hand, Gemini accurately mentioned that it was not recommended to stay in bed as early ambulation was crucial for recovery. However, it did not say why and then contradicted itself by recommending 2 days of strict bed rest followed by short walks and light activity. While low Likert scores do not necessarily mean that the responses might be harmful to the patient, encourage risky behaviors, or provide misinformation, these inaccuracies make them unfit as independent tools.

Although medical accuracy is paramount, LLMs' responses must be readable to successfully serve their purpose as patient resources. The average adult in the United States reads at approximately a 7th-grade reading level [33]. Additionally, one study identified that in plastic surgery, 50.2% of patients had an education level lower than high school and that 48% of attendings, residents, and PAs said it was challenging to make patients follow postoperative instructions [34]. Moreover, patient materials in plastic surgery are often above the recommended average reading level of 6th to 8th grade and may be too difficult for the average patient [34–37].

Vallurupalli et al. [37] successfully used ChatGPT-3.5 to significantly simplify traditional patient education materials for craniofacial surgery by 3 FKGL points. Interestingly, in our study, ChatGPT-3.5 and 4's average FKGL scores were far superior to the recommended reading level. This was consistent with the results of Momenaei et al. [38], where ChatGPT-4's FKGL and FRE scores averaged at 14.3 and 31.6, respectively. Conversely, Gemini proved to be significantly superior in terms of readability, with responses at an average reading level of 10th grade and an average FRE score 10 points higher than that of the other models. Al-Sharif et al. [28] identified similar results, with GPT having a higher analytical reading inventory (ARI) score than BARD, indicating that a higher level of education was required to understand its responses. Perhaps providing tailored prompts requesting a specific reading level might consistently improve the readability of the answers. However, this might risk oversimplifying the responses and missing essential information.

Gemini also outperformed both ChatGPT models in providing understandable answers. This was because the PEMAT contemplates the use of visual aids as part of its score. Gemini created images for three responses, two of which helped improve understandability. Additionally, in a question about breast augmentation complications, it provided a link to the FDA information website. While ChatGPT-4 also has the ability to create images due to its integration with DALL-E, it only does so when specifically asked to. The ability to think when it would be appropriate to include images for an explanation instead of waiting to be asked to is what determined Gemini's superiority. Nevertheless, both GPT models scored above 85%, proving that they provide understandable answers. Similar to readability, tailoring the prompt so that it provides helpful images may improve further ChatGPT-4's understandability.

Overall, the three models performed poorly in actionability, scoring less than 60% on average. This was a consequence of the format in which the models presented their responses. A minimum of two out of the seven questions were not applicable, and while most of the time they provided clear, broken down actions, they rarely provided tangible tools such as checklists. As visual aids were also part of the actionability section, both GPT models could only score as high as 80%. Although Gemini did provide images, they were not useful for inspiring actionability, hence not showing any difference between the models.

## 5. Strengths and Limitations

To our knowledge, this is the first study comparing the two versions of ChatGPT and Gemini in terms of providing postoperative care recommendations to patients who have undergone cosmetic plastic surgery procedures. However, our study has some limitations. First are the limited number of questions prompted per procedure. This limited the depth in which we could analyze the models' capacity to provide accurate, readable, understandable, and actionable responses for any particular procedure, limiting their clinical applicability. Furthermore, our findings may not generalize to other LLMs or fields within or outside of plastic surgery and are limited by the current training data of the models. Further research into the newest, more potent versions of Gemini may be paramount, especially considering the current version's superiority to ChatGPT models. Moreover, with additional research constraining the LLMs to provide good-quality information, either through RAG, functional tuning, prompt engineering, or parameterization, we can leverage language understanding but restrict the answers to good, accurate information. Notably, as LLMs evolve rapidly and constantly, our results will likely differ from those obtained in the near future. Nevertheless, a continuous evaluation of model performance is crucial at all stages of development. The limitations and weaknesses highlighted by our study can provide valuable insights to guide future development and practice, especially toward specialty-specific models.

The present study evaluated the LLMs' responses based on their textual contents without considering the patient–physician interaction and feedback. The impact on patient understanding, satisfaction, subsequent behavior, and real-life clinical settings remains unexplored. Lastly, our study primarily focused on English-language responses, demanding further research on the performance across different languages and cultural contexts.

## 6. Conclusions

Our study provides valuable insights into the efficacy of LLMs in delivering postoperative care recommendations to patients who have undergone cosmetic plastic surgery. Although ChatGPT-4 is the most effective and latest updated version of OpenAI, the publicly available 3.5 version and Google's Gemini public version provided equally accurate medical advice. However, Gemini proved to be superior in providing understandable and more readable responses. While all three models demonstrated their potential as adjunctive tools in postoperative patient care, their shortcomings in providing actionable and concise guidance highlight the need for additional refinement and research to enable their evolution into comprehensive standalone resources. Further experimentation is necessary to evaluate the performance of a retrieval-augmented generation technique.

**Supplementary Materials:** The following supporting information can be downloaded at: https://www.mdpi.com/article/10.3390/healthcare12111083/s1, Supplementary File S1. Questions provided to LLMs; Supplementary File S2. LLMs Responses.

**Author Contributions:** Conceptualization, A.J.F., A.S. and C.A.G.-C.; methodology, C.A.G.-C. and S.B.; software, C.A.G.-C. and S.A.H.; formal analysis, C.A.G.-C., S.M.P. and S.B.; validation, S.A.H., S.B. and S.M.P.; investigation, C.A.G.-C., S.M.P. and S.A.H.; writing—original draft, C.A.G.-C. and S.B.; writing—review and editing, S.B., S.M.P., S.A.H., B.C.L., A.S. and A.J.F.; supervision, A.J.F., A.S. and B.C.L.; project administration, A.J.F., A.S. and B.C.L. All authors have read and agreed to the published version of the manuscript.

**Funding:** This research received no external funding.

**Institutional Review Board Statement:** Not applicable.

**Informed Consent Statement:** Not applicable.

**Data Availability Statement:** The raw data supporting the conclusions of this article will be made available by the authors upon request.

**Conflicts of Interest:** The authors declare no conflicts of interest.

## References

1. Hadi, M.U.; Al-Tashi, Q.; Qureshi, R.; Shah, A.; Muneer, A.; Irfan, M.; Zafar, A.; Shaikh, M.B.; Akhtar, N.; Al-Garadi, M.A.; et al. Large Language Models: A Comprehensive Survey of Applications, Challenges, Limitations, and Future Prospects. *TechRxiv* **2023**. [CrossRef]
2. Abi-Rafeh, J.; Henry, N.; Xu, H.H.; Bassiri-Tehrani, B.; Arezki, A.; Kazan, R.; Gilardino, M.S.; Nahai, F. Utility and Comparative Performance of Current Artificial Intelligence Large Language Models as Postoperative Medical Support Chatbots in Aesthetic Surgery. *Aesthet. Surg. J.* **2024**, sjae025. [CrossRef] [PubMed]
3. Seth, I.; Cox, A.; Xie, Y.; Bulloch, G.; Hunter-Smith, D.J.; Rozen, W.M.; Ross, R.J. Evaluating Chatbot Efficacy for Answering Frequently Asked Questions in Plastic Surgery: A ChatGPT Case Study Focused on Breast Augmentation. *Aesthet. Surg. J.* **2023**, *43*, 1126–1135. [CrossRef] [PubMed]
4. Gupta, R.; Pande, P.; Herzog, I.; Weisberger, J.; Chao, J.; Chaiyasate, K.; Lee, E.S. Application of ChatGPT in Cosmetic Plastic Surgery: Ally or Antagonist? *Aesthet. Surg. J.* **2023**, *43*, NP587–NP590. [CrossRef] [PubMed]
5. American Society of Plastic Surgeons. American Society of Plastic Surgeons Reveals 2022's Most Sought-After Procedures. Available online: https://www.plasticsurgery.org/news/press-releases/american-society-of-plastic-surgeons-reveals-2022s-most-sought-after-procedures (accessed on 12 February 2024).
6. Humar, P.; Asaad, M.; Bengur, F.B.; Nguyen, V. ChatGPT Is Equivalent to First-Year Plastic Surgery Residents: Evaluation of ChatGPT on the Plastic Surgery In-Service Examination. *Aesthet. Surg. J.* **2023**, *43*, NP1085–NP1089. [CrossRef] [PubMed]
7. Pan, W.; Liu, D.; Fang, J. An Examination of Factors Contributing to the Acceptance of Online Health Misinformation. *Front. Psychol.* **2021**, *12*, 630268. [CrossRef] [PubMed]
8. Yun, J.Y.; Kim, D.J.; Lee, N.; Kim, E.K. A comprehensive evaluation of ChatGPT consultation quality for augmentation mammoplasty: A comparative analysis between plastic surgeons and laypersons. *Int. J. Med. Inform.* **2023**, *179*, 105219. [CrossRef] [PubMed]
9. Aliyeva, A.; Sari, E.; Alaskarov, E.; Nasirov, R. Enhancing Postoperative Cochlear Implant Care With ChatGPT-4: A Study on Artificial Intelligence (AI)-Assisted Patient Education and Support. *Cureus* **2024**, *16*, e53897. [CrossRef] [PubMed]

10. Ayers, J.W.; Poliak, A.; Dredze, M.; Leas, E.C.; Zhu, Z.; Kelley, J.B.; Faix, D.J.; Goodman, A.M.; Longhurst, C.A.; Hogarth, M.; et al. Comparing Physician and Artificial Intelligence Chatbot Responses to Patient Questions Posted to a Public Social Media Forum. *JAMA Intern. Med.* **2023**, *183*, 589–596. [CrossRef]
11. Clusmann, J.; Kolbinger, F.R.; Muti, H.S.; Carrero, Z.I.; Eckardt, J.N.; Laleh, N.G.; Loffler, C.M.L.; Schwarzkopf, S.C.; Unger, M.; Veldhuizen, G.P.; et al. The future landscape of large language models in medicine. *Commun. Med.* **2023**, *3*, 141. [CrossRef]
12. Dias, P.; Clerc, D.; da Rocha Rodrigues, M.G.; Demartines, N.; Grass, F.; Hubner, M. Impact of an Operating Room Nurse Preoperative Dialogue on Anxiety, Satisfaction and Early Postoperative Outcomes in Patients Undergoing Major Visceral Surgery-A Single Center, Open-Label, Randomized Controlled Trial. *J. Clin. Med.* **2022**, *11*, 1895. [CrossRef] [PubMed]
13. Putterman, A.M. Patient satisfaction in oculoplastic surgery. *Ophthalmic Surg. Lasers Imaging Retin.* **1990**, *21*, 15–21. [CrossRef]
14. Cox, A.; Seth, I.; Xie, Y.; Hunter-Smith, D.J.; Rozen, W.M. Utilizing ChatGPT-4 for Providing Medical Information on Blepharoplasties to Patients. *Aesthet. Surg. J.* **2023**, *43*, NP658–NP662. [CrossRef] [PubMed]
15. Soto-Galindo, G.A.; Capelleras, M.; Cruellas, M.; Apaydin, F. Effectiveness of ChatGPT in Identifying and Accurately Guiding Patients in Rhinoplasty Complications. *Facial Plast. Surg.* 2023. *online ahead of print*. [CrossRef]
16. Atkinson, C.J.; Seth, I.; Xie, Y.; Ross, R.J.; Hunter-Smith, D.J.; Rozen, W.M.; Cuomo, R. Artificial Intelligence Language Model Performance for Rapid Intraoperative Queries in Plastic Surgery: ChatGPT and the Deep Inferior Epigastric Perforator Flap. *J. Clin. Med.* **2024**, *13*, 900. [CrossRef] [PubMed]
17. American Society of Plastic Surgeons. What are the Risks of Eyelid Surgery? Available online: https://www.plasticsurgery.org/cosmetic-procedures/eyelid-surgery/safety?_gl=1*4kj7fz*_ga*OTU4NTgxOTM3LjE3MDc5NDcwOTY.*_ga_2N9PTXXTDN*MTcxMDM0ODc1MC44LjEuMTcxMDM0ODkwOC41Ny4wLjA (accessed on 2 February 2024).
18. American Society of Plastic Surgeons. What are the Risks of Breast Augmentation? Available online: https://www.plasticsurgery.org/cosmetic-procedures/breast-augmentation/safety?_gl=1*aa45id*_ga*OTU4NTgxOTM3LjE3MDc5NDcwOTY.*_ga_2N9PTXXTDN*MTcxMDk0NjQwOC4xMS4xLjE3MTA5NDY2OTEuMTYuMC4w%20 (accessed on 2 February 2024).
19. American Society of Plastic Surgeons. What Are the Risks of Breast Lift Surgery? Available online: https://www.plasticsurgery.org/cosmetic-procedures/breast-lift/safety?_gl=1*1xicxp8*_ga*OTU4NTgxOTM3LjE3MDc5NDcwOTY.*_ga_2N9PTXXTDN*MTcxMDk0NjQwOC4xMS4xLjE3MTA5NDY4MDEuNTkuMC4w (accessed on 2 February 2024).
20. American Society of Plastic Surgeons. What Are the Risks of Liposuction? Available online: https://www.plasticsurgery.org/cosmetic-procedures/liposuction/safety?_gl=1*xsqaqz*_ga*OTU4NTgxOTM3LjE3MDc5NDcwOTY.*_ga_2N9PTXXTDN*MTcxMDk0NjQwOC4xMS4xLjE3MTA5NDY5MjcuNTkuMC4w (accessed on 2 February 2024).
21. American Society of Plastic Surgeons. What Are the Risks of Tummy Tuck Surgery? Available online: https://www.plasticsurgery.org/cosmetic-procedures/tummy-tuck/safety?_gl=1*n5pmbf*_ga*OTU4NTgxOTM3LjE3MDc5NDcwOTY.*_ga_2N9PTXXTDN*MTcxMDk0NjQwOC4xMS4xLjE3MTA5NDcwODYuNTIuMC4w (accessed on 2 February 2024).
22. *The Art of Aesthetic Surgery: Principles & Techniques*, 3rd ed.; Nahai, F.; Nahai, F. (Eds.) Thieme: New York, NY, USA, 2020. [CrossRef]
23. *Essentials of Plastic Surgery*, 3rd ed.; Janis, J.E. (Ed.) Thieme: New York, NY, USA, 2022.
24. Readable. Flesch Reading Ease and the Flesch Kincaid Grade Level. Available online: https://readable.com/readability/flesch-reading-ease-flesch-kincaid-grade-level/ (accessed on 12 February 2024).
25. Weis, B. *Health Literacy: A Manual for Clinicians*; American Medical Association, American Medical Foundation: Chicago, IL, USA, 2003.
26. Rooney, M.K.; Santiago, G.; Perni, S.; Horowitz, D.P.; McCall, A.R.; Einstein, A.J.; Jagsi, R.; Golden, D.W. Readability of Patient Education Materials From High-Impact Medical Journals: A 20-Year Analysis. *J. Patient Exp.* **2021**, *8*, 2374373521998847. [CrossRef] [PubMed]
27. Shoemaker, S.J.; Wolf, M.S.; Brach, C. Development of the Patient Education Materials Assessment Tool (PEMAT): A new measure of understandability and actionability for print and audiovisual patient information. *Patient Educ. Couns.* **2014**, *96*, 395–403. [CrossRef] [PubMed]
28. Al-Sharif, E.M.; Penteado, R.C.; Dib El Jalbout, N.; Topilow, N.J.; Shoji, M.K.; Kikkawa, D.O.; Liu, C.Y.; Korn, B.S. Evaluating the Accuracy of ChatGPT and Google BARD in Fielding Oculoplastic Patient Queries: A Comparative Study on Artificial versus Human Intelligence. *Ophthalmic Plast. Reconstr. Surg.* **2024**, *40*, 303–311. [CrossRef] [PubMed]
29. BioRender. Available online: https://www.biorender.com/ (accessed on 16 February 2024).
30. Pressman, S.M.; Borna, S.; Gomez-Cabello, C.A.; Haider, S.A.; Haider, C.; Forte, A.J. AI and Ethics: A Systematic Review of the Ethical Considerations of Large Language Model Use in Surgery Research. *Healthcare* **2024**, *12*, 825. [CrossRef]
31. Leslie, D.; Mazumder, A.; Peppin, A.; Wolters, M.K.; Hagerty, A. Does "AI" stand for augmenting inequality in the era of covid-19 healthcare? *BMJ* **2021**, *372*, n304. [CrossRef]
32. Zaidi, D.; Miller, T. Implicit Bias and Machine Learning in Health Care. *South. Med. J.* **2023**, *116*, 62–64. [CrossRef] [PubMed]
33. Ricci, J.A.; Vargas, C.R.; Chuang, D.J.; Lin, S.J.; Lee, B.T. Readability assessment of online patient resources for breast augmentation surgery. *Plast. Reconstr. Surg.* **2015**, *135*, 1573–1579. [CrossRef] [PubMed]
34. Barton, N.; Janis, J.E. Missing the Mark: The State of Health Care Literacy in Plastic Surgery. *Plast. Reconstr. Surg. Glob. Open* **2020**, *8*, e2856. [CrossRef] [PubMed]
35. Chen, A.D.; Ruan, Q.Z.; Bucknor, A.; Chattha, A.S.; Bletsis, P.P.; Furnas, H.J.; Lee, B.T.; Lin, S.J. Social Media: Is the Message Reaching the Plastic Surgery Audience? *Plast. Reconstr. Surg.* **2019**, *144*, 773–781. [CrossRef] [PubMed]

36. Fanning, J.E.; Okamoto, L.A.; Levine, E.C.; McGee, S.A.; Janis, J.E. Content and Readability of Online Recommendations for Breast Implant Size Selection. *Plast. Reconstr. Surg. Glob. Open* **2023**, *11*, e4787. [CrossRef] [PubMed]
37. Vallurupalli, M.; Shah, N.D.; Vyas, R.M. Validation of ChatGPT 3.5 as a Tool to Optimize Readability of Patient-facing Craniofacial Education Materials. *Plast. Reconstr. Surg. Glob. Open* **2024**, *12*, e5575. [CrossRef]
38. Momenaei, B.; Wakabayashi, T.; Shahlaee, A.; Durrani, A.F.; Pandit, S.A.; Wang, K.; Mansour, H.A.; Abishek, R.M.; Xu, D.; Sridhar, J.; et al. Appropriateness and Readability of ChatGPT-4-Generated Responses for Surgical Treatment of Retinal Diseases. *Ophthalmol. Retin.* **2023**, *7*, 862–868. [CrossRef]

healthcare

MDPI

Article

# Beyond the Clinic Walls: Examining Radiology Technicians' Experiences in Home-Based Radiography

Graziano Lepri [1], Francesco Oddi [2], Rosario Alfio Gulino [2] and Daniele Giansanti [3,*]

1 Azienda Unità Sanitaria Locale Umbria 1, Via Guerriero Guerra 21, 06127 Perugia, Italy; graziano.lepri@uslumbria1.it
2 Facoltà di Ingegneria, Università di Tor Vergata, Via del Politecnico, 1, 00133 Rome, Italy; francesco.oddi@alumni.uniroma2.eu (F.O.); gulino@disp.uniroma2.it (R.A.G.)
3 Centro Nazionale TISP, Istituto Superiore di Sanità, Viale Regina Elena 299, 00161 Rome, Italy
* Correspondence: daniele.giansanti@iss.it; Tel.: +39-0649902701

**Abstract:** In recent years, the landscape of diagnostic imaging has undergone a significant transformation with the emergence of home radiology, challenging the traditional paradigm. This shift, bringing diagnostic imaging directly to patients, has gained momentum and has been further accelerated by the global COVID-19 pandemic, highlighting the increasing importance and convenience of decentralized healthcare services. This study aims to offer a nuanced understanding of the attitudes and experiences influencing the integration of in-home radiography into contemporary healthcare practices. The research methodology involves a survey administered through Computer-Aided Web Interviewing (CAWI) tools, enabling real-time engagement with a diverse cohort of medical radiology technicians in the health domain. A second CAWI tool is submitted to experts to assess their feedback on the methodology. The survey explores key themes, including perceived advantages and challenges associated with domiciliary imaging, its impact on patient care, and the technological intricacies specific to conducting radiologic procedures outside the conventional clinical environment. Findings from a sample of 26 medical radiology technicians (drawn from a larger pool of 186 respondents) highlight a spectrum of opinions and constructive feedback. Enthusiasm is evident for the potential of domiciliary imaging to enhance patient convenience and provide a more patient-centric approach to healthcare. Simultaneously, this study suggests areas of intervention to improve the diffusion of home-based radiology. The methodology based on CAWI tools proves instrumental in the efficiency and depth of data collection, as evaluated by 16 experts from diverse professional backgrounds. The dynamic and responsive nature of this approach allows for a more allocated exploration of technicians' opinions, contributing to a comprehensive understanding of the evolving landscape of medical imaging services. Emphasis is placed on the need for national and international initiatives in the field, supported by scientific societies, to further explore the evolving landscape of teleradiology and the integration of artificial intelligence in radiology. This study encourages expansion involving other key figures in this practice, including, naturally, medical radiologists, general practitioners, medical physicists, and other stakeholders.

**Keywords:** radiology; home radiology; CAWI; technology assessment

## 1. Introduction

### 1.1. Background

Within the transformative realm of domiciliary radiology, illuminated by the exhaustive scoping review led by Toppemberg et al. [1], a profound shift in healthcare delivery is discernible. Spanning from the pioneering initiatives of Losev in 1958 [2] to contemporary endeavors exemplified by Mark et al.'s establishment of a domiciliary-based X-ray response team in 2022 [3], a palpable evolution toward a patient-centric ethos in radiological practices unfolds. While an array of studies illuminates promising outcomes, encompassing noteworthy cost-effectiveness [4], intricate operational dynamics [5], and a resounding positive reception from patients [6], a compelling necessity emerges for a meticulous exploration into the experiential landscape of professionals within this dynamically evolving field.

The landmark survey conducted by Sawyer et al. in 1995 [7], resonating with the unanimous acknowledgment among practitioners regarding the paramount significance of domiciliary radiography, triggers a critical examination of the nuanced challenges encountered by these professionals. Recent inquiries led by Andersen et al. [5] and Dollard et al. [6], offering invaluable insights into the operational nuances and patient perspectives, further illuminate the multifaceted nature of assimilating radiological services into the fabric of non-clinical settings. While economic analyses by Kjelle et al. [4] present commendable evidence of cost reduction, Aldridge et al.'s scrupulous study [8] underscores the need for qualitative investigations to glean a comprehensive understanding. The exhaustive analysis conducted by Kjelle and Lysdahl [9], reaffirming the potential advantages of domiciliary radiology, accentuates reductions in hospital transfers and the assurance of timely diagnoses. In a broader societal context, public–private partnerships, as exemplified by Datta et al. (2017) [10], illustrate the potential impact of collaborative efforts in addressing healthcare gaps. The success of this specific initiative in detecting pulmonary TB highlights the broader role such partnerships can play in scaling up and designing impactful interventions. This small sample of recent studies (although a specific review study would undoubtedly provide an even broader perspective) already serves as an illustration of how domiciliary radiology can be conducted in various locations and settings, each with a different focus, as outlined in Table 1.

**Table 1.** An example of the locations/focuses of application of home radiology.

| Study | Location | Focus |
|---|---|---|
| Andersen et al. (2023) [5] | Community settings | Implementation initiatives for patient-centered care through setting up a mobile X-ray unit in the community |
| Dollard et al. (2022) [6] | Residential aged care facility | Residents' perspectives on mobile X-ray services supporting healthcare-in-place in aged care facilities |
| Kjelle et al. (2019) [4] | Nursing homes in Southeast Norway | Cost analysis of mobile radiography services for nursing home residents |
| Aldridge et al. (2015) [8] | Homeless hostels | Effectiveness of peer educators on the uptake of mobile X-ray tuberculosis screening |
| Kjelle and Lysdahl (2017) [9] | Nursing homes | Investigation on services in nursing homes, examining residents' and societal outcomes |
| Datta et al. (2017) [10] | Public–private partnership | Detection of sputum-negative pulmonary TB through digital chest X-ray conducted via a mobile van |

In navigating these intricately woven dimensions, it becomes imperatively clear that a comprehensive technology assessment is not merely a desirable but an essential undertaking. The narrative, gracefully meandering through historical foundations, the intertwined perspectives of practitioners and patients, the intricacies of operational challenges, economic considerations, and collaborative models, resoundingly underscores the transformative potential embedded within domiciliary radiology. This evocative landscape underscores the need for a meticulous investigation into the experiences and perspectives of professionals operating within this evolving field, as has been conducted in other fields of digital radiology in several applications, including teleradiology and the integration of artificial intelligence [11–27]. An overview of surveys provides a nuanced understanding of various aspects of the field. Starting with a snapshot of teleradiology practice in Turkey, Dicle et al. delve into the practicalities and challenges faced by radiologists [11]. Transitioning to Ghana, Dzefi-Tettey et al. explore the perceptions of clinical medical students regarding a career in radiology, shedding light on the factors influencing future professionals in the field [12]. Vabo et al.'s survey focuses on patient-reported outcomes after fracture treatment in primary healthcare, providing insights into the impact of initial conservative approaches [13]. On the technological front, Macedo et al. evaluate the usability and efficiency of an application in orthopedics, emphasizing the integration of technology into diagnostic processes [14]. The socio-economic and psychological repercussions of the COVID-19 outbreak on radiologists are investigated by Florin et al., offering a glimpse into the challenges faced by practitioners [15]. In Japan, Yamashiro et al. present survey results on work-style reform and technology utilization among diagnostic radiologists, reflecting the evolving landscape of radiological practices [16]. A comprehensive survey encompassing radiologists, medical students, and surgeons by van Hoek et al. underscores skepticism about artificial intelligence and the potential evolution of the radiology field [17]. Turning to the realm of teleradiology, Coppola et al. present Italian survey results, while Jacobs et al. explore patient satisfaction with teleradiology services in general practice [18,19]. The on-call service of neurosurgeons in Germany is investigated by Brenke et al., revealing organizational aspects and the acceptance of modern technologies [20]. Meanwhile, Kim et al. gauge the attitude of Korean primary care family physicians toward telehealth, offering insights into the acceptance and perspectives of telehealth services [21]. Examining factors influencing clinician satisfaction with radiology services, Lindsay et al. contribute to the discourse on service quality [22]. Winblad et al.'s nationwide survey in Finland sheds light on the positive aspects found in healthcare information and communication technology implementation [23]. Finally, Ninos et al. focus on the development and evaluation of a PDA-based teleradiology terminal, emphasizing advancements in technology and diagnostic capabilities [24]. CAWI tools could be a valid aid, as demonstrated under the COVID-19 pandemic [25] and in the investigation of the acceptance of the integration with artificial intelligence [26,27]. Collectively, these surveys weave a narrative that encompasses technological advancements, practitioner perspectives, patient outcomes, and the evolving landscape of radiological practices. The discourse not only underscores the current state of the field but also hints at potential future directions, emphasizing the need for continuous adaptation and innovation in the dynamic field of radiology. The application of surveys in home/domiciliary radiology could provide a nuanced understanding of various aspects of this specialized field. Such an exploration is not merely an academic endeavor but a crucial undertaking to comprehend the intricate challenges, gain unique insights, and consider the pragmatic aspects confronted by these professionals. A dedicated investigation into their experiences could not only enhance our understanding but also shape strategies and policies aligned with the dynamic nuances of domiciliary radiology. This, in turn, contributes to fostering its seamless integration into contemporary healthcare practices. Overall, the brief literature analysis highlights the need for targeted surveys among professionals directly involved in home radiology practice to gather valuable and structured information for enhancing and promoting this approach. From a healthcare perspective, this practice can bring numerous advantages, as seen in this brief review, by shifting the practice to the patient's home and avoiding complex hospital visits. Fragile and/or significantly disabled patients, for instance, can benefit significantly from the spread of home radiology. The healthcare system can also gain several advantages, as it prevents potential risks of worsening for these patient categories.

### 1.2. The Rationale for the Study and Purpose

Exploring home radiology involves addressing pivotal questions spanning logistical, training, patient care, and technological aspects. Key inquiries include optimizing logistical challenges, defining essential skills for technicians, assessing patient care impact, understanding technological requirements, implementing quality control, gauging technician opinions, tracking industry evolution, leveraging patient feedback, and identifying specific populations or scenarios where domiciliary imaging excels or faces challenges. This comprehensive framework sheds light on the inherent opportunities and obstacles in the dynamic field of home radiology.

The aim of the study is to conduct a *pilot study* facing a comprehensive investigation into home radiology by scrutinizing the experiences, challenges, and perceptions of medical radiology technicians, with the overarching goal of informing strategies for the optimal integration of domiciliary radiology into modern healthcare practices.

## 2. Methods

The research methodology hinged upon the deployment of a comprehensive questionnaire facilitated by a cutting-edge CAWI tool. This instrument was strategically disseminated not only to citizens but also to other professionals potentially engaged in the realm of home radiology practices in the *health domain*.

The participants in the pilot study were contacted using peer-to-peer methods, which leveraged messenger/chatting groups and social media platforms. These methods were used to select participants based on professions and on their affiliations with professional associations. Throughout this outreach process, utmost care was taken both to ensure the privacy of the participants was respected during all interactions and to reach the entire national territory.

To facilitate the data-collection process, Computer-Assisted Web Interviewing (CAWI) tools were employed. These tools were customized with different menus and sets of questions, which were tailored to the specific professions declared by the participants in the initial survey questions. This customization ensured that the questions were relevant and appropriate for each participant group. The development of the CAWI tools was executed utilizing Microsoft Forms, a deliberate choice owing to its seamless integration with the Office 365 (Version 2024) suite provided to the Tor Vergata University staff. Notably, Microsoft Forms boasts certification for compliance with prevailing IT security regulations from a systems perspective.

This choice was, therefore, influenced by the tool's integration within the university's Office 365 suite and its official approval for research purposes. Selecting an alternative external tool would have necessitated additional approval processes, which were not guaranteed and would have entailed a significant expenditure of time and resources.

Overall, these strategic decisions regarding participant outreach and data collection tools were made to ensure the efficiency, reliability, and ethical integrity of the research process.

Within the confines of this pilot study, our analytical focus has been steadfastly directed toward scrutinizing the outcomes derived from the detected perspectives of medical radiology technicians (MRTs). As the linchpin figures in the delivery of home radiology practices, their insights carry paramount significance. It is pertinent to note that our ongoing efforts extend beyond this specific cohort, encompassing a broader spectrum of stakeholders. Furthermore, we introduced a secondary CAWI tool tailored for experts affiliated with national scientific societies and the national associations of professionals integral to this phase of the project.

The dissemination of both CAWI instruments occurred in a peer-to-peer fashion, ensuring anonymity, and leveraged social networks and other channels affiliated with the scientific societies and associations involved. This approach was meticulously crafted to uphold the utmost standards of privacy and confidentiality. The following modules were used in the CAWI:

- Single choice questions;
- Multiple choice questions;
- Evaluation (graded) questions (with a 6-level psychometric scale);
- Likert questions with a 6-level scale;
- Open-ended questions (in a few cases).

The *principal CAWI tool is the electronic survey (ES),* which allows the collection of feedback from the actors related to the home radiology practice.

The link and the QR code for the electronic survey are as follows: https://forms.office.com/e/fW1w6YbwNr (accessed on 15 March 2024) (see Figure 1).

**Figure 1.** The QR code of ES.

The *second tool*, the CAWI tool, is the *electronic feedback form* (EFF) dedicated to the experts of the scientific societies/scientific associations.

Below, we report the link and the QR code for the EFF: https://forms.office.com/e/MW9M7aykWP (accessed on 15 March 2024) (see Figure 2).

**Figure 2.** The QR code of the EFF.

## 3. Results

The results are organized into sections and subsections.

Section 3.1, *"The Outcome from the Electronic Survey"*, presents the results of administering the electronic survey to radiologic healthcare technicians. This section consists of three subsections.

Section 3.1.1, *"Insights into the Study Participants: Unveiling Characteristics of the Sample"*, characterizes the sample.

Section 3.1.2, *"Findings from Graded, Multiple-Choice, and Likert Scale Questions"*, reports the outcome of quantitative data obtained from numerical responses (single-choice questions, multiple-choice questions, graded questions, and Likert questions with a 6-level scale).

The last section, Section 3.1.3, *"Unveiling Insights from Open-Ended Responses: A Dual Perspective on Feedback and the Future of Home Radiology"*, reports the outcome of open-ended responses.

Section 3.2, *"The Outcome from the Electronic Feedback Form"*, presents the results of administering the CAWI to experts to gather feedback on the devised tool. It is divided into two subsections.

Section 3.2.1, *"Identification of the Expert Observer Group"*, identifies the group of experts involved in this CAWI.

Section 3.2.2, *"In-Depth Feedback Through the Electronic Feedback Form"*, reports the outcome of the administration of the second CAWI:

Finally, Section 3.3, *"Comprehensive Insights Summary"*, provides a synthesis of the results for the two CAWI administrations, organized into two corresponding subsections: Section 3.3.1, *"Insight summary from the Electronic survey"*, and Section 3.3.2, *"Insight summary from the Electronic Feedback Form"*.

### 3.1. The Outcome of the Electronic Survey

#### 3.1.1. Insights into the Study Participants: Unveiling Characteristics of the Sample

One significant outcome derived from this study is the development of the CAWI product, a result of careful consideration given to multiple perspectives. The individuals involved in this endeavor comprised *Bioengineers, Medical Engineers, and experts with a background in health professions and diagnostic techniques, including training in medical radiology techniques. Additionally, experts in economics and the development of Medical Devices* were part of this collaborative effort, with these first five competencies being among the authors of the work. Furthermore, contributors from the fields of *medical physics and radiological medicine* also played integral roles. Notably, no critical issues were identified across any of the submissions. It is noteworthy that the survey was completed swiftly, with participants taking an average of 79.7 s to open and complete it, never exceeding 120 s in the entire process. After the survey was opened, every participant willingly provided their responses. Notably, there are no inquiries related to cybersecurity, as the team has carefully evaluated the incorporation of the Virtual Private Network (VPN) in this context, deeming the security measures equivalent to those achievable within a local hospital setting. Consequently, the examination of cyber risks, a well-recognized concern in the hospital domain, falls outside the initial focus of this investigation.

The two tables (Tables 2 and 3) provide details on the overall sample of interviewed Medical Radiology Technologists (MRTs) (Table 1) and the subset of those who, in some capacity, have been involved with home radiology (HR) matters (Table 2). The first table presents a comprehensive overview of the entire MRT sample interviewed, while the second table specifically focuses on those within the sample who have encountered or dealt with HR-related aspects.

**Table 2.** Sample of MRTs interviewed using the CAWI ES.

| Participants | Males/Females | Min Age/Max Age | Mean Age |
|---|---|---|---|
| 186 | 80/106 | 34/59 | 45.6 |

**Table 3.** Subsample with experience in HR.

| Experience in HR | Males/Females | Min Age/Max Age | Mean Age |
|---|---|---|---|
| 26 | 16/10 | 33/58 | 46.3 |

#### 3.1.2. Findings from Graded, Multiple-Choice, and Likert Scale Questions

In the assessment, individually graded and Likert responses were employed, with a scale ranging from a maximum score of 5 to a minimum of 1. An average score surpassing $3.0 = \frac{1+5}{2}$ signified a positive evaluation, with a higher score approaching 5 indicating a more favorable response. Conversely, a score falling below 3.0 signaled a negative evaluation, with a lower score approaching 1 indicating a more critical stance.

The following three multiple-choice questions (with four choices each) yielded comparable outcomes, as depicted in Figures 3–5:

- *"Do you believe that the examination conducted at home complies with the safety requirements regarding exposure to ionizing radiation?"*
- *"Are the means and technologies (vehicle, PC, radiological equipment, etc.) provided by the Health Authority suitable for delivering the service?"*

- *"Do you believe it is important for the MRT to be part of the Integrated Home Care team?"*

None of the three questions received negative responses. All three exhibited a preference for the response "Yes, enough", followed closely by "Yes very much". The $\chi^2$ test indicated high significance ($p < 0.01$) in all three cases.

The graded question

- *"How important do you consider listening to the problems of the patient or family/caregivers?"*

received an average score of 4.83 (STD $\pm$ 0.21), with only 1 vote coinciding with 3 (neither positive nor negative), while all other votes were higher.

The graded question

- *"Overall, how satisfied are you with the Home Radiology service?"*

achieved an average score of 4.93 (STD $\pm$ 0.13), with all votes being $\geq$ 4.

Figures 6–8 show the outcome from the three module-Likert:

Giving a comprehensive view, the Butterfly diagrams vividly highlight the overall minimal presence of the tail below 0% across all options. This observation signifies a consistently high level of positive appraisal for each presented choice. Furthermore, an approach was adopted by applying the $\chi^2$ test option by option, assessing the significance in the frequency of positive and non-negative ratings in comparison to negative ones. Across every option, the $\chi^2$ test yielded notably high significance levels ($p < 0.01$), reinforcing the statistical robustness of positive evaluations over negative counterparts.

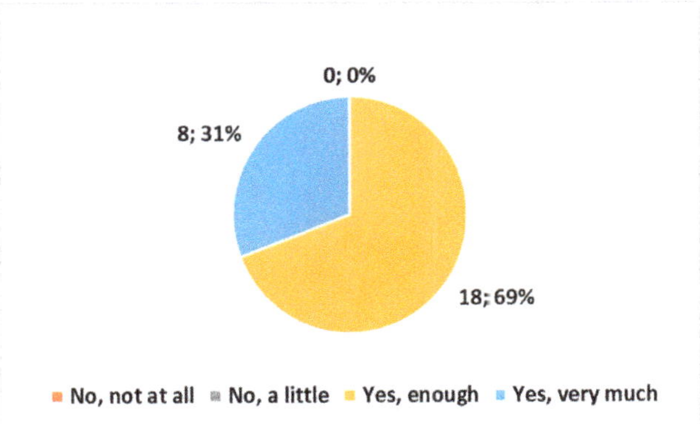


**Figure 3.** Answer to the multiple choice question, "Do you believe that the examination conducted at home complies with the safety requirements regarding exposure to ionizing radiation?".

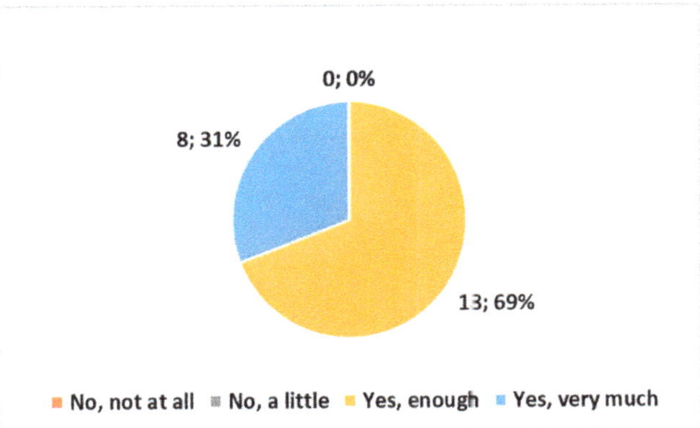


**Figure 4.** Answer to the multiple choice question, "Are the means and technologies (vehicle, PC, radiological equipment, etc.) provided by the Health Authority suitable for delivering the service?".

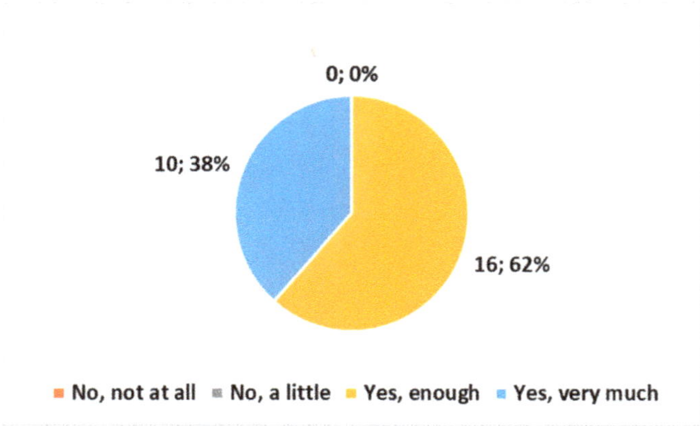


**Figure 5.** Answer to the multiple choice question, "Do you believe it is important for the MRT to be part of the Integrated Home Care team?".

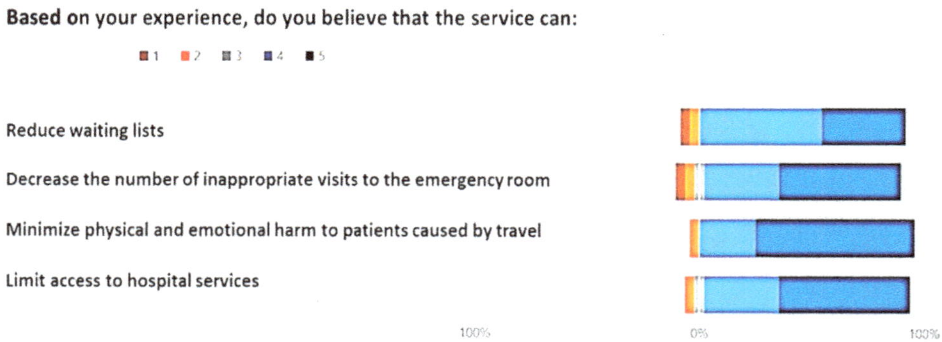


**Figure 6.** Answer to the Likert, "Based on your experience, do you believe that the service can?".

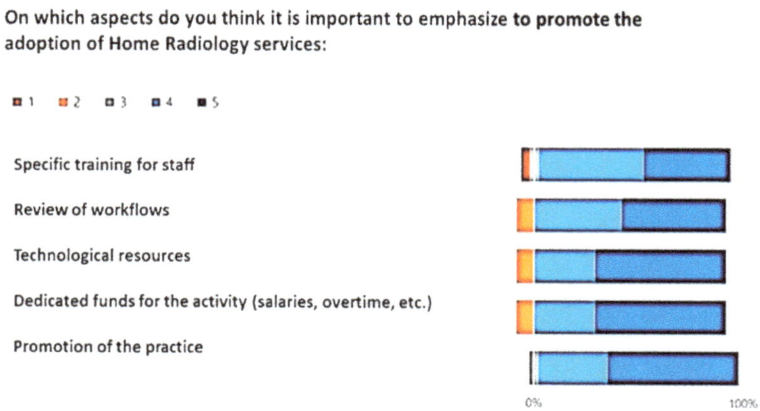


**Figure 7.** Answer to the Likert, "On which aspects do you think it is important to emphasize to promote the adoption of Home Radiology services:?".

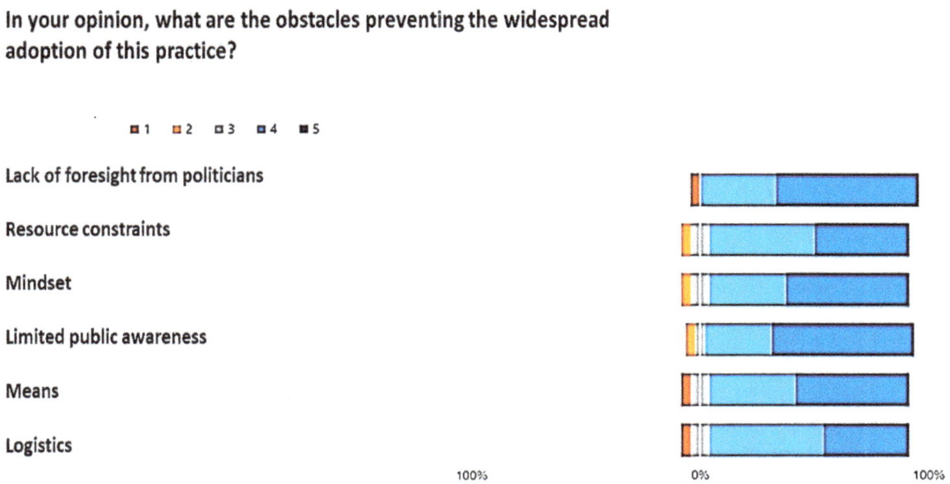


**Figure 8.** Answer to the Likert, "In your opinion, what are the obstacles preventing the widespread adoption of this practice?".

Details:

Within the Likert scale associated with the set of options for *"Based on your experience, do you believe that the service can:"*, the most favored choice was *"Minimize physical and emotional harm to patients caused by travel"*, garnering the highest average rating of 4.3 (STD $\pm$ 0.50)

Within the Likert scale associated with the set of options for "On which aspects do you think it is important to emphasize to promote the adoption of Home Radiology services:", the most favored choice was "Promotion of the practice", garnering the highest average rating of 4.5 (STD $\pm$ 0.33)

Within the Likert scale associated with the set of options for "In your opinion, what are the obstacles preventing the widespread adoption of this practice?", the most favored choice was "lack of foresight from politicians", garnering the highest average rating of 4.4 (STD $\pm$ 0.42).

#### 3.1.3. Unveiling Insights from Open-Ended Responses: A Dual Perspective on Feedback and the Future of Home Radiology

We also present the insights derived from a global perspective through open-ended questions. In this exploration, we delve into the valuable feedback gleaned from open-ended responses, shedding light not only on the challenges and triumphs of home radiology but also on the potential applications of surveys in shaping its future landscape.

Open Question: What types of challenges have you encountered?

In the realm of home radiology, challenges manifest as nuanced facets of our commitment to providing quality healthcare. When working with individuals with significant disabilities and/or frailties, several important challenges may arise and have been reported, including communication, mobility, emotional sensitivity, accessibility, interaction with the caregiver, and cultural sensitivity. However, all those who submitted open-ended questions regarding these issues did not report any critical problems and stated that they felt prepared to face the challenge, considering it a personal reason for professional and human growth.

Open Question: What are the positive aspects that you have identified in providing the service at the patient's home?

The provision of home radiology services brings forth a spectrum of positive aspects that profoundly impact both patients and healthcare practitioners. Conducting examinations in the familiar setting of a patient's home, especially for those in fragile conditions, is a transformative benefit. Beyond the inherent convenience, this approach ensures a higher level of patient care by eliminating the need for them to traverse to a diagnostic center, concurrently contributing to the reduction in healthcare costs.

Moreover, the unique rapport established during home visits fosters a sense of hospitality and appreciation reminiscent of a bygone era. This not only enriches the patient's experience but also aligns with the broader mission of combatting disability, creating a more holistic and patient-centric healthcare model.

Open Question: If you deem it appropriate, you can leave a comment on the topic of home radiology.

The comments highlight that the potential of home radiology services remains untapped without a comprehensive census, both in public and private spheres. A centralized survey is imperative to gauge the extent of utilization and, consequently, unlock the full potential of this diagnostic tool. With data-driven insights from a thorough census, home radiology can be strategically harnessed, catering to the specific needs of the healthcare landscape.

Open Question: Respecting the patient's privacy, share an experience of home radiology that you consider significant.

As we collect data for a comprehensive report on home radiology's contributions to the national healthcare system, the experiences gathered during the COVID-19 pandemic stand out as indelible markers. The challenges posed by the pandemic highlighted the critical role of home radiology in ensuring healthcare continuity. The stories we are assembling serve not only as a testament to the service's importance but also as a guide for future enhancements, solidifying its role in the ever-evolving healthcare landscape.

### 3.2. *The Outcome of the Electronic Feedback Form*

#### 3.2.1. Identification of the Expert Observer Group

For the purposes of this investigation, we enlisted the expertise of a group consisting of 16 observers chosen for their experience in the field. They were selected based on their background in the sciences of diagnostic technical professions (training for a coordinating role in this field) and with various primary professional focuses. This deliberate and thorough selection process aimed to incorporate a diverse range of qualified perspectives, ensuring a comprehensive and well-rounded evaluation of our research.

#### 3.2.2. In-Depth Feedback through the Electronic Feedback Form

In the assessment, individually graded and Likert responses were employed, with a scale ranging from a maximum score of 6 to a minimum of 1. An average score surpassing $3.5 = \frac{1+6}{2}$ signified a positive evaluation, with a higher score approaching 6 indicating a more favorable response. Conversely, a score falling below 3.5 signaled a negative evaluation, with a lower score approaching 1 indicating a more critical stance.

The response to the question "*Please indicate your level of familiarity with the topic of home radiology*" received an average rating of 5.3, with a minimum of 4 and a maximum of 6 (STD $\pm$ 0.41).

The answer to the question "*Provide your overall assessment of the proposed tool*" received an average rating of 5.1, with a minimum of 4 and a maximum of 6 (STD $\pm$ 0.52).

An intriguing aspect emerges in the responses to a question offering three distinct choices, "*I think that the proposed tool is:*". The graphical representation (Figure 9) highlights a unanimous positive sentiment toward the ES, with every option reflecting a favorable opinion. Notably, the most favored choice, selected by 88% of respondents, expressed that the survey was "Valuable and efficient, serving as an excellent foundation for scientific societies". This overwhelming preference holds substantial significance, as demonstrated by the $\chi^2$ test ($p < 0.01$), underlining a robust consensus among participants regarding the commendable nature of the ES.

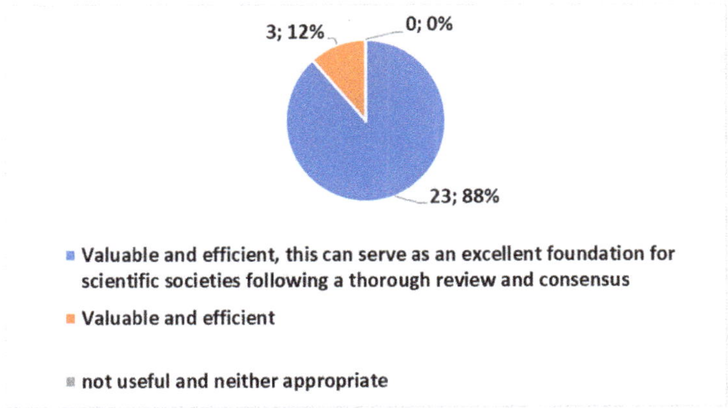


**Figure 9.** Answer to the multiple choice question, *"I think that the proposed tool is:"*.

The Likert scale, in its findings (Figure 10), notably showcased a remarkably high level of acceptance, consistently yielding ratings never falling below 5.1 on each individual item. The Butterfly diagram further accentuates this positive trend by illustrating a complete absence of ratings below 4 percent. This absence of lower ratings obviates the necessity of applying the $\chi^2$ test, as it becomes apparent that the overwhelming majority of responses align positively with the subject matter, reinforcing the robust acceptance of the surveyed elements.

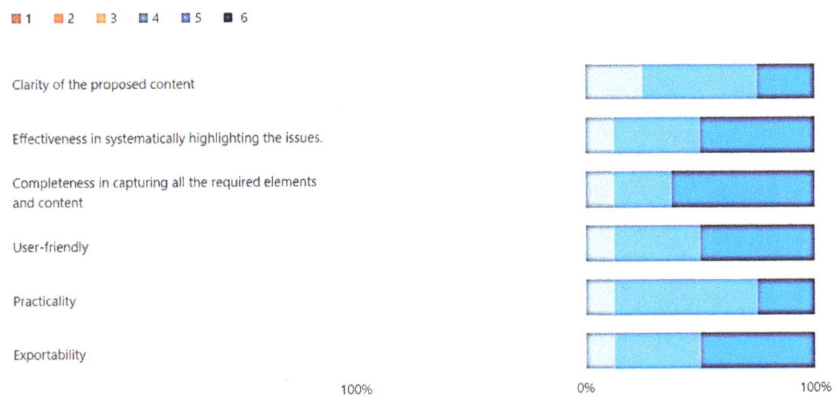


**Figure 10.** Answer to the Likert, "Provide a detailed evaluation of the following points concerning the tool".

### 3.3. *Comprehensive Insights Summary*

A study with two polarities was conducted using two CAWI tools. Through the first CAWI tool, it was possible to capture feedback from medical radiology technicians familiar with the practice. The second CAWI tool allowed for obtaining feedback on the methodology used and its related perspectives.

#### 3.3.1. Insight Summary from the Electronic Survey

The assessment, utilizing graded and Likert responses on a scale of 1 to 5, unveils a favorable perspective for home radiology, where an average score exceeding 3.0 indicates positive sentiments. Multiple-choice questions consistently received affirmative responses, statistically significant at $p < 0.01$, reflecting a widespread positive perception.

Graded inquiries about the importance of listening to patient concerns and overall satisfaction garnered high average scores (4.83 and 4.93, respectively), underscoring their pivotal role. Butterfly diagrams illustrating Likert scale responses showcased a unanimous positive outlook. Specific emphasis on minimizing harm during patient travel and promoting home radiology services received high average ratings of 4.3 and 4.5.

Within the Likert scale, the question exploring obstacles to the widespread adoption of home radiology services provided valuable insights. Respondents favored the option *"lack of foresight from politicians"*, with a high average rating of 4.4, highlighting its significance in the context of adoption challenges.

Open-ended responses delved into nuanced challenges, such as physical demands and occasional biases, emphasizing the necessity for inclusivity. Conversely, positive aspects highlighted the transformative benefits of home examinations, contributing not only to patient comfort but also yielding cost reductions.

This study underscores the urgency of a comprehensive census to unlock the full potential of home radiology. Insights from the COVID-19 pandemic underscore the service's indispensable role in maintaining healthcare continuity, offering valuable guidance for future enhancements.

In summation, the findings offer a compelling narrative of home radiology's positive reception, supported by a blend of quantitative and qualitative assessments. These holistic insights provide a robust understanding of the service's strengths, challenges, and avenues for continual improvement.

#### 3.3.2. Insight Summary from the Electronic Feedback Form

Engaging 16 seasoned observers with diverse expertise, our study meticulously represented crucial roles in the medical field. This deliberate selection process enriched the evaluation with a comprehensive range of qualified perspectives.

Utilizing a 1 to 6 scale, an average score above 3.5 indicated positive evaluations. The responses demonstrated a high level of familiarity with home radiology (average rating: 5.3) and a positive overall assessment of the proposed tool (average rating: 5.1). Notably, a unanimous 88% consensus favored the tool's value and efficiency, emphasizing its excellence as a foundation for scientific societies, as confirmed by the $\chi^2$ test.

Consistently high ratings, never falling below 5.1, were observed across all Likert scale items. The Butterfly diagram underscored the absence of ratings below 4, affirming overwhelming positive consensus without the need for the $\chi^2$ test. In summary, seasoned observers validate the commendable nature of the Evaluation Survey, highlighting its efficiency and value. The consensus positions it as an excellent foundation for scientific societies, showcasing robust acceptance and positive feedback.

## 4. Discussion

### *4.1. Key Discoveries: Opportunities, Challenges, and Issues*

This study delved into the pivotal role of investigating professionals' experiences and opinions regarding home/domiciliary radiology within the health domain. A specific CAWI-based tool was employed and submitted in a peer-to-peer mode to both citizens and professionals. The focus of this work specifically concerns medical radiology technicians involved in this radiology practice. Given the inherent complexity and heterogeneity of the domains, the survey addressed various aspects. In a broader sense, this study has illuminated how an expansive electronic questionnaire within this realm can emerge as a valuable and indispensable tool. Expanding on the distinct values, this study brings forth the following results:

- *The CAWI ES Tool:*

The first contribution of this study lies in the careful design of the CAWI ES tool itself. This tool has been meticulously crafted to explore the intricacies of daily radiology practices, allowing for a detailed examination of key points and the collection of valuable feedback. Its construction ensures that it serves as a potential instrument for understanding and potentially improving the efficiency of radiological procedures in HR.

- *High Acceptance Level of the ES CAWI tool:*

Another significant aspect revealed by the study is the remarkably high acceptance level of the ES tool. This finding comes from the perspectives of a panel consisting of 16 experts who not only recognize its current utility but also see its potential as a valuable instrument in future applications. The unanimous agreement among these experts underscores the perceived credibility and effectiveness of the ES tool in the field of radiology.

- *CAWI Tools:*

Another noteworthy feature is the introduction of two CAWI tools, encompassing both the ES and the EFF. This dual-tool approach represents a substantial and final enhancement to the research methodology. Beyond their evident usefulness, these tools demonstrate a commendable level of adaptability, being easily exportable. This not only adds to the convenience of the research process but also emphasizes the practicality and versatility of the applied methodology.

- *Specific Outcome:*

This study's last contribution is the in-depth evaluation of outcomes derived from interviews with medical radiology technicians. This thorough examination provides insights into the practical implications of the implemented methodologies and sheds light on the tangible impact on the daily practices of these healthcare professionals.

Regarding the outcome, it is essential to note that the obtained sample is not small, considering the following factors. The health domain in Italy is organized on a regional model, with the country divided into 20 regions. The use of Health Radiography (HR) varies across these regions, with some utilizing it while others do not. According to a survey [28], only four regions offered HR services in 2018. However, this landscape changed post-pandemic, with more regions, including Umbria [29], adopting this service. It is crucial to recognize that Italian regions are further divided into provinces, where HR usage may vary. For example, in Umbria (approximately 1/50 of the entire national population), HR is only used in the province of Perugia, involving an Opertavive Unit [29]. Considering these aspects, the identified sample of 26 Medical Radiology Technicians (MRTs) is entirely reasonable. An indirect suggestion to the Ministry of Health, responsible for mapping healthcare activities, is to initiate a census in this domain. A census, coupled with raising awareness through scientific societies/associations, could collectively boost both the monitoring and practice of HR. The feedback from MRTs reflects the enthusiasm and, simultaneously, significant expectations surrounding this practice, which is viewed as having promising and motivating prospects on a personal level. However, MRTs acknowledge the need for various strategic initiatives (e.g., specific personnel training, workflow revisions, technological resources, dedicated funds for activities such as salaries and overtime, and the promotion of the practice). The lack of foresight among politicians is considered an obstacle. Additionally, it is crucial to focus on the citizen and caregiver and on all the key working figures involved in this practice. Notably, medical radiologists emerge as central figures, bearing the responsibility in the medical act and playing a key role in the overall medical process. From those overseeing remote diagnostics to general practitioners managing complex eligibility identification procedures and medical physicists ensuring radiological safety, each contributes indispensably to other key individuals organizing the work, including stakeholders associated with HR practice.

It is also helpful to interpret these results in light of some historical studies in this field focused on surveying the experiences. The uniqueness and innovation of our study lie in its targeted exploration of the experiences of medical radiology technicians involved in home radiology, achieved through the application of a Computer-Assisted Web Interviewing (CAWI) survey method. From a general perspective, our approach continues that proposed by Sawyer et al. in 1995 [7] to gather feedback on this practice, but now utilizing a methodology (CAWI) that was not available in 1995. We focus on the individuals actively involved in the field, addressing new developments that have occurred over three decades. In comparison to a broader overview of surveys [11–24] that focus on teleradiology in general, of which home radiology can, in a sense, be considered an integral part, our study specifically delves into the intricacies of this particular professional group and their engagement with home radiology practices.

The other referenced overview of surveys encompasses a diverse range of investigations within the broader field of radiology but has not addressed home radiology. These include examinations of teleradiology practices in Turkey [11], perceptions of clinical medical students toward radiology careers in Ghana [12], patient-reported outcomes after fracture treatment in primary healthcare [13], usability and efficiency evaluations of an application in orthopedics [14], socio-economic and psychological impacts of the COVID-19 outbreak on radiologists [15], work-style reform and technology utilization among diagnostic radiologists in Japan [16], skepticism about artificial intelligence in the radiology field [17], patient satisfaction with teleradiology services in Italy [18], patient satisfaction with teleradiology services in general practice [19], on-call service of neurosurgeons in Germany [20], attitudes of Korean primary care family physicians toward telehealth [21], factors influencing clinician satisfaction with radiology services [22], and positive aspects found in healthcare information and communication technology implementation in Finland [23]. In contrast, our study focuses specifically on the experiences of medical radiology technicians in the context of home radiology. The use of the CAWI as a survey method provides a modern and efficient approach to gathering insights directly from this professional group, allowing for detailed feedback on their perspectives, challenges, and contributions in this evolving field. By narrowing the scope to this specific demographic, our study adds a targeted and specialized dimension to the broader landscape of radiology research [11–24]. In common with these studies, our research highlights the importance of targeted questionnaire proposals rather than standardized ones. This is evident when analyzing questionnaires proposed to investigate the introduction of innovative technologies in radiology, such as artificial intelligence. Various surveys have been proposed [30–40] to explore the perspectives of diverse stakeholders in this field, including radiologists, radiographers, primary care providers (PCPs), students, and patients. Research focused on patients [30–32] has shed light on their curiosity and general acceptance of these techniques, emphasizing the need for awareness campaigns and educational efforts and addressing cybersecurity concerns in tandem with eHealth and mHealth integration. Among students [39], prevalent curiosity and optimism were observed, but in tandem with dissatisfaction surfaced regarding the inadequacy of training, prompting a call for the integration of specific modules into their training programs. Investigations into radiologists and radiographers [34–38] uncovered a widespread openness to these innovative solutions. Moreover, there was a strong desire among these professionals to actively contribute to future workflow modifications, contingent upon receiving adequate training. In almost all studies, with only rare exceptions like [32], researchers opted for free and non-standardized questionnaires, employing validation processes. This implies that, in the current historical context, scholars are leveraging their creativity to construct increasingly innovative and adaptable survey instruments. Other standardized and more widely used instruments, such as the Technology Acceptance Model, have seen more limited utilization [40]. Another aspect that emerges when comparing studies conducted on teleradiology [11–24] and on the integration of artificial intelligence in radiology [30–40] is the need to activate national and international initiatives of this kind sponsored by societies and/or scientific federations in the field and to focus more on the entire working domain [26].

### 4.2. Takeaway Message

This study, through the application of a CAWI survey method, specifically explores the experiences of medical radiology technicians engaged in home radiology. The use of CAWI tools is highlighted as a significant innovation, providing meticulous design, high acceptance levels, and a comprehensive impact evaluation. This study's focus on the specific professional group of MRTs, utilizing a modern approach, adds a targeted dimension to the broader landscape of HR research. The need for national and international initiatives in the field, supported by scientific societies, is emphasized to further explore the evolving landscape of the integration of HR in the health domain.

### 4.3. Work in Progress

Future work will focus on the citizen and caregiver and on all the key working figures involved in this practice, from radiologists engaged in remote diagnostics, general practitioners involved in complex eligibility identification procedures, and medical physicists ensuring radiological safety to other key individuals organizing the work, including stakeholders associated with HR practice. Concurrently, we will initiate a structured transition process with the following objectives: effectively transferring our findings and key insights to relevant scientific societies and raising awareness among key institutions regarding census initiatives. This transition is vital to ensure that the wealth of information we've gathered becomes an integral part of the broader scientific discourse. By fostering collaboration with scientific societies, we envision a dynamic exchange of ideas, methodologies, and best practices that will contribute to the advancement of the field. This work in progress signifies our commitment to not only conducting a comprehensive analysis but also actively participating in the knowledge-sharing ecosystem. Through this dual approach, we aspire to make meaningful contributions to both public understanding and the scientific community, fostering a continuous dialogue that propels the field of home radiology forward.

### 4.4. Key Recommendations for Advancing Further Research

We have proposed a *pilot study* that we hope will serve as a catalyst for future developments. Our envisioned direction for upcoming research recommends a focused exploration of citizens, caregivers, and key figures within the field of home radiology. Notably, medical radiologists emerge as central figures, bearing the responsibility in the medical act and playing a key role in the overall medical process. From those overseeing remote diagnostics to general practitioners managing complex eligibility identification procedures and medical physicists ensuring radiological safety, each contributes indispensably.

Additionally, we aspire for this pilot study to inspire all scientific societies of the involved professionals to continue in this direction. Among the suggestions indirectly arising is the encouragement to persist through these initiatives, concurrently working on refining and building consensus on these Computer-Assisted Web Interviewing (CAWI) tools. Simultaneously, we aim to motivate and support institutions in targeted and precise census initiatives.

## 5. Conclusions

In conclusion, this pilot study delves into the experiences and perspectives of medical radiology technicians engaged in home radiology, utilizing a CAWI survey method. The use of CAWI tools represents a significant innovation, providing a meticulously designed approach with high acceptance levels and a comprehensive impact evaluation. The study's focused exploration of this specific professional group adds a targeted dimension to the broader landscape of HR research.

This study acknowledges the need for strategic initiatives to optimize HR integration. It suggests recommendations for advancing further research by focusing on citizens, caregivers, and key figures in home radiology. Medical radiologists are highlighted as central figures, bearing responsibility in the medical act and playing a key role in the overall medical process. From those overseeing remote diagnostics to general practitioners managing complex eligibility identification procedures and medical physicists ensuring radiological safety, each contributes indispensably. This pilot study aims to inspire scientific societies to continue in this direction, encouraging the persistence and refinement of tools.

Simultaneously, census initiatives are suggested. This transition is crucial for integrating the findings into the scientific discourse and aligns with our desire for our study to actively contribute to the knowledge-sharing ecosystem.

**Author Contributions:** Conceptualization, G.L. and D.G.; Methodology, F.O., R.A.G. and D.G.; Software, D.G.; Validation, G.L. and D.G.; Formal analysis, F.O. and D.G.; Investigation, R.A.G. and D.G.; Resources, G.L. and D.G.; Data curation, F.O. and D.G.; Writing—original draft, D.G.; Writing—review & editing, G.L., F.O., R.A.G. and D.G.; Project administration, D.G. All authors have read and agreed to the published version of the manuscript.

**Funding:** This research received no external funding.

**Data Availability Statement:** Data are contained within the article.

**Conflicts of Interest:** The authors declare no conflict of interest.

## References

1. Toppenberg, M.D.; Christiansen, T.E.M.; Rasmussen, F.; Nielsen, C.P.; Damsgaard, E.M. Mobile X-ray outside the hospital: A scoping review. *BMC Health Serv. Res.* **2020**, *20*, 767. [CrossRef]
2. LOSEV, I.K. Improvement of quality of roentgenological work in villages by improvement of mobile x-ray units. *Vestn. Rentgenol. Radiol.* **1958**, *33*, 86–87. (In Russian)
3. Mark, S.; Henderson, D.; Brealey, J. Taking acute medical imaging to the patient, the domiciliary based X-ray response team. *Radiography* **2022**, *28*, 550–552. [CrossRef]
4. Kjelle, E.; Kleven, L.; Olerud, H.M.; Melberg, H.O. Cost analysis of mobile radiography services for nursing home residents in Southeast Norway. *J. Eval. Clin. Pract.* **2019**, *25*, 275–281. [CrossRef]
5. Andersen, P.A.B.; Precht, H.; McEntee, M.F.; Pedersen, M.R.V. How to set up a mobile X-ray unit in the community—Implementation initiatives for patient-centred care. *Radiography* **2023**, *29* (Suppl. S1), S148–S151. [CrossRef]
6. Dollard, J.; Edwards, J.; Yadav, L.; Gaget, V.; Tivey, D.; Inacio, M.; Maddern, G.; Visvanathan, R. Residents' perspectives of mobile X-ray services in support of healthcare-in-place in residential aged care facilities: A qualitative study. *BMC Geriatr.* **2022**, *22*, 525. [CrossRef]
7. Sawyer, R.H.; Patel, U.; Horrocks, A.W. Domiciliary radiography: An important service? *Clin. Radiol.* **1995**, *50*, 51–55. [CrossRef]
8. Aldridge, R.W.; Hayward, A.C.; Hemming, S.; Possas, L.; Ferenando, G.; Garber, E.; Lipman, M.; McHugh, T.D.; Story, A. Effectiveness of peer educators on the uptake of mobile X-ray tuberculosis screening at homeless hostels: A cluster randomised controlled trial. *BMJ Open* **2015**, *5*, e008050. [CrossRef]
9. Kjelle, E.; Lysdahl, K.B. Mobile radiography services in nursing homes: A systematic review of residents' and societal outcomes. *BMC Health Serv. Res.* **2017**, *17*, 231. [CrossRef] [PubMed]
10. Datta, B.; Hazarika, A.; Shewade, H.D.; Ayyagari, K.; Kumar, A.M. Digital chest X-ray through a mobile van: Public private partnership to detect sputum negative pulmonary TB. *BMC Res. Notes* **2017**, *10*, 96. [CrossRef]
11. Dicle, O.; Şenol, U.; Özmen, M.N.; Aydıngöz, Ü. A snapshot of teleradiology practice in Turkey: The results of a survey among radiologists. *Diagn. Interv. Radiol.* **2023**, *29*, 46–52. [CrossRef] [PubMed]
12. Dzefi-Tettey, K.; Kobina Mesi Edzie, E.; Brakohiapa, E.K.; Gorleku, P.N.; Amankwa, A.T.; Abdulai, A.B.; Yabasin, I.B.; Kekessie, K.K.; Idun, E.A.; Ntiamoah-Koufie, C.E.; et al. Career in radiology; the Ghanaian clinical medical Student's perception. *Heliyon* **2022**, *8*, e12603. [CrossRef] [PubMed]
13. Vabo, S.; Steen, K.; Brudvik, C.; Hunskaar, S.; Morken, T. Patient-reported outcomes after initial conservative fracture treatment in primary healthcare—A survey study. *BMC Prim. Care* **2022**, *23*, 191. [CrossRef] [PubMed]
14. Macedo, F.S.; Silva, P.G.B.; Marçal, E.B.F.; Rolim, J.P.M.L. Evaluation of Usability, Perception of Usefulness, and Efficiency of an Application in Interpreting Imaging Examinations and Supporting Decision-Making in Orthopedics. *Telemed. e-Health* **2021**, *27*, 561–567. [CrossRef] [PubMed]
15. Florin, M.; Pinar, U.; Chavigny, E.; Bouaboula, M.; Jarboui, L.; Coulibaly, A.; Lemogne, C.; Fournier, L. Socio-economic and psychological impact of the COVID-19 outbreak on private practice and public hospital radiologists. *Eur. J. Radiol.* **2020**, *132*, 109285. [CrossRef] [PubMed]
16. Yamashiro, T.; Kumamaru, K.K.; Kido, A.; Namoto Matsubayashi, R.; Ota, H.; Ida, M.; Aoki, S. Joint Committee for Diversity Promotion and Work-Style Reform of the Japan Radiological Society and the Japanese College of Radiology. Work-style reform and use of information and communication technology among diagnostic radiologists in Japan: Results of the 2018 JRS/JCR joint survey. *Jpn. J. Radiol.* **2020**, *38*, 636–642. [CrossRef] [PubMed]
17. van Hoek, J.; Huber, A.; Leichtle, A.; Härmä, K.; Hilt, D.; von Tengg-Kobligk, H.; Heverhagen, J.; Poellinger, A. A survey on the future of radiology among radiologists, medical students and surgeons: Students and surgeons tend to be more skeptical about artificial intelligence and radiologists may fear that other disciplines take over. *Eur. J. Radiol.* **2019**, *121*, 108742. [CrossRef] [PubMed]

18. Coppola, F.; Bibbolino, C.; Grassi, R.; Pierotti, L.; Silverio, R.; Lassandro, F.; Neri, E.; Regge, D. Results of an Italian survey on teleradiology. *La Radiol. Medica* **2016**, *121*, 652–659. [CrossRef]
19. Jacobs, J.J.W.M.; Ekkelboom, R.; Jacobs, J.P.A.M.; van der Molen, T.; Sanderman, R. Patient satisfaction with a teleradiology service in general practice. *BMC Fam. Pract.* **2016**, *17*, 17. [CrossRef]
20. Brenke, C.; Lassel, E.A.; Terris, D.; Kurt, A.; Schmieder, K.; Schoenberg, S.O.; Weisser, G. On-call service of neurosurgeons in Germany: Organization, use of communication services, and personal acceptance of modern technologies. *J. Neurol. Surg. Part A Cent. Eur. Neurosurg.* **2013**, *75*, 217–223. [CrossRef]
21. Kim, J.E.; Song, Y.M.; Park, J.H.; Lee, J.R. Attitude of korean primary care family physicians towards telehealth. *Korean J. Fam. Med.* **2011**, *32*, 341–351. [CrossRef]
22. Lindsay, R.; McKinstry, S.; Vallely, S.; Thornbury, G. What influences clinician's satisfaction with radiology services? *Insights Imaging* **2011**, *2*, 425–430. [CrossRef]
23. Winblad, I.; Hämäläinen, P.; Reponen, J. What is found positive in healthcare information and communication technology implementation?-the results of a nationwide survey in Finland. *Telemed. e-Health* **2011**, *17*, 118–123. [CrossRef]
24. Ninos, K.; Spiros, K.; Glotsos, D.; Georgiadis, P.; Sidiropoulos, K.; Dimitropoulos, N.; Kalatzis, I.; Cavouras, D. Development and evaluation of a PDA-based teleradiology terminal in thyroid nodule diagnosis. *J. Telemed. Telecare* **2010**, *16*, 232–236. [CrossRef]
25. Giansanti, D.; Di Basilio, F. The Artificial Intelligence in Digital Radiology: Part 1: The Challenges, Acceptance and Consensus. *Healthcare* **2022**, *10*, 509. [CrossRef] [PubMed]
26. Di Basilio, F.; Esposisto, G.; Monoscalco, L.; Giansanti, D. The Artificial Intelligence in Digital Radiology: *Part 2*: Towards an Investigation of *acceptance* and *consensus* on the Insiders. *Healthcare* **2022**, *10*, 153. [CrossRef] [PubMed]
27. Giansanti, D.; Rossi, I.; Monoscalco, L. Lessons from the COVID-19 Pandemic on the Use of Artificial Intelligence in Digital Radiology: The Submission of a Survey to Investigate the Opinion of Insiders. *Healthcare* **2021**, *9*, 331. [CrossRef] [PubMed]
28. Papi, R.; Grosso, M.; Cardelli, D.; Nocentini, C.; Lorenzini, C.; Messina, G.; Nante, N. Sperimentazione di un servizio di Radiologia Domiciliare per non deambulanti nell'Azienda USL Toscana Sud Est. *Mondo Sanit.* **2018**, *25*, 1–18.
29. Lepri, G.; Pentiricci, A.; Ferranti, A.; Abbritti, E.; Rossi, G.; Nappini, M.; Fiordelli, P.; Papa, V. La Radiologia Domiciliare, alla luce dell'applicazione del D.M. 77/2022: Modelli e Standard per lo sviluppo, dell'Assistenza nel Territorio. In *"Sfide e Opportunità per il S.S.N. I Professionisti Della Salute Leva per il Cambiamento" Supplemento Sanità 4.0*; Pubblicazione dei Forum di Federsanità; Confederazione Federsanità ANCI Regionali: Torino, Italy, 2023; pp. 234–237.
30. Lennartz, S.; Dratsch, T.; Zopfs, D.; Persigehl, T.; Maintz, D.; Hokamp, N.G.; Dos Santos, D.P. Use and Control of Artificial Intelligence in Patients Across the Medical Workflow: Single-Center Questionnaire Study of Patient Perspectives. *J. Med. Internet Res.* **2021**, *23*, e24221. [CrossRef] [PubMed]
31. Zhang, Z.; Citardi, D.; Wang, D.; Genc, Y.; Shan, J.; Fan, X. Patients' perceptions of using artificial intelligence (AI)-based technology to comprehend radiology imaging data. *Health Inform. J.* **2021**, *27*, 14604582211011215. [CrossRef]
32. Ongena, Y.P.; Haan, M.; Yakar, D.; Kwee, T.C. Patients' views on the implementation of artificial intelligence in radiology: Development and validation of a standardized questionnaire. *Eur. Radiol.* **2020**, *30*, 1033–1040. [CrossRef] [PubMed]
33. Hendrix, N.; Hauber, B.; Lee, C.I.; Bansal, A.; Veenstra, D.L. Artificial intelligence in breast cancer screening: Primary care provider preferences. *J. Am. Med. Inform. Assoc.* **2021**, *28*, 1117–1124. [CrossRef]
34. Abuzaid, M.M.; Elshami, W.; McConnell, J.; Tekin, H.O. An extensive survey on radiographers from the Middle East and India on artificial intelligence integration in radiology practice. *Health Technol.* **2021**, *11*, 1045–1050. [CrossRef] [PubMed]
35. Abuzaid, M.M.; Tekin, H.O.; Reza, M.; Elhag, I.R.; Elshami, W. Assessment of MRI technologists in acceptance and willingness to integrate artificial intelligence into practice. *Radiography* **2021**, *27*, S83–S87. [CrossRef] [PubMed]
36. Abuzaid, M.M.; Elshami, W.; Tekin, H.; Issa, B. Assessment of the Willingness of Radiologists and Radiographers to Accept the Integration of Artificial Intelligence into Radiology Practice. *Acad. Radiol.* **2020**, *29*, 87–94. [CrossRef] [PubMed]
37. Alelyani, M.; Alamri, S.; Alqahtani, M.S.; Musa, A.; Almater, H.; Alqahtani, N.; Alshahrani, F.; Alelyani, S. Radiology Community Attitude in Saudi Arabia about the Applications of Artificial Intelligence in Radiology. *Healthcare* **2021**, *9*, 834. [CrossRef] [PubMed]
38. European Society of Radiology (ESR). Impact of artificial intelligence on radiology: A EuroAIM survey among members of the European Society of Radiology. *Insights Imaging* **2019**, *10*, 105. [CrossRef]
39. Galán, G.C.; Portero, F.S. Medical students' perceptions of the impact of artificial intelligence in Radiology. *Radiologia*, 2021; *in press*.
40. Aldosari, B. User acceptance of a picture archiving and communication system (PACS) in a Saudi Arabian hospital radiology department. *BMC Med. Inform. Decis. Mak.* **2012**, *12*, 44. [CrossRef]

healthcare

MDPI

Review

# Effects of Telerehabilitation on Pain and Disability in Patients with Chronic Neck Pain: A Systematic Review and Meta-Analysis

Geraldine Valenza-Peña [1], Andrés Calvache-Mateo [1], Marie Carmen Valenza [1,*], María Granados-Santiago [2], Julia Raya-Benítez [2], Irene Cabrera-Martos [1] and Esther Díaz-Mohedo [3]

1 Department of Physiotherapy, Faculty of Health Sciences, University of Granada, 60 Av. Ilustración, 18016 Granada, Spain; geraldinevalenza@ugr.es (G.V.-P.); andrescalvache@ugr.es (A.C.-M.); irenecm@ugr.es (I.C.-M.)
2 Department of Nursing, Faculty of Health Sciences, University of Granada, 60 Av. Ilustración, 18016 Granada, Spain; mariagranados@ugr.es (M.G.-S.); juliarb@ugr.es (J.R.-B.)
3 Department of Physiotherapy, University of Málaga, 29071 Málaga, Spain; estherdiaz@uma.es
* Correspondence: cvalenza@ugr.es; Tel.: +34-95-824-8035

**Abstract:** (1) *Background*: This systematic review and meta-analysis explores the effectiveness of telerehabilitation in patients suffering from chronic neck pain, specifically on pain and disability. The research delves into an area of growing significance within the realm of healthcare, aiming to understand the impact of digital interventions on the rehabilitation process for individuals with prolonged neck pain. (2) *Methods*: The comprehensive review encompasses a wide array of studies evaluating the collective outcomes of numerous trials focused on telerehabilitation strategies. In this systematic review, PubMed/MEDLINE, Scopus, and Web of Science databases were systematically searched to identify studies on telerehabilitation's impact on pain. (3) *Results*: Eight studies met the inclusion criteria. Using the Downs and Black quality assessment, three studies were classified as good and five as fair. The authors identify specific modalities within telerehabilitation, such as remote exercise programs and virtual consultations, that contribute significantly to positive patient outcomes. Meta-analysis indicated a significant overall effect of telerehabilitation on pain reduction (MD = −1.27; 95% CI = −2.06; −0.47; $p = 0.002$). These findings support telerehabilitation's efficacy in pain management. (4) *Conclusions*: The synthesis of evidence presented in this systematic review and meta-analysis underscores the potential of telerehabilitation as an effective and accessible means of managing chronic neck pain, offering valuable insights for both healthcare practitioners and policymakers in advancing patient-centered care.

**Keywords:** telerehabilitation; chronic neck pain; disability; review; meta-analysis

## 1. Introduction

Neck pain represents a significant health issue, affecting millions of individuals worldwide and imposing a substantial burden in terms of disability and healthcare costs [1]. A significant number of individuals grappling with neck pain find that a full recovery remains elusive. Among patients experiencing neck pain, a mere 6.3% perceive their discomfort as persistently chronic. This highlights the enduring and often challenging nature of neck pain, underlining the need for comprehensive and sustained approaches to address the diverse factors contributing to its prolonged impact on individuals' well-being [1]. This disorder, characterized by persistent pain in the cervical region over an extended period, negatively impacts the quality of life and functionality of those affected [2].

Moreover, persistent and/or chronic pain is characterized by its continuous presence for at least three out of the preceding six months. The origins of non-specific neck pain remain elusive, with the onset and recurrence of such pain being acknowledged as multifactorial [3]. While the precise mechanisms initiating pain are not fully understood, certain influences may be modifiable, whereas others may be attributed to personal and environmental factors [4]. These factors encompass aspects such as occupation, headaches, emotional issues, low job satisfaction, sedentary work postures, and a suboptimal physical work environment [5].

The importance of understanding and addressing chronic neck pain lies in its pervasive nature, often leading to disability and reduced quality of life for affected individuals [6]. Persistent neck pain can restrict mobility, hinder daily activities, and contribute to emotional distress [7]. The presence of disability in chronic neck pain underscores the need for comprehensive approaches to pain management, focusing not only on symptom relief but also on enhancing functional capabilities and minimizing the long-term impact on a person's ability to engage in normal activities [8].

It has been previously stated that although pain and disability are interrelated, they should be assessed separately and considered as two distinct aspects of pain [9]. Pain is defined as a subjective experience, and the assessment tools are focused on what the person reports about their pain. These assessment tools include the visual analog scale, which is the most frequently used pain measure, and the numeric rating scale, which allows better discrimination of small changes in pain or pain questionnaires that are reported to be sensitive in detecting health improvement [10]. Regarding disability due to neck pain, the most widely used tool is the neck disability index, published in 1991 [11]. This index has appropriate psychometric properties and has been used in clinical and research settings [12].

In the current landscape of healthcare [13], telerehabilitation has emerged as an innovative strategy to address various chronic health conditions, including neck pain. The convergence of information and communication technology with rehabilitation practices offers new opportunities to deliver effective interventions remotely, overcoming geographical barriers and enhancing access to care [14]. Exploring the potential of telerehabilitation can modify a paradigm shift in how rehabilitation services can be delivered. By leveraging the capabilities of telecommunication technologies [15], healthcare professionals can extend their reach, providing timely and personalized interventions to individuals dealing with chronic neck pain.

The premise that telerehabilitation [16] can not only provide a convenient approach to rehabilitation service delivery but also has the potential to empower patients by enabling active participation in their recovery process has been in the middle of controversy when applied to chronic pathologies [17]. In this line, telerehabilitation has been defined as a branch of telehealth and is set up as a system for the control or monitoring of remote rehabilitation using telecommunications technologies. The purpose of telerehabilitation is to increase accessibility and improve continuity of care in vulnerable, geographically remote populations with disabilities, with the potential to save time and resources in health care [18]. The detailed exploration of this treatment modality is essential to inform healthcare professionals, patients, and policymakers about its viability and effectiveness in the context of chronic neck pain. The relevance of telerehabilitation in transforming healthcare delivery requires a growing and meaningful body of evidence for its effects that go beyond the traditional boundaries of healthcare [18]. Specifically, the available evidence can elucidate the results of telerehabilitation interventions, offering a comprehensive perspective on their impact on pain management and functional outcomes.

At a time when healthcare is undergoing an accelerated digital transformation, understanding how telerehabilitation can contribute to the successful management of chronic neck pain is crucial for optimizing care, improving patient outcomes, and ensuring accessible and efficient healthcare [19]. However, it has not yet been demonstrated for chronic neck pain. Furthermore, the up-to-date evidence base about the use of telerehabilitation for chronic neck pain rehabilitation has not been reviewed. Therefore, this systematic review and meta-analysis investigate the effects of telerehabilitation in patients with chronic neck pain to improve pain and disability.

## 2. Materials and Methods

### *2.1. Design*

A systematic review and meta-analyses were performed to identify randomized clinical trials reviewing the effects of telerehabilitation on pain and disability in patients with chronic neck pain. The guidelines of the Preferred Reporting Items for Systematic Reviews and Meta-Analyses (PRISMA) were used [20]. The Cochrane Collaboration guidelines for reviewing interventions were also closely followed [21]. We previously registered the protocol of this systematic review on PROSPERO (CRD42023402445).

### *2.2. Search Strategy*

A wide search of the literature was conducted for randomized controlled trials indexed on PubMed/MEDLINE, Scopus, and Web of Science databases from their inception to June 2023 in English (Figure 1). The following search strategy was developed for the PubMed/MEDLINE database ((“Telerehabilitation” OR “telerehabilitation program” OR “Telemedicine” OR ”telemedicine program” OR “telehealth” OR “Telehealthcare” OR “telehealth program” OR “telecare” OR “telecare program” OR “electronic health” OR “electronic health program” OR “Virtual Physical Therapy” OR “Tele-physical therapy” OR “home exercise” OR “home exercise program”) AND (“Neck Pain” OR “Chronic Neck Pain” OR “Chronic Pain” OR “Cervical Pain” OR “Cervical Chronic Pain”)). Then, this strategy was adapted to the other databases. Additionally, we screened the reference lists of relevant reviews related to the terms and considered non-English language studies for inclusion if the translation was possible.

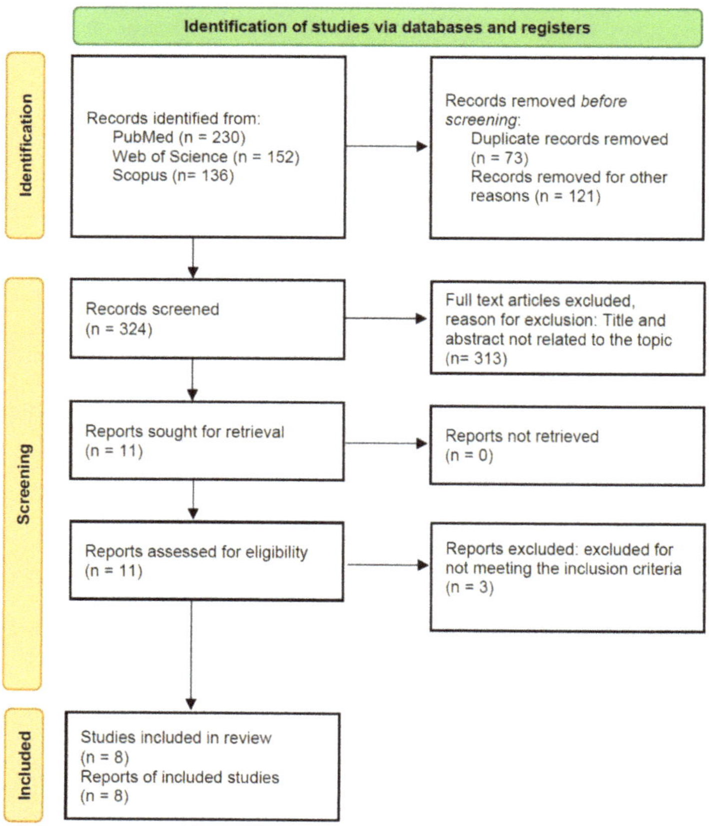


**Figure 1.** Flow chart of literature search and study selection [20].

### 2.3. Study Selection

We applied the PICOS (participants, interventions, comparisons, outcome, and study design) model to define the research question. The inclusion criteria were as follows: (1) adult patients with chronic neck pain not related to a traumatic trauma or head and neck cancer; (2) telerehabilitation programs as described by Seron et al. [18]; (3) no intervention or a control intervention without telerehabilitation will be included; (4) pain and disability were the main outcomes, but other pain-related variables will be extracted as secondary outcomes when available; and (5) randomized controlled clinical trials and pilot randomized clinical trials were included.

To reduce potential selection bias, two authors (G.V.-P. and M.C.V.) independently performed the literature search, and the disagreements were resolved by further consultation with a third author (A.C.-M.). The search process included removing duplicates and screening titles, abstracts, and eligible full texts.

### 2.4. Data Extraction

The following data from the studies included were recorded: author, year of publication, sample size, age (years), gender (percentage of women), disease etiology, and pain characteristics. The full information is summarized in Table 1. Information about the characteristics of interventions containing experimental group interventions, control group interventions, session duration, frequency, program duration, outcome instrument, and main results is summarized in Table 2.

When information was lacking or ambiguous, we tried to contact the study's corresponding author through email. If data remained unclear or if communication was not possible, we analyzed the available data. The data extraction was independently conducted by two independent reviewers (G.V.-P. and A.C.-M.).

**Table 1.** Characteristics of the studies.

| Study (Year) | Study Design/Groups | Sample Size per Group *n* (% Women) | Age Years Mean ± SD | Duration of Pain Months Mean ± SD | Pain Intensity Mean (0–10) ± SD | Downs and Black Score |
|---|---|---|---|---|---|---|
| **Gialanella et al. (2017)** [22] | RCT/2 Groups | **TG:** 47 (89.3)<br>**CG:** 47 (89.3) | **TG:** 56.0 ± 14.0<br>**CG:** 60.1 ± 11.0 | NR | **TG:** 6.8 ± 1.3<br>**CG:** 6.6 ± 1.5 | 23 |
| **Lee et al. (2017)** [23] | Pilot RCT/2 Groups | **TG:** 11 (55)<br>**CG:** 9 (45) | **TG:** 27.09 ± 4.83<br>**CG:** 27.56 ± 4.67 | **TG:** 50.81 ± 71.72<br>**CG:** 35.33 ± 18.11 | **TG:** 5.20 ± 2.19<br>**CG:** 4.02 ± 1.75 | 16 |
| **Thongtipmak et al. (2020)** [24] | RCT/2 Groups | **TG:** 50 (82)<br>**CG:** 50 (76) | **TG:** 22.86 ± 1.99<br>**CG:** 22.68 ± 2.23 | NR | **TG:** 3.97 ± 0.74<br>**CG:** 4.06 ± 0.68 | 18 |
| **Abadiyan et al. (2021)** [25] | RCT/3 Groups | **TG:** 20 (50)<br>**CG:** 20 (50) | **TG:** 41.3 ± 8.1<br>**CG:** 37.4 ± 9.8 | NR | **TG:** 7.3 ± 0.9<br>**CG:** 6.4 ± 1.8 | 21 |
| **Ozel et al. (2022)** [26] | RTC/3 Groups | **TG1:** 22 (72.7)<br>**TG2:** 22 (77.3)<br>**CG:** 22 (59.1) | **TG1:** 36.23 ± 12.45<br>**TG2:** 34.18 ± 13.03<br>**CG:** 39.2 7 ± 15.46 | NR | **TG1:** 6.77<br>**TG2:** 4.86<br>**CG:** 5.55 | 18 |
| **Pach et al. (2022)** [27] | RTC/2 Groups | **TG:** 110 (67.3)<br>**CG:** 110 (71.8) | **TG:** 37.9 ± 11<br>**CG:** 39.8 ± 11.6 | **TG:** 79.2 ± 74.8<br>**CG:** 86.4 ± 97.7 | **TG:** 5.7 ± 1.4<br>**CG:** 5.8 ± 1.3 | 20 |
| **Onan et al. (2023)** [28] | RCT/2 Groups | **TG:** 15 (73.3)<br>**CG:** 16 (68.7) | **TG:** 37.4 ± 10.58<br>**CG:** 39.5 ± 10.96 | **TG:** 36<br>**CG:** 60 | **TG:** 7.13 ± 1.92<br>**CG:** 6.75 ± 1.98 | 16 |
| **Peterson et al. (2023)** [29] | RTC/2 Groups | **TG:** 70 (79)<br>**CG:** 70 (79) | **TG:** 40.4 ± 11.6<br>**CG:** 40.5 ± 11.4 | **TG:** 27.4 ± 21.0<br>**CG:** 25.2 ± 15.5 | **TG:** 5.77 ± 1.87<br>**CG:** 5.86 ± 1.70 | 19 |

SD: standard deviation; RCT: Randomized controlled trial; *n*: number; TG: telehealth group; CG: Control group; NR: not reported.

**Table 2.** Characteristics of the interventions.

| Study (Year) | Experimental Intervention Design and Support | Telerehabilitation Components | Intervention Duration and Frequency Weeks Days/Week | Telehealth Setting, and Supervision | Comparator Group | Main Results |
|---|---|---|---|---|---|---|
| **Gialanella et al. (2017)** [22] | Telerehabilitation isolated via phone calls | -Education content<br>-Symptom and mood monitoring<br>-Physical activity monitoring and personalized feedback<br>-Education in self-management skills<br>-Tele-consultation with healthcare professionals<br>-Remote decision support system<br>-Therapeutic exercise program | 24 w<br>5 d/w<br>20 min | Home<br>Fortnightly scheduled phone calls | Exercise recommendation | Pain (VAS):<br>TG ** > CG ** ($p < 0.001$)<br>Disability (NDI):<br>TG ** > CG ** ($p < 0.001$) |
| **Lee et al. (2017)** [23] | Telerehabilitation isolated via smartphone app + phone calls | -Education content<br>-Symptom and mood monitoring<br>-Physical activity monitoring and personalized feedback<br>-Therapeutic exercise program | 8 w<br>2 d/w<br>10–15 min | Work setting<br>Supervised | Brochure to correct the posture | Pain (VAS):<br>TG * > CG ($p < 0.05$)<br>Disability (NDI):<br>TG * > CG ($p < 0.05$)<br>Fear-avoidance belief (FABQ):<br>-Physical activity: TG vs. CG (NSD)<br>-Work: TG vs. CG * ($p < 0.05$)<br>-Health-related quality of life (SF-36):<br>TG vs. CG (NSD) |
| **Thongtipmak et al. (2020)** [24] | Telerehabilitation isolated via a smartphone app | -Education content<br>-Symptom and mood monitoring<br>-Tele-education in self-management skills<br>-Therapeutic exercise program | 15–20 min | Home<br>Supervised | No intervention | Pain (VAS):<br>TG ** > CG * ($p < 0.001$) |
| **Abadiyan et al. (2021)** [25] | Telerehabilitation via smartphone app combined with a presential exercise program | -Physical activity monitoring and personalized feedback<br>-Therapeutic exercise program | 8 w<br>4 d/w<br>50 min | Home<br>Supervised | Usual care | TG-CG<br>Pain (VAS):<br>TG > CG *; $p < 0031$<br>Disability (NDI):<br>TG vs. CG (NSD)<br>Quality of life (SF-36):<br>TG > CG *; $p < 0.001$ |

**Table 2.** *Cont.*

| Study (Year) | Experimental Intervention Design and Support | Telerehabilitation Components | Intervention Duration and Frequency Weeks Days/Week | Telehealth Setting, and Supervision | Comparator Group | Main Results |
|---|---|---|---|---|---|---|
| **Ozel et al. (2022)** [26] | Telerehabilitation via videoconference | -Physical activity monitoring and personalized feedback<br>-Education in self-management skills<br>-Tele-consultation with healthcare professionals<br>-Therapeutic exercise program | 4 w<br>4 d/w<br>20 min | Home<br>Bi-weekly individual online sessions | No intervention | TG1 vs. CG:<br>Pain (VAS):<br>TG1 ** > CG ($p < 0.001$)<br>Disability (NDI):<br>TG1 ** vs. CG (NSD)<br>TG2 vs. CG:<br>Pain (VAS):<br>TG2 ** > CG ($p < 0.001$)<br>Disability (NDI):<br>TG2 ** > CG ($p < 0.001$) |
| **Pach et al. (2022)** [27] | Telerehabilitation via smartphone app | -Symptom and mood monitoring<br>-Education in self-management skills<br>-Therapeutic exercise program | 7 d/w<br>15 min | Home<br>Supervised | Usual care and app for data entry only | Pain intensity (NRS):<br>TG ** > CG ($p < 0.05$)<br>Neck Disability (NDI):<br>TG ** vs. CG (NSD)<br>General and physical health (WHOQOL-BREF):<br>TG ** vs. CG (NSD) |
| **Onan et al. (2023)** [28] | Telerehabilitation via videoconference | -Physical activity monitoring and personalized feedback<br>-Tele-consultation with healthcare professionals<br>-Therapeutic exercise program | 8 w<br>3 d/w<br>45 min | Home<br>Supervised | Supervised presential exercises | Pain (VAS):<br>TG vs. CG (NSD)<br>Neck Disability (NDI):<br>TG vs. CG (NSD) |
| **Peterson et al. (2023)** [29] | Telerehabilitation via videoconference | -Physical activity monitoring and personalized feedback<br>-Education in self-management skills<br>-Therapeutic exercise program | 4 w<br>4 d/w<br>20 min | Home<br>Unsupervised | Supervised presential exercises | Pain (NRS):<br>TG ** > CG (NSD)<br>Neck Disability (NDI):<br>TG ** > CG (NSD)<br>General and physical health status (WHOQOL-BREF):<br>TG ** vs. CG (NSD) |

* $p < 0.05$; ** $p < 0.001$

### 2.5. Methodological Quality of Included Studies

After obtaining the eligible articles, data extraction and methodological quality assessment were carried out by two independent reviewers (G.V. and A.C.). Methodological quality assessment was evaluated using the Downs and Black Checklist [30], one of the most used methodological quality assessment scales for clinical trials. This tool consists of 27 items, including five subscales, which are as follows: reporting, external validity, internal validity (study bias and confounding), selection bias, and study power. Poor quality is considered when a score of 14 or less is achieved, fair quality between 15 and 19, good between 20 and 25, and excellent quality when the score is higher or equal to 26 [31,32].

### 2.6. Risk of Bias of Included Studies

The risk of bias for the included randomized controlled trials was assessed using the Cochrane Risk-of-Bias tool version 2.0 (RoB-2) [33]. This tool consists of five domains that focus on the randomization process, deviations from the intended interventions, missing outcome data, measurement of the outcome, and the selection of the reported result. The methodological quality depends on the risk of each of the following subscales: high quality (low risk in all domains), fair quality (high risk in one domain or two unclear domains), and poor quality (two or more unclear domains or there are important limitations that could invalidate the results) [34].

### 2.7. Statistical Analysis

A quantitative synthesis of studies presenting means and standard deviations of pain and disability was carried out using Review Manager (RevMan) software (Version 5.0. The Cochrane Collaboration. Available at revman.cochrane.org). Quantitative data, including the number of patients assessed, mean values, and standard deviations for each treatment arm, was extracted to estimate the overall mean differences between the experimental and control arms. When the studies did not present sufficient data to calculate the effect size (e.g., no means provided, no standard deviation provided), the authors were contacted. We calculated the missing standard deviations when n, $p$-values, or 95% confidence intervals were given via the embedded Review Manager calculator.

We assumed to measure the same underlying symptom or condition, and therefore, standardized mean differences were used as all the scales. The overall mean effect sizes were estimated using random effect models or fixed effect models according to statistical heterogeneity $I_2$ tests (for sizes of less than 50%, fixed effect models were used) [35]. We also undertook a visual inspection of the forest plots for outlier studies, explored sources of heterogeneity, and conducted sensitivity analyses by excluding trials that were at a high risk of detection or attrition bias.

## 3. Results

Figure 1 presents the process of the search, screening, and selection of studies. We collected a total of 518 studies from the three electronic databases and 73 duplicate records were removed before screening.

### 3.1. Search Selection

After that, 445 reports were assessed for eligibility. A total of 121 records were excluded as they did not meet the inclusion criteria specified in our study. After screening the titles and abstracts, 313 records unrelated to this review's topic were also deleted (specifically, population and intervention were not related to the PICOS strategy). Finally, 11 records were full-text screened, and three were excluded due to the control intervention. Finally, eight manuscripts were included in the review [22–29].

### 3.2. Characteristics of Studies

The characteristics of the sample and the methodological evaluation of the included studies are shown in Table 1. The studies, published between 2017 and 2023, included randomized clinical trial designs [22,24–29] and a pilot randomized trial study [23]. The total sample of patients included in the studies was 689, with a gender distribution in the combined sample of 61.92% female. The mean age of the participants ranged from 22.68 to 60.1 years, with a mean duration of pain reported between 4.02 and 86.4 months. The mean pain intensity reported ranged from 3.97 to 7.3 on a scale of 0–10. These results suggest significant diversity in the demographic and clinical characteristics of the participants included in the studies analyzed.

Regarding the methodological quality of the studies evaluated using the Downs and Black quality assessment method, three articles were classified as good [22,25,26], while five were classified as fair [23,24,26,28,29]. Additionally, the risk of bias in all the studies [22–29] was assessed using the RoB-2 tool (Figure 2), which concluded that three of the articles had a high risk of bias [22,24,28], and the remaining had some concerns [23,25–27,29].

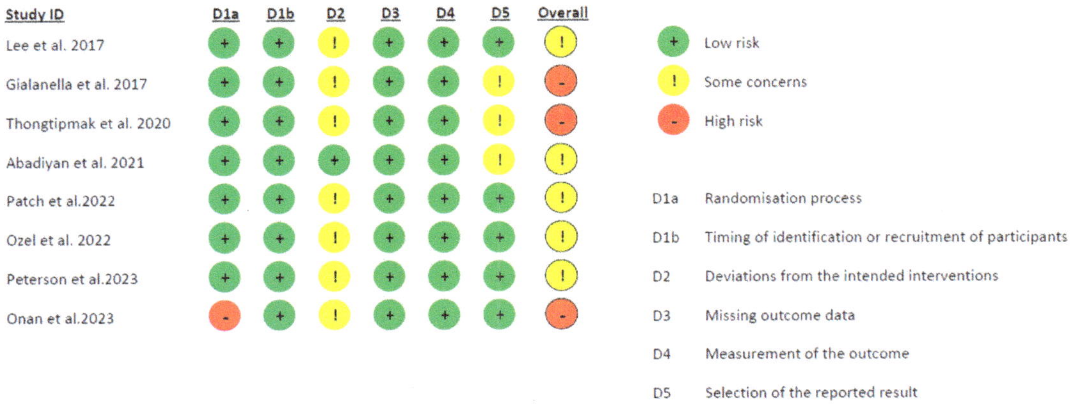


**Figure 2.** Cochrane Risk-of-Bias tool version 2.0 scores [22–29].

The characteristics of the interventions carried out in the different studies are shown in Table 2. This table includes information about the description of the different interventions, their components, their duration and frequency, the modality, setting, and supervision, as well as the comparator group and the main results found.

The most commonly used interventions are telerehabilitation programs based on therapeutic exercise [22,23,25,26,28,29]. The intervention proposed by Thongtipmak et al. [24] was based on stretching and breathing exercises. In addition, the intervention by Pach et al. [27] consisted of relaxation exercises.

The most frequently repeated telerehabilitation components include tele-education content, symptom, and mood monitoring, as well as physical activity monitoring with personalized feedback to the patient. These elements suggest comprehensive care that addresses both physical and psychosocial aspects of the patient.

The duration and frequency of interventions vary between studies, but on average, interventions last about 8 weeks with a frequency of 4 days per week and a duration of 20 min per session. This indicates consistency in the duration and frequency of interventions that may be optimal for meaningful results.

The most commonly used modality of telerehabilitation intervention is through smartphone apps [23–25,27], followed by phone calls [23] and videoconferencing [26,29]. These results suggest a trend toward mobile technology for the delivery of telerehabilitation services. Only Peterson et al. [29] used email as a communication method with patients.

In terms of setting, all the interventions were conducted in the patient's home [22–29], suggesting significant convenience and accessibility for participants. In addition, most interventions were delivered under supervision [22–28], either through scheduled calls, videoconferences, or online consultations with healthcare professionals. Only Peterson et al. [29] conducted an unsupervised telerehabilitation program.

The most common comparator group is non-intervention [24,26] or usual care, [27] allowing for an assessment of the specific impact of telerehabilitation interventions compared with standard care. Other studies used a brochure to correct the posture [23], exercise recommendations [22], physiotherapy, postural reeducation [25], and supervised presential exercises as comparator groups [28,29].

Overall, the results suggest that telerehabilitation interventions have a positive effect on reducing pain [22–25,27,29] and disability [22,23,25,29] compared with control groups. This is evidenced in several studies where the telerehabilitation group showed significant improvement in pain and disability compared with the control group, as indicated by VAS and NDI scores. However, it is important to keep in mind that the results may vary depending on the specific components of the intervention and the study population.

### 3.3. Results Obtained in Meta-Analysis

The results obtained in the meta-analysis concerning pain were analyzed as shown in Figure 3. The pooled mean difference (MD) showed a significant overall effect of telerehabilitation compared with the comparator groups (MD = −1.27; 95% CI = −2.06; −0.47; $p = 0.002$). The results showed heterogeneity, detecting a significant variability of $I_2 = 92\%$, not attributable to chance.

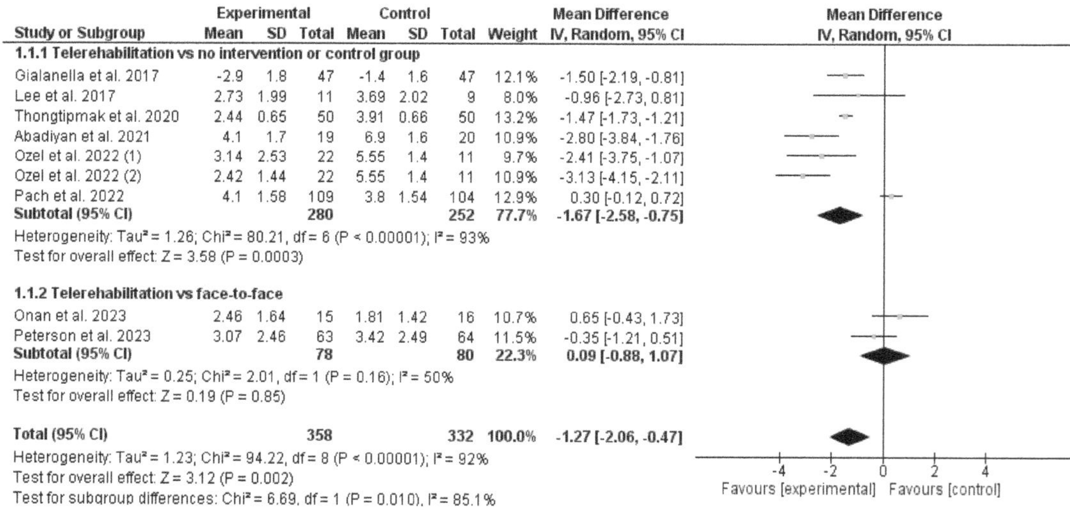


**Figure 3.** Results of pain [22–29].

A subgroup analysis was carried out. The first subgroup aimed to determine whether telerehabilitation obtained better results than the no-intervention or control group. The pooled MD showed a significant overall effect of telerehabilitation compared with the no-intervention or control groups (MD = −1.67; 95% CI = −2.58; −0.75; $p = 0.0003$). The second subgroup aimed to determine whether performing a treatment through telerehabilitation was not inferior to performing the same treatment in a face-to-face modality. The pooled MD showed a non-significant overall effect of telerehabilitation compared with face-to-face interventions (MD = 0.09; 95% CI = −0.88; 1.07; $p = 0.85$).

The results obtained in the meta-analysis concerning disability were analyzed, as shown in Figure 4. The pooled MD showed a significant overall effect of telerehabilitation compared with the comparator groups (MD = −5.04; 95% CI = −9.69; −0.39; $p = 0.03$). The results showed heterogeneity, detecting a significant variability of $I_2 = 92\%$, not attributable to chance.

| Study or Subgroup | Experimental Mean | Experimental SD | Experimental Total | Control Mean | Control SD | Control Total | Weight | Mean Difference IV, Random, 95% CI |
|---|---|---|---|---|---|---|---|---|
| **1.2.1 Telerehabilitation vs no intervention or control group** | | | | | | | | |
| Gialanella et al. 2017 | -7.4 | 5.3 | 47 | -2.5 | 3.1 | 47 | 15.8% | -4.90 [-6.66, -3.14] |
| Lee et al. 2017 | 17.25 | 8.34 | 11 | 15.92 | 8.67 | 9 | 11.4% | 1.33 [-6.18, 8.84] |
| Abadiyan et al. 2021 | 19.3 | 6 | 19 | 39.3 | 6.4 | 20 | 14.5% | -20.00 [-23.89, -16.11] |
| Ozel et al. 2022 (1) | 8.73 | 7.53 | 22 | 12.68 | 5.46 | 22 | 14.5% | -3.95 [-7.84, -0.06] |
| Ozel et al. 2022 (2) | 5.23 | 4.74 | 22 | 12.68 | 5.46 | 22 | 15.1% | -7.45 [-10.47, -4.43] |
| **Subtotal (95% CI)** | | | **121** | | | **120** | **71.3%** | **-7.32 [-12.93, -1.70]** |
| Heterogeneity: Tau² = 36.42; Chi² = 55.44, df = 4 (P < 0.00001); I² = 93% | | | | | | | | |
| Test for overall effect: Z = 2.55 (P = 0.01) | | | | | | | | |
| **1.2.2 Telerehabilitation vs face-to-face** | | | | | | | | |
| Onan et al. 2023 | 6.8 | 4.85 | 15 | 6.93 | 3.62 | 16 | 15.1% | -0.13 [-3.16, 2.90] |
| Peterson et al. 2023 | 30.5 | 15.2 | 63 | 29 | 13.8 | 64 | 13.6% | 1.50 [-3.55, 6.55] |
| **Subtotal (95% CI)** | | | **78** | | | **80** | **28.7%** | **0.30 [-2.30, 2.90]** |
| Heterogeneity: Tau² = 0.00; Chi² = 0.29, df = 1 (P = 0.59); I² = 0% | | | | | | | | |
| Test for overall effect: Z = 0.23 (P = 0.82) | | | | | | | | |
| **Total (95% CI)** | | | **199** | | | **200** | **100.0%** | **-5.04 [-9.69, -0.39]** |
| Heterogeneity: Tau² = 34.89; Chi² = 78.56, df = 6 (P < 0.00001); I² = 92% | | | | | | | | |
| Test for overall effect: Z = 2.12 (P = 0.03) | | | | | | | | |
| Test for subgroup differences: Chi² = 5.82, df = 1 (P = 0.02), I² = 82.8% | | | | | | | | |

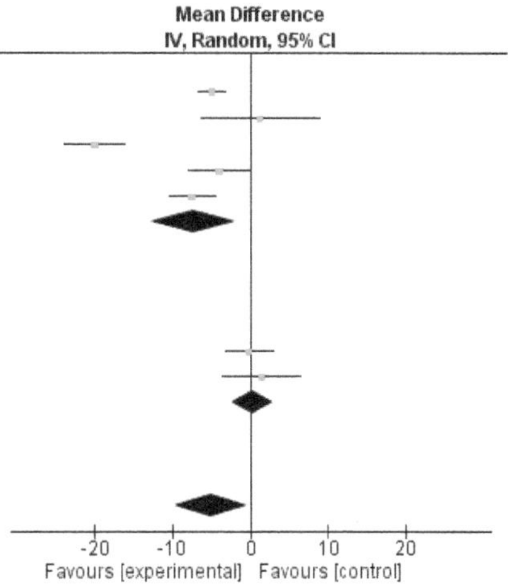


**Figure 4.** Results of disability [22,23,25,26,28,29].

A subgroup analysis was carried out. The first subgroup aimed to determine whether telerehabilitation obtained better results than the no-intervention or control group. The pooled MD showed a significant overall effect of telerehabilitation compared with the no-intervention or control groups (MD = −7.32; 95% CI = −12.93; −1.70; $p = 0.01$). The second subgroup aimed to determine whether performing a treatment through telerehabilitation was not inferior to performing the same treatment in a face-to-face modality. The pooled MD showed a non-significant overall effect of telerehabilitation compared with face-to-face interventions (MD = 0.30; 95% CI = −2.30; 2.90; $p = 0.82$).

## 4. Discussion

This systematic review and meta-analysis aimed to investigate the effects of telerehabilitation on pain and disability in patients with chronic neck pain. Our results show positive effects on pain and disability when considering telerehabilitation compared with other interventions. However, our results should be interpreted with caution due to the number of strategies implemented and the dosage of experimental interventions in the studies analyzed.

This systematic review includes eight studies [22–29] that address the effects of telerehabilitation on pain and disability in patients with chronic neck pain. This set of studies provides valuable information on the utility and effectiveness of telerehabilitation in this population, contributing significantly to the current knowledge about treatment options for chronic neck pain.

The results obtained reveal significant findings that have important implications for clinical practice and public health policy. The findings of this review indicate that telerehabilitation interventions have a positive effect on reducing pain and disability associated with chronic neck pain. Specifically, patients who received telerehabilitation interventions were observed to experience a significant decrease in pain intensity and a reduction in disability compared with control groups. These results support the idea that telerehabilitation may be an effective and convenient option for the treatment of chronic neck pain.

In addition, we found that telerehabilitation did not show a significant difference in effectiveness compared with traditional face-to-face interventions. This suggests that telerehabilitation can show no significant differences in its effects from conventional in-person interventions in reducing pain and disability associated with chronic neck pain. A possible reason is the focus on telerehabilitation components. For instance, in the study of Onen et al. [28] the intervention was focused on muscle modifications, and the study of Petersen and Peolsson [29] was focused on self-management skills. Additionally, when comparing face-to-face vs. telerehabilitation programs, the studies included have different components for the intervention and control groups.

Regarding the characteristics of the sample included in the review, it is important to highlight that the selected studies presented considerable variability in terms of the participants' age, pain duration, and pain intensity. Most of the included studies had a high proportion of women in the sample, which is consistent with the reported prevalence of chronic neck pain in the general population [36]. Compared with other reviews in the field, this sample presents similar heterogeneity in terms of demographic and clinical characteristics, allowing for better interpretation of the results [37,38].

The results of this review are consistent with the existing literature supporting the efficacy of telerehabilitation in a variety of chronic health conditions [39–41]. In particular, and due to the high prevalence of this symptom, telerehabilitation is increasingly important in the management of chronic pain [17,42,43]. However, to the authors' knowledge, this is the first systematic review focused on evaluating the effect of telerehabilitation in the management of patients with chronic neck pain.

If we compare the results of this review with those of other reviews in the field, several consistent trends and findings are observed. First, most of the studies included in this review reported significant improvements in pain and disability in the telerehabilitation group compared with the control group. These findings are in line with previous reviews that have highlighted the potential benefit of telerehabilitation in chronic pain management [17,37,42]. However, it is important to consider that results may vary depending on the specific components of the intervention and the study population. For example, the duration and intensity of the intervention, as well as the participant's ability to use the technology, may influence the results [44,45].

Concerning disability, the results of this review demonstrate that telerehabilitation has beneficial effects in reducing disability levels in patients with chronic neck pain. These results are in line with those of other reviews previously conducted in other populations [46–52].

Telerehabilitation interventions were studied and separated according to the different components they offered to patients [51,52]. The most highlighted components among the different interventions included in this systematic review were tele-education content, symptom and mood monitoring, as well as physical activity monitoring with personalized feedback to the patient. These elements suggest comprehensive care that addresses both the physical and psychosocial aspects of the patient. The results obtained in pain and disability in favor of telerehabilitation are positive, but at the same time, we cannot assume the best delivery method or the effects in the mid/long term due to the diversity among studies.

The results of this review have important clinical and public health policy implications. First, they support the feasibility of telerehabilitation as an effective treatment option for chronic neck pain. The ability to perform therapeutic exercises, monitor symptoms, and receive personalized feedback from the comfort of home may significantly improve accessibility and adherence to treatment for this population.

Furthermore, the findings of this study suggest that telerehabilitation may be a comparable alternative to traditional in-person interventions. The lack of a significant difference between the outcomes of telerehabilitation and face-to-face interventions in terms of pain and disability reduction supports the validity and efficacy of this treatment approach. This is particularly relevant in the context of the COVID-19 pandemic, where social constraints have been applied that limit access to in-person health services, leading to increased interest in remote health interventions [53–57].

Despite the promising results, it is important to consider several limitations of this study. First, heterogeneity among the studies included in the review may affect the generalizability of the results. Variability in the intervention methods, duration, and frequency of telerehabilitation may influence the observed effects. In addition, despite the effort to search for and select relevant studies, there is a possibility that some relevant studies may have been omitted due to restrictions in the inclusion criteria or data availability.

The exclusion of unpublished studies or studies in languages other than English could also introduce bias into the results. In addition, the duration of follow-up in some studies was limited, making it difficult to assess the long-term sustainability of the effects of telerehabilitation on chronic neck pain.

Considering the limitations identified, further research is needed to consolidate and extend the findings of this study. Future studies could further explore the specific components of telerehabilitation that contribute to pain relief and decreased disability in patients with chronic neck pain. Longitudinal studies evaluating the long-term effects of telerehabilitation on chronic neck pain, as well as investigating patients' experiences and preferences regarding this treatment approach, would be beneficial.

## 5. Conclusions

In conclusion, this systematic review and meta-analysis show that telerehabilitation is superior to other interventions to improve pain and disability in patients with chronic neck pain. Specifically, the results were significant when compared with the no/control intervention. No significant differences were found when compared with a face-to-face intervention. These results suggest that telerehabilitation may be a useful alternative for patients with chronic neck pain and no access to face-to-face approaches. However, more high-quality research and studies with long-term follow-up are needed to confirm these findings and establish clear guidelines for the implementation of telerehabilitation in clinical practice.

Concerning the clinical implications of this systematic review, telerehabilitation may be an effective and convenient option for the treatment of chronic neck pain, especially in situations where access to in-person medical care is limited. Healthcare professionals should consider integrating telerehabilitation interventions into their clinical practice to improve accessibility and treatment adherence for this patient population. Health policymakers should consider integrating telerehabilitation into healthcare systems to improve access and quality of care for patients with chronic neck pain. Policies and programs that promote the adoption and implementation of telerehabilitation as a viable treatment option in the management of chronic neck pain are needed.

**Author Contributions:** M.C.V. had full access to all the data in the study and takes responsibility for the integrity of the data and the accuracy of the data analysis. G.V.-P. and A.C.-M. contributed substantially to the study design, data analysis, interpretation, and the writing of the manuscript. I.C.-M. had full access to all the data in the study and took responsibility for the integrity of the data and the accuracy of the data analysis. M.C.V. contributed substantially to the study design, data analysis, and interpretation, and the writing of the manuscript. J.R.-B. contributed substantially to the study design, data analysis, interpretation, and the writing of the manuscript. M.G.-S. and E.D.-M. had full access to all of the data in the study and took responsibility for the integrity. All authors have read and agreed to the published version of the manuscript.

**Funding:** This work was supported by the Spanish Ministry of Education (Grant numbers FPU:19/02609).

**Institutional Review Board Statement:** Not applicable.

**Informed Consent Statement:** Not applicable.

**Data Availability Statement:** No new data were created or analyzed in this study. Data sharing is not applicable to this article.

**Conflicts of Interest:** The authors declare no conflict of interest.

## References

1. Kazeminasab, S.; Nejadghaderi, S.A.; Amiri, P.; Pourfathi, H.; Araj-Khodaei, M.; Sullman, M.J.M.; Kolahi, A.A.; Safiri, S. Neck pain: Global epidemiology, trends and risk factors. *BMC Musculoskelet. Disord.* **2022**, *23*, 26. [CrossRef] [PubMed]
2. Ris Hansen, I.; Barbero, M.; Falla, D.; Larsen, M.H.; Kraft, M.N.; Søgaard, K.; Juul-Kristensen, B. The relation between pain extent and quality-of-life, psychological factors and neck function in patients with chronic neck pain. *Man. Ther.* **2016**, *25*, e73–e74. [CrossRef]

3. Asiri, F.; Reddy, R.S.; Tedla, J.S.; Al Mohiza, M.A.; Alshahrani, M.S.; Govindappa, S.C.; Sangadala, D.R. Kinesiophobia and its correlations with pain, proprioception, and functional performance among individuals with chronic neck pain. *PLoS ONE* **2021**, *16*, e0254262. [CrossRef] [PubMed]
4. Arribas-Romano, A.; Fernández-Carnero, J.; González-Zamorano, Y.; Rodríguez-Lagos, L.; Gurdiel-Álvarez, F.; Molina-Álvarez, M.; Morales Tejera, D.; Mercado, F. Conditioned pain modulation and psychological factors in young adults with recurrent or chronic neck pain. *Pain Pract.* **2023**, *24*, 419–430. [CrossRef] [PubMed]
5. Farrell, S.F.; de Zoete, R.M.J.; Cabot, P.J.; Sterling, M. Systemic inflammatory markers in neck pain: A systematic review with meta-analysis. *Eur. J. Pain* **2020**, *24*, 1666–1686. [CrossRef] [PubMed]
6. Ortego, G.; Lluch, E.; Herrero, P.; Boudreau, S.A.; Doménech-garcía, V. Profiling and Association over Time between Disability and Pain Features in Patients with Chronic Nonspecific Neck Pain: A Longitudinal Study. *J. Clin. Med.* **2022**, *11*, 1346. [CrossRef] [PubMed]
7. Multanen, J.; Häkkinen, A.; Kautiainen, H.; Ylinen, J. Associations of neck muscle strength and cervical spine mobility with future neck pain and disability: A prospective 16-year study. *BMC Musculoskelet. Disord.* **2021**, *22*, 911. [CrossRef] [PubMed]
8. Weigl, M.; Letzel, J.; Angst, F. Prognostic factors for the improvement of pain and disability following multidisciplinary rehabilitation in patients with chronic neck pain. *BMC Musculoskelet. Disord.* **2021**, *22*, 330. [CrossRef]
9. Fejer, R.; Hartvigsen, J. Neck pain and disability due to neck pain: What is the relation? *Eur. Spine J.* **2008**, *17*, 80–88. [CrossRef] [PubMed]
10. Misailidou, V.; Malliou, P.; Beneka, A.; Karagiannidis, A.; Godolias, G. Assessment of patients with neck pain: A review of definitions, selection criteria, and measurement tools. *J. Chiropr. Med.* **2010**, *9*, 49–59. [CrossRef]
11. Vernon, H. The Neck Disability Index: State-of-the-art, 1991–2008. *J. Manip. Physiol. Ther.* **2008**, *31*, 491–502. [CrossRef]
12. Saltychev, M.; Mattie, R.; McCormick, Z.; Laimi, K. Psychometric properties of the neck disability index amongst patients with chronic neck pain using item response theory. *Disabil. Rehabil.* **2018**, *40*, 2116–2121. [CrossRef] [PubMed]
13. Mahtta, D.; Daher, M.; Lee, M.T.; Sayani, S.; Shishehbor, M.; Virani, S.S. Promise and Perils of Telehealth in the Current Era. *Curr. Cardiol. Rep.* **2021**, *23*, 115. [CrossRef] [PubMed]
14. Shachar, C.; Engel, J.; Elwyn, G. Implications for Telehealth in a Postpandemic Future: Regulatory and Privacy Issues. *JAMA J. Am. Med. Assoc.* **2020**, *323*, 2375–2376. [CrossRef] [PubMed]
15. Perimal-Lewis, L.; Williams, P.A.H.; Mudd, G.; Gunasekara, G. Virtual care: The future for telehealth. *Telehealth Innov. Remote Healthc. Serv. Deliv. Glob. Telehealth* **2021**, *277*, 106–113. [CrossRef]
16. Haque, S.N. Telehealth beyond COVID-19. *Psychiatr. Serv.* **2021**, *72*, 100–103. [CrossRef] [PubMed]
17. de Araújo Vieira, L.M.S.M.; de Andrade, M.A.; de Oliveira Sato, T. Telerehabilitation for musculoskeletal pain—An overview of systematic reviews. *Digit. Health* **2023**, *9*, 20552076231164242. [CrossRef]
18. Seron, P.; Oliveros, M.J.; Gutierrez-Arias, R.; Fuentes-Aspe, R.; Torres-Castro, R.C.; Merino-Osorio, C.; Nahuelhual, P.; Inostroza, J.; Jalil, Y.; Solano, R.; et al. Effectiveness of Telerehabilitation in Physical Therapy: A Rapid Overview. *Phys. Ther.* **2021**, *101*, pzab053. [CrossRef] [PubMed]
19. Timurtaş, E.; Selçuk, H.; Uğur Canöz, E.; Inceer, M.; Batar, S.; Demirbüken, İ.; Polat, M.G. Synchronous and asynchronous telerehabilitation methods produce similar benefits in individuals with non-specific neck pain. *Arch. Orthop. Trauma Surg.* **2024**, *144*, 559–566. [CrossRef] [PubMed]
20. Page, M.J.; Moher, D.; Bossuyt, P.M.; Boutron, I.; Hoffmann, T.C.; Mulrow, C.D.; Shamseer, L.; Tetzlaff, J.M.; Akl, E.A.; Brennan, S.E.; et al. PRISMA 2020 explanation and elaboration: Updated guidance and exemplars for reporting systematic reviews. *BMJ* **2021**, *372*, n71. [CrossRef] [PubMed]
21. Higgins, J.P.T.; Green, S. (Eds.) *Cochrane Handbook for Systematic Reviews of Interventions Version 5.1.0*; Updated March 2011; The Cochrane Collaboration: London, UK, 2015; Available online: www.cochrane-handbook.org (accessed on 14 October 2023).
22. Gialanella, B.; Ettori, T.; Faustini, S.; Baratti, D.; Bernocchi, P.; Comini, L.; Scalvini, S. Home-Based Telemedicine in Patients with Chronic Neck Pain. *Am. J. Phys. Med. Rehabil.* **2017**, *96*, 327–332. [CrossRef] [PubMed]
23. Lee, J.; Lee, M.; Lim, T.; Kim, T.; Kim, S.; Suh, D.; Lee, S.; Yoon, B. Effectiveness of an application-based neck exercise as a pain management tool for office workers with chronic neck pain and functional disability: A pilot randomized trial. *Eur. J. Integr. Med.* **2017**, *12*, 87–92. [CrossRef]
24. Thongtipmak, S.; Buranruk, O.; Eungpinichpong, W.; Konharn, K. Immediate Effects and Acceptability of an Application-Based Stretching Exercise Incorporating Deep Slow Breathing for Neck Pain Self-management. *Healthc. Inform. Res.* **2020**, *26*, 50–60. [CrossRef]
25. Abadiyan, F.; Hadadnezhad, M.; Khosrokiani, Z.; Letafatkar, A.; Akhshik, H. Adding a smartphone app to global postural re-education to improve neck pain, posture, quality of life, and endurance in people with nonspecific neck pain: A randomized controlled trial. *Trials* **2021**, *22*, 274. [CrossRef] [PubMed]
26. Özel, M.; Kaya Ciddi, P. The effectiveness of telerehabilitation-based structured exercise therapy for chronic nonspecific neck pain: A randomized controlled trial. *J. Telemed. Telecare* **2022**, 1357633X221095782. [CrossRef] [PubMed]
27. Pach, D.; Blödt, S.; Wang, J.; Keller, T.; Bergmann, B.; Rogge, A.A.; Barth, J.; Icke, K.; Roll, S.; Witt, C.M. App-Based Relaxation Exercises for Patients with Chronic Neck Pain: Pragmatic Randomized Trial. *JMIR mHealth uHealth* **2022**, *10*, e31482. [CrossRef] [PubMed]

28. Onan, D.; Ulger, O.; Martelletti, P. Effects of spinal stabilization exercises delivered using telerehabilitation on outcomes in patients with chronic neck pain: A randomized controlled trial. *Expert Rev. Neurother.* **2023**, *23*, 269–280. [CrossRef] [PubMed]
29. Peterson, G.; Peolsson, A. Efficacy of Neck-Specific Exercise With Internet Support Versus Neck-Specific Exercise at a Physiotherapy Clinic in Chronic Whiplash-Associated Disorders: Multicenter Randomized Controlled Noninferiority Trial. *J. Med. Internet Res.* **2023**, *25*, e43888. [CrossRef] [PubMed]
30. Downs, S.H.; Black, N. The feasibility of creating a checklist for the assessment of the methodological quality both of randomised and non-randomised studies of health care interventions. *J. Epidemiol. Community Health* **1998**, *52*, 377. [CrossRef] [PubMed]
31. Deeks, J.J.; Dinnes, J.; D'Amico, R.; Sowden, A.J.; Sakarovitch, C.; Song, F.; Petticrew, M.; Altman, D.G. Evaluating non-randomised intervention studies. *Health Technol. Assess.* **2003**, *7*, iii-173. [CrossRef] [PubMed]
32. Saunders, L.D.; Soomro, G.M.; Buckingham, J.; Jamtvedt, G.; Raina, P. Assessing the methodological quality of nonrandomized intervention studies. *West. J. Nurs. Res.* **2003**, *25*, 223–237. [CrossRef] [PubMed]
33. Sterne, J.A.C.; Savović, J.; Page, M.J.; Elbers, R.G.; Blencowe, N.S.; Boutron, I.; Cates, C.J.; Cheng, H.Y.; Corbett, M.S.; Eldridge, S.M.; et al. RoB 2: A revised tool for assessing risk of bias in randomised trials. *BMJ* **2019**, *366*, l4898. [CrossRef] [PubMed]
34. Higgins, J.; Altman, D.G.; Gøtzsche, P.C.; Jüni, P.; Moher, D.; Oxman, A.D.; Savović, J.; Schulz, J.K.F.; Weeks, L.; Sterneet, J.A.C. The Cochrane Collaboration's tool for assessing risk of bias in randomised trials. *BMJ* **2011**, *343*, d5928. [CrossRef] [PubMed]
35. Dwan, K.; Kirkham, J.; Paton, R.W.; Morley, E.; Newton, A.W.; Perry, D.C. Splinting for the non-operative management of developmental dysplasia of the hip (DDH) in children under six months of age. *Cochrane Database Syst. Rev.* **2022**, *10*, CD012717. [CrossRef] [PubMed]
36. Fejer, R.; Kyvik, K.O.; Hartvigsen, J. The prevalence of neck pain in the world population: A systematic critical review of the literature. *Eur. Spine J.* **2006**, *15*, 834–848. [CrossRef] [PubMed]
37. Moreno-Ligero, M.; Moral-Munoz, J.A.; Salazar, A.; Failde, I. mHealth Intervention for Improving Pain, Quality of Life, and Functional Disability in Patients with Chronic Pain: Systematic Review. *JMIR mHealth uHealth* **2023**, *11*, e40844. [CrossRef] [PubMed]
38. Pfeifer, A.C.; Uddin, R.; Schröder-Pfeifer, P.; Holl, F.; Swoboda, W.; Schiltenwolf, M. Mobile application-based interventions for chronic pain patients: A systematic review and meta-analysis of effectiveness. *J. Clin. Med.* **2020**, *9*, 3557. [CrossRef] [PubMed]
39. Isernia, S.; Pagliari, C.; Morici, N.; Toccafondi, A.; Banfi, P.I.; Rossetto, F.; Borgnis, F.; Tavanelli, M.; Brambilla, L.; Baglio, F. Telerehabilitation Approaches for People with Chronic Heart Failure: A Systematic Review and Meta-Analysis. *J. Clin. Med.* **2023**, *12*, 64. [CrossRef] [PubMed]
40. Hwang, R.; Bruning, J.; Morris, N.; Mandrusiak, A.; Russell, T. A systematic review of the effects of telerehabilitation in patients with cardiopulmonary diseases. *J. Cardiopulm. Rehabil. Prev.* **2015**, *35*, 380–389. [CrossRef] [PubMed]
41. Cottrell, M.A.; Galea, O.A.; O'Leary, S.P.; Hill, A.J.; Russell, T.G. Real-time telerehabilitation for the treatment of musculoskeletal conditions is effective and comparable to standard practice: A systematic review and meta-analysis. *Clin. Rehabil.* **2017**, *31*, 625–638. [CrossRef] [PubMed]
42. Lee, A.Y.L.; Wong, A.K.C.; Hung, T.T.M.; Yan, J.; Yang, S. Nurse-led Telehealth Intervention for Rehabilitation (Telerehabilitation) Among Community-Dwelling Patients With Chronic Diseases: Systematic Review and Meta-analysis. *J. Med. Internet Res.* **2022**, *24*, e40364. [CrossRef] [PubMed]
43. Tchero, H.; Teguo, M.T.; Lannuzel, A.; Rusch, E. Telerehabilitation for stroke survivors: Systematic review and meta-analysis. *J. Med. Internet Res.* **2018**, *20*, e10867. [CrossRef] [PubMed]
44. Lara-Palomo, I.C.; Gil-Martínez, E.; Ramírez-García, J.D.; Capel-Alcaraz, A.M.; García-López, H.; Castro-Sánchez, A.M.; Antequera-Soler, E. Efficacy of e-Health Interventions in Patients with Chronic Low-Back Pain: A Systematic Review with Meta-Analysis. *Telemed. e-Health* **2022**, *28*, 1734–1752. [CrossRef] [PubMed]
45. Wu, Y.Q.; Long, Y.; Peng, W.J.; Gong, C.; Liu, Y.Q.; Peng, X.M.; Zhong, Y.B.; Luo, Y.; Wang, M.Y. The Efficacy and Safety of Telerehabilitation for Fibromyalgia: Systematic Review and Meta-analysis of Randomized Controlled Trials. *J. Med. Internet Res.* **2023**, *25*, e42090. [CrossRef] [PubMed]
46. Niknejad, N.; Ismail, W.; Bahari, M.; Nazari, B. Understanding Telerehabilitation Technology to Evaluate Stakeholders' Adoption of Telerehabilitation Services: A Systematic Literature Review and Directions for Further Research. *Arch. Phys. Med. Rehabil.* **2021**, *102*, 1390–1403. [CrossRef] [PubMed]
47. Pramuka, M.; Van Roosmalen, L. Telerehabilitation Technologies: Accessibility and Usability. *Int. J. Telerehabil.* **2009**, *1*, 85. [CrossRef] [PubMed]
48. Amatya, B.; Galea, M.P.; Kesselring, J.; Khan, F. Effectiveness of telerehabilitation interventions in persons with multiple sclerosis: A systematic review. *Mult. Scler. Relat. Disord.* **2015**, *4*, 358–369. [CrossRef] [PubMed]
49. Moulaei, K.; Sheikhtaheri, A.; Nezhad, M.S.; Haghdoost, A.A.; Gheysari, M.; Bahaadinbeigy, K. Telerehabilitation for upper limb disabilities: A scoping review on functions, outcomes, and evaluation methods. *Arch. Public Health* **2022**, *80*, 196. [CrossRef] [PubMed]
50. Appleby, E.; Gill, S.T.; Hayes, L.K.; Walker, T.L.; Walsh, M.; Kumar, S. Effectiveness of telerehabilitation in the management of adults with stroke: A systematic review. *PLoS ONE* **2019**, *14*, e0225150. [CrossRef] [PubMed]
51. Hailey, D.; Roine, R.; Ohinmaa, A.; Dennett, L. Evidence of benefit from telerehabilitation in routine care: A systematic review. *J. Telemed. Telecare* **2011**, *17*, 281–287. [CrossRef] [PubMed]

52. Solomon, R.M.; Dhakal, R.; Halpin, S.J.; Hariharan, R.; O'Connor, R.J.; Allsop, M.; Sivan, M. Telerehabilitation for individuals with spinal cord injury in low-and middle-income countries: A systematic review of the literature. *Spinal Cord* **2022**, *60*, 395–403. [CrossRef] [PubMed]
53. Kuijpers, W.; Groen, W.G.; Aaronson, N.K.; Van Harten, W.H. A systematic review of web-based interventions for patient empowerment and physical activity in chronic diseases: Relevance for cancer survivors. *J. Med. Internet Res.* **2013**, *15*, e2281. [CrossRef] [PubMed]
54. Gregersen, T.L.; Green, A.; Frausing, E.; Ringbæk, T.; Brøndum, E.; Ulrik, C.S. Do telemedical interventions improve quality of life in patients with COPD? A systematic review. *Int. J. Chronic Obstr. Pulm. Dis.* **2016**, *11*, 809–822. [CrossRef]
55. de Moraes, É.B.; Santos Garcia, J.B.; de Macedo Antunes, J.; Daher, D.V.; Seixas, F.L.; Muniz Ferrari, M.F. Chronic Pain Management during the COVID-19 Pandemic: A Scoping Review. *Pain Manag. Nurs.* **2021**, *22*, 103–110. [CrossRef] [PubMed]
56. Emerick, T.; Alter, B.; Jarquin, S.; Brancolini, S.; Bernstein, C.; Luong, K.; Morrisseyand, S.; Wasan, A. Telemedicine for Chronic Pain in the COVID-19 Era and beyond. *Pain Med.* **2020**, *21*, 1743–1748. [CrossRef] [PubMed]
57. El-Tallawy, S.N.; Nalamasu, R.; Pergolizzi, J.V.; Gharibo, C. Pain Management during the COVID-19 Pandemic. *Pain Ther.* **2020**, *9*, 453–466. [CrossRef] [PubMed]

*healthcare* MDPI

*Systematic Review*

# Exploring the Role of Voice Assistants in Managing Noncommunicable Diseases: A Systematic Review on Clinical, Behavioral Outcomes, Quality of Life, and User Experiences

**Alessia Bramanti [1], Angelo Corallo [2], Gennaro Clemente [3], Luca Greco [4], Marina Garofano [1,*], Massimo Giordano [1,*], Claudio Pascarelli [2], Gianvito Mitrano [2], Maria Pia Di Palo [1], Federica Di Spirito [1], Massimo Amato [1], Marianna Bartolomeo [1], Rosaria Del Sorbo [1], Michele Ciccarelli [1], Placido Bramanti [5] and Pierluigi Ritrovato [4]**

1 Department of Medicine, Surgery and Dentistry, University of Salerno, Via S. Allende, 84081 Baronissi, Italy; abramanti@unisa.it (A.B.); mariapia140497@gmail.com (M.P.D.P.); fdispirito@unisa.it (F.D.S.); mamato@unisa.it (M.A.); mbartolomeo@unisa.it (M.B.); rdelsorbo@unisa.it (R.D.S.); mciccarelli@unisa.it (M.C.)
2 Department of Engineering for Innovation, University of Salento, 73100 Lecce, Italy; angelo.corallo@unisalento.it (A.C.); claudio.pascarelli@unisalento.it (C.P.); gianvito.mitrano@unisalento.it (G.M.)
3 Department of Diabetology, University Hospital "San Giovanni di Dio e Ruggi d'Aragona", Via San Leonardo, 84125 Salerno, Italy; gennaro.clemente@sangiovannieruggi.it
4 Department of Information Engineering, Electrical Engineering, and Applied Mathematics, University of Salerno, Via Giovanni Paolo II, 132, 84084 Fisciano, Italy; lgreco@unisa.it (L.G.); pritrovato@unisa.it (P.R.)
5 Faculty of Psychology, University eCampus, 22060 Novedrate, Italy; bramanti.dino@gmail.com
* Correspondence: mgarofano@unisa.it (M.G.); masgiordano@unisa.it (M.G.)

**Abstract:** Background: Non-communicable diseases (NCDs) represent a leading cause of global mortality, demanding innovative approaches to management. Voice assistants (VAs) have emerged as promising tools in healthcare, offering support for self-management, behavioral engagement, and patient care. This systematic review evaluates the role of VAs in NCD management, analyzing their impact on clinical and behavioral outcomes, quality of life, usability, and user experiences while identifying barriers to their adoption. Methods: A systematic search was conducted in PubMed, Scopus, and Web of Science from January 2014 to October 2024. Studies were selected based on predefined inclusion and exclusion criteria using the PRISMA guidelines. Data extraction focused on outcomes such as usability, acceptability, adherence, clinical metrics, and quality of life. The risk of bias was assessed using the Cochrane Risk of Bias (RoB) 2 and ROBINS-I tools. Results: Eight studies involving 541 participants were included, examining VAs across various NCD contexts such as diabetes, cardiovascular diseases, and mental health. While VAs demonstrated good usability and moderate adherence, their clinical and quality-of-life outcomes were modest. Behavioral improvements, such as increased physical activity and problem-solving skills, were noted in some interventions. Key challenges included privacy concerns, speech recognition errors, and accessibility issues. Conclusions: VAs show potential as supportive tools in NCD management, especially for enhancing patient engagement and self-management, and their impact on clinical outcomes and long-term usability requires further investigation. Future research should focus on diverse populations, standardized metrics, and comparative studies with alternative technologies.

**Keywords:** voice assistants; non-communicable diseases (NCDs); healthcare technology; artificial intelligence; chronic disease management; digital health tools

## 1. Introduction

Noncommunicable diseases (NCDs) are responsible for 41 million deaths annually, representing 74% of global mortality [1]. Each year, the deaths related to NCDs account for 17 million before the age of 70, and 86% occur in low- and middle-income countries [1,2]. Cardiovascular diseases are associated with the highest number of deaths among NCDs, amounting to 17.9 million deaths annually, followed by cancers (9.3 million), chronic respiratory diseases (4.1 million), and diabetes (2 million, including kidney disease linked to diabetes) [1,2]. Together, these four diseases account for over 80% of premature deaths caused by NCDs. Risk factors such as tobacco use, physical inactivity, harmful alcohol consumption, unhealthy diets, and air pollution significantly increase the risk of NCD-related deaths [3,4]. Addressing NCDs requires a comprehensive approach that includes early detection, screening, treatment, and palliative care. In light of these considerations, both the healthcare system and patients have begun to benefit from emerging technologies, including voice assistants, particularly in telemedicine and telerehabilitation [5,6] Voice assistant (VAs) gained popularity in commerce due to their usability; in fact, digital voice assistants have become an essential part of everyday life [7]. By 2018, 15.4% of the United States population and 5.9% of the German population owned an Amazon Echo, reflecting the rapid adoption of voice assistants in private households, with smart home purchases increasing by 116% in the third quarter of 2018 compared to the previous year [8].

Beyond commercial applications, VAs have emerged as valuable tools in healthcare providing real-time medication reminders, virtual care, and e-monitoring, enhancing patient engagement and self-management [9]. Studies have demonstrated the reliability of commercial VAs, such as Amazon Alexa, Apple Siri, and Google Assistant, in responding to health-related queries pertinent to NCD management. These VAs can provide accurate information, supporting patients in making informed health decisions, and can be utilized to augment health service delivery, particularly during times when traditional healthcare access may be limited [10,11].

VAs are part of a broader category of conversational agents (CAs), which include artificial intelligence-driven chatbots capable of engaging in dynamic and interactive conversations. Unlike VAs, which primarily rely on voice commands and responses, CAs can incorporate text-based interactions and more advanced dialogue management to provide tailored healthcare support [5,12]. These technologies have gained significant attention in healthcare, supporting telemedicine, self-management of chronic diseases, and mental health interventions [13,14]. Integrating VAs and CAs into healthcare systems has the potential to enhance patient engagement, improve access to health information, and support behavioral change strategies, especially for individuals with NCDs [15].

Elderly individuals frequently face isolation, anxiety, and a feeling of helplessness, both in their homes and in care facilities, which can have a substantial effect on their physical and mental well-being [16]. Speech-based assistants can serve as a valuable tool for individuals who struggle to use other technology-driven services requiring manual dexterity, mobility, or good vision [17]. These systems have the potential to improve the independence of individuals with chronic conditions and enhance their quality of life (QoL), even in the presence of physical or cognitive impairments [18,19]. The aim of this systematic review is to explore the integration of VAs in healthcare, particularly their use in managing NCDs. By analyzing evidence from the included studies, this review aims to assess the impact of VAs on clinical and behavioral outcomes, quality of life, and user experiences, identifying the benefits and challenges associated with their adoption, including usability, acceptability, and readiness to use these technologies. Furthermore, this review provides insights into how VAs contribute to enhancing patient engagement, supporting self-management practices, and addressing broader healthcare needs across different populations.

## 2. Materials and Methods

### *2.1. Study Protocol*

This systematic review was performed according to the Preferred Reporting Items for Systematic Review and Meta-Analyses (PRISMA) statement [20]; before starting the literature search and data analysis, the related study protocol was registered in the International Prospective Register of Systematic Reviews (PROSPERO) database of systematic review (identification number: CRD42024604358).

The search strategy, research question, and study selection criteria were designed using the PICO model, with the research question framed as follows [21]:

- Population (P): Subjects with NCDs;
- Intervention (I): Voice Assistants for healthcare support;
- Comparison (C): Digital Twins/Avatars or Textual Chatbots for healthcare support;
- Outcome (O): Outcomes related to QoL, Cost–benefit, Rehospitalizations, Adherence, Accessibility, and any healthcare outcome measures.

### *2.2. Search Strategy and Study Selection*

A literature search was conducted by three reviewers (AB, Massimo Giordano, Marina Garofano) independently, across PubMed/MEDLINE, Scopus, and Web of Science (WOS), systematically searched from January 2014 to October 2024 using the following keywords combined by Boolean operators: voice assistant, virtual assistant, speech assistant, healthcare, health services. The selected keywords were chosen to ensure a comprehensive search strategy, capturing relevant studies regardless of indexing with standardized MeSH terms. This approach maximizes search sensitivity by including various terminologies used to describe voice assistants and digital health technologies, thereby reducing the risk of missing pertinent literature. Complete search strategies are provided in Table 1.

**Table 1.** Search Strategy.

| Database | Search Terms | Filters Applied | Date of Search |
|---|---|---|---|
| PubMed | "Voice Assistant" OR "Virtual Assistant" OR "Vocal Assistant" OR "Speech Assistant" OR "Voice-Activated Assistant" OR "AI Assistant" OR "Digital Assistant" OR "Conversational Agent" OR "Intelligent Personal Assistant" OR "Smart Assistant" OR "Speech Recognition System" AND "Healthcare" OR "Health Services" OR "Health Care Quality" OR "Public Health" OR "Health Care" OR "Health Policy" | Publication years: 2014–2024, Article type: RCT, Clinical Trial, Species: Humans, Language: English, Age: 19+ | 28 October 2024 |
| Scopus | "Voice Assistant" OR "Virtual Assistant" OR "Vocal Assistant" OR "Speech Assistant" OR "AI Assistant" OR "Digital Assistant" AND "Healthcare" OR "Health Services" OR "Public Health" | Publication years: 2014–2024, Article type: Research articles, Others | 28 October 2024 |
| Web of Science | "Voice Assistant" OR "Virtual Assistant" OR "Vocal Assistant" OR "Speech Assistant" OR "Voice-Activated Assistant" OR "AI Assistant" OR "Digital Assistant" OR "Conversational Agent" OR "Intelligent Personal Assistant" OR "Smart Assistant" OR "Speech Recognition System" AND "Healthcare" OR "Health Services" OR "Health Care Quality" OR "Public Health" OR "Health Care" OR "Health Policy" | Publication years: 2014–2024, Document types: Article, Language: English | 28 October 2024 |

Citations obtained through the literature search were recorded, duplicates were eliminated using EndNote, and titles and abstracts were independently screened by three reviewers (Massimo Giordano, Marina Garofano, AB). Available full texts, compliant with inclusion and exclusion criteria, detailed below, were also independently reviewed for potentially eligible studies (see Figure 1 for the study selection process). Any disagreement between the reviewers was solved by discussion and consensus.

The inclusion criteria were as follows:

- Source: studies published in the English language from January 2014 to 28 October 2024;
- Study design: randomized controlled trial (RCT), observational studies, feasibility studies;
- Study population: subjects with NCDs (no age or gender restrictions);
- Study intervention: use of a voice assistant;
- Study outcomes: behavioral and clinical outcomes, quality of life, user experiences (usability, readiness, acceptability), cost-effectiveness, rehospitalizations rate, adherence, accessibility.

The exclusion criteria were as follows:

- Source: studies published before 2014 and after 28 October 2024;
- Study intervention: studies that do not involve the use of a voice assistant as the primary intervention;
- Study outcomes: studies that do not report on at least one of the following outcomes, behavioral and clinical outcomes, quality of life, user experiences (usability, readiness, acceptability), cost-effectiveness, rehospitalization rate, adherence, accessibility, or studies that lack any form of quantitative or qualitative measurement of these outcomes.

### 2.3. Data Extraction

Two authors (Massimo Giordano, AB) independently reviewed the titles and abstracts extracted from the database searches to assess their alignment with the inclusion criteria. In cases where they agreed, studies were either included or excluded based on mutual assessment. When discrepancies arose regarding the inclusion or exclusion of a manuscript based on abstract evaluation, these were resolved through discussion and consensus. If consensus could not be reached, a third reviewer (MPDP) was consulted to make the final decision. The data extraction process was structured based on established methodologies and tailored to the research questions of this review. Extracted information included (a) author, year, country; (b) study design; (c) participants; d sample size, mean age; (e) intervention and control group; (f) outcomes; (g) key results.

This systematic approach ensured a comprehensive and consistent collection of critical data, enabling a thorough synthesis of evidence to address the research questions.

### 2.4. Quality Assessment

The risk of bias in the studies included in this systematic review was assessed by two independent reviewers (Marina Garofano, AB), with assistance from another reviewer (FDS) if necessary in case of disagreement to resolve the issue by discussion and achieve consensus. The Cochrane risk-of-bias tool (RoB 2) [22] was used for the RCTs, evaluating the following domains: bias arising from the randomization process, bias due to deviations from intended interventions, bias due to missing outcome data, bias in the measurement of the outcome, and bias in the selection of the reported result. The risk of bias was classified as "low", "high", or "unclear" (Table 2).

The ROBINS-I Tool [25] was used for the non-RCTs to evaluate the following domains: bias due to confounding, bias in the selection of participants, bias in the classification of interventions, bias due to deviations from intended interventions, bias due to missing data, bias in the measurement of outcomes, and bias in the selection of reported results. The risk of bias for these studies was classified as "low", "moderate", or "high" (Table 3).

**Table 2.** Cochrane risk of bias tool for the risk of bias in individual studies.

| | Glavas C. et al., 2024 [23] | Kannampallil T. et al., 2024 [24] |
|---|---|---|
| Bias arising from the randomization process | Low Risk Of Bias | Low Risk Of Bias |
| Bias due to deviations from intended interventions | Low Risk Of Bias | Low Risk Of Bias |
| Bias due to missing outcome data | Low Risk Of Bias | Low Risk Of Bias |
| Bias in measurement of the outcome | Unclear Risk Of Bias | Unclear Risk Of Bias |
| Bias in selection of the reported result | Low Risk Of Bias | Low Risk Of Bias |
| Overall | Unclear Risk Of Bias | Unclear Risk Of Bias |

: Low Risk Of Bias; : Unclear Risk Of Bias; : High Risk Of Bias.

**Table 3.** ROBINS-I Tool for non-RCTs; abbreviations: PY (Probably Yes), P (Possibly), NY (Probably No), N (No).

| Article | Bias Due to Confounding | Bias in Selection of Participants | Bias in Classification of Interventions | Bias Due to Deviations from Intended Interventions | Bias Due to Missing Data | Bias in Measurement of Outcomes | Bias in Selection of Reported Results | Overall Risk of Bias |
|---|---|---|---|---|---|---|---|---|
| Balsa J. et al., 2019 [26] | PY | P | P | P | NY | PY | N | MODERATE |
| Baptista S. et al., 2020 [27] | PY | P | P | NY | NY | PY | N | MODERATE |
| Barbaric A. et al., 2022 [28] | PY | P | P | NY | N | PY | N | MODERATE |
| Kowalska M. et al., 2020 [29] | PY | P | P | NY | NY | PY | N | MODERETE |
| Roca S. et al., 2021 [30] | PY | P | P | NY | NY | PY | N | MODERATE |
| Smith E. et al., 2023 [31] | PY | P | P | P | NY | PY | N | MODERATE |

## 3. Results

### *3.1. Study Selection and Characteristics*

The study selection process followed the PRISMA 2020 guidelines [20]. A total of 1410 records were identified through database searches, including PubMed (66 records), Scopus (427 records), and Web of Science (929 records). After removing 46 duplicate records with EndNote, 1376 records remained for screening. Following the screening, 1348 records were excluded based on relevance, leaving 28 reports for retrieval. All reports were successfully retrieved and assessed for eligibility. Of these, 17 were excluded for various reasons, including the absence of non-communicable diseases [14], being review articles [2], and lacking clinical trials [8]. Ultimately, eight studies met the inclusion criteria and were included in the systematic review. These studies were critically appraised to ensure they aligned with the research objectives and provided relevant data for analysis. This selection process is summarized in the PRISMA flow diagram (Figure 1), and in Table 4, there are the descriptive characteristics of the eight included studies, with a focus on (a) author, year, country; (b) study design; (c) participants; (d) sample size, mean age; (e) intervention and control group; (f) outcomes; (g) key results.

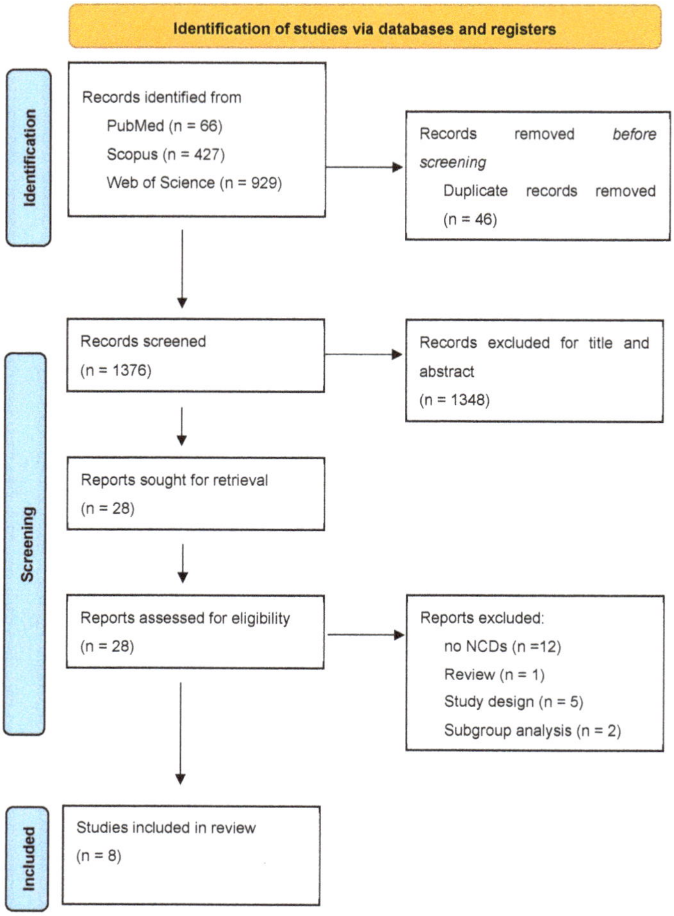


**Figure 1.** Flow diagram of study selection.

### 3.2. Participant Demographics

The total sample consisted of 541 participants, including diverse populations:

Diabetes management: 178 participants across four studies [23,26,27,30];

Cardiovascular diseases and heart failure (HF): 257 participants across two studies [28,29];

Depression and anxiety: 63 participants across one study [24,28];

Intellectual disabilities: 44 participants across one study [31].

Participants varied in age, gender, and baseline health status, but all the studies included NCDs management with VAs.

### 3.3. Outcome Measures

Studies specifically investigating cost–benefit analyses, rehospitalizations, and accessibility concerning the use of VAs in the management of individuals with NCDs were not identified in the literature. The studies included in this review assessed a variety of outcomes, grouped into behavioral measures, clinical and medical outcomes, quality of life, usability, acceptability, readiness, and adherence (Table 4).

**Table 4.** Descriptive characteristics of the included studies.

| Author, Year, Country | Study Design | Participants | Sample Size, Mean Age | Intervention and Control Group | Outcome Measures | Key Results |
|---|---|---|---|---|---|---|
| Balsa J. et al., 2020, Portugal [26] | Observational | Older adults with Type 2 diabetes | N = 20 (11 users: 3 F, 8 M; 9 experts: 8 F, 1 M) | Virtual assistant 'Vitória' for medication adherence, physical activity, and diet. Uses behavior change techniques. | - Usability: SUS, qualitative feedback<br>- Acceptability: Feedback on user experience | - Usability: SUS: 76.6 (users), 70.2 (experts) (Good–excellent usability)<br>- Acceptability: Positive aspects: easy to use; Suggested improvements: reduce repetitions, better interface, more features |
| Baptista S. et al., 2020, Australia [27] | Mixed methods | Adults with Type 2 diabetes | N = 93 (49 M, 44 F), mean age 55 | ECA-based app ("Laura") for diabetes self-management, emotional support, and education. | - Clinical or Medical Outcomes: HbA1c<br>- Usability: Survey<br>- Acceptability: Survey | - Clinical or Medical Outcomes: decrease in HbA1c levels ↓ (7.3% → 7.1%)<br>- Acceptability: 86% found it useful, 44% felt motivated, 20% frustrated<br>- Usability: Issues: monotonous voice, mismatched gestures |
| Barbaric A. et al., 2022, Canada [28] | Observational | Patients with HF | N = 8 | A voice app version of Medly for HF management, daily monitoring, and feedback. | - Usability: SUS, interviews<br>- Acceptability: Preferences for voice app vs. smartphone | - Usability: SUS: 92/100 (Excellent usability)<br>- Acceptability: 75% preferred voice app over smartphone, 25% had privacy concerns |
| Glavas C. et al., 2024, Australia [23] | RCT | Adults with obesity and diabetes | N = 50 (29 M, 21 F); IG = 25 (mean age 65), CG = 25 (mean age 67.3) | IG: Alexa Echo Show 8 + "Buddy Link" for personalized exercise and diet reminders.<br>CG: Generic physical activity and diet info via email. | - Behavioral Measures: Physical activity (accelerometer)<br>- Clinical or Medical Outcomes: Diabetes self-care (DSMQ)<br>- Quality of Life: EQ-5D-5L<br>- Usability: SUS | - Behavioral Measures: Decrease in Sedentary time ↓67 min/day ($p$ = 0.006), Increase in Moderate activity ↑24.7 min/day ($p$ = 0.04)<br>- Usability: SUS: 70.4/100 (Good usability)<br>- Quality of Life: No significant changes |
| Kannampallil T. et al., 2023, USA [24] | Pilot RCT | Adults with mild-to-moderate depression/anxiety | N = 63 (20 M, 43 F); IG = 42, CG = 21, mean age 37.8 | IG: 'Lumen' voice coach on Alexa for Problem-Solving Therapy (PST) with 8 sessions and reminders.<br>CG: Waitlist control. | - Behavioral Measures: Problem-solving (SPSI-R:S, PPO, NPO, RPS, ICS, AS)<br>- Clinical or Medical Outcomes: Neural markers (Amygdala, dlPFC)<br>- Quality of Life: Penn State Worry, affect scores<br>- Acceptability: Dysfunctional Attitudes Scale | - Behavioral Measures: Small improvements in problem solving<br>- Clinical or Medical Outcomes: Limited neural changes<br>- Acceptability: ↓ Decrease in Dysfunctional attitudes (d = 0.6, moderate) |

**Table 4.** *Cont.*

| Author, Year, Country | Study Design | Participants | Sample Size, Mean Age | Intervention and Control Group | Outcome Measures | Key Results |
|---|---|---|---|---|---|---|
| Kowalska M. et al., 2020, Poland [29] | Observational (cross-sectional) | Patients with cardiovascular diseases | N = 249 (158 M, 91 F), mean age 65.3 | Voice assistants + telemedicine services for remote cardiologist contact and monitoring. | - Readiness: Survey on telemedicine and voice assistant adoption | - Readiness: 83.9% readiness for telemedicine, 66.7% for voice technology<br>- Key factors: prior healthcare access issues, urban living, higher education |
| Roca S. et al., 2021, Spain [30] | Observational | Patients with diabetes mellitus and depressive disorders | N = 13 (9 F, 4 sM), mean age 63.8 | Virtual assistant on the Signal platform for medication reminders, appointment scheduling, and feedback on adherence. | - Clinical or Medical Outcomes: HbA1c, PHQ-9<br>- Adherence: Medication adherence<br>- Usability: Acceptance, real use | - Clinical or Medical Outcomes: HbA1c ↓ ($p = 0.02$), PHQ-9 ↓ ($p = 0.002$)<br>- Adherence: 74.4% responded to reminders<br>- Acceptability: 69% planned continued use |
| Smith E. et al., 2023, UK [31] | Mixed-methods semi-RCT | Individuals with mild-to-moderate intellectual disabilities | N = 44 (IG = 22, CG = 22); IG mean age 45.3, CG mean age 48.6 | IG: Alexa/Google Home for increased independence and well-being.<br>CG: No device provided. | - Quality of Life: WEBWMS<br>- Behavioral Measures: Independence<br>- Usability: Ease of use, challenges<br>- Readiness: Technology awareness, training needs<br>- Acceptability: User satisfaction, frustration<br>- Adherence: Feature utilization, perseverance | - Quality of Life: No significant improvement<br>- Behavioral Measures: 80% felt more independent<br>- Usability: 73% found it easy, but 41% needed frequent assistance<br>- Acceptability: 79% enjoyed it, 25% frustrated (speech issues)<br>- Adherence: Most-used feature: music (90%) |

Abbreviations: AS, Avoidance Style; BCTs, Behavior Change Techniques; CG, Control Group; DAS, Dysfunctional Attitudes Scale; dlPFC, Dorsolateral Prefrontal Cortex; DSMQ, Diabetes Self-Management Questionnaire; ECA, Embodied Conversational Agent; EQ-5D-5L, EuroQol-5 Dimensions-5 Levels; F, female; HbA1c, Hemoglobin A1c; IG, Intervention Group; ICS, Impulsivity in Problem Solving; M, male; N, number; NPO, Negative Problem Orientation; PHQ-9, Patient Health Questionnaire-9; PPO, Positive Problem Orientation; PST, Problem-Solving Therapy; RPS, Rational Problem Solving; SPSI-R:S, Social Problem-Solving Index-Revised Short Form; SUS, System Usability Scale; WEBWMS, Warwick–Edinburgh Mental Wellbeing Scale.

### 3.3.1. Behavioral Measures

Two studies analyzed behavioral changes, including physical activity and problem-solving skills. For example, in an RCT by Glavas et al. [23], participants in the intervention group showed a significant reduction in sedentary time (−67 min/day, $p = 0.006$) and an increase in moderate activity (+24.7 min/day, $p = 0.04$) compared to the control group. Kannampallil et al. [24] reported minor improvements in problem-solving behaviors, measured through problem-solving indices, with small effect sizes and limited clinical significance (Table 5).

**Table 5.** Behavioral measures.

| Study | Behavioral Outcome | Measurement Tool | Key Findings |
|---|---|---|---|
| Glavas et al., 2024 [23] | Physical activity | ActiGraph GT9XLink (accelerometer) | ↓ Decrease in Sedentary time: -67 min/day ($p = 0.006$)<br>↑ Increase in Mod. activity: +24.7 min/day ($p = 0.04$)<br>↑ Increase in MVPA: +30.9 min/day ($p = 0.046$) |
| Kannampallil et al., 2023 [24] | Problem-solving skills | SPSI-R:S, PPO, NPO, RPS, ICS, AS | Minor improvements, Cohen's d = 0.0–0.3<br>No clinically meaningful differences |

Abbreviations: MVPA, Moderate to Vigorous Physical Activity; SPSI-R:S, Social Problem-Solving Index-Revised Short Form; PPO, Positive Problem Orientation; NPO, Negative Problem Orientation; RPS, Rational Problem Solving; ICS, Impulsivity in Problem Solving; AS, Avoidance Style.

### 3.3.2. Clinical and Medical Outcomes

Four studies evaluated clinical outcomes such as Hemoglobin A1c (HbA1c) levels, depressive symptoms, and neural activity changes. Baptista et al. [27] observed a slight reduction, not statistically significant, in HbA1c levels from 7.3% ± 1.5 at baseline to 7.1% ± 1.4 at 6-month follow-up ($n = 66$), also Glavas et al. [23] observed potential benefits of the VA on glycemic management with a moderate effect size. Roca et al. [30] reported significant improvements in both HbA1c ($p = 0.02$) and depressive symptoms ($p = 0.002$), with high medication adherence (MPR ≥ 100% for several participants). Kannampallil [24] et al. examined neural activity changes but found only minor, statistically insignificant differences (Table 6).

**Table 6.** Clinical and medical outcomes.

| Study | Clinical Outcome | Measurement Tool | Key Findings |
|---|---|---|---|
| Baptista et al., 2020 [27] | HbA1c | Lab tests | ↓ Decrease in HbA1c levels:<br>7.3% ± 1.5 → 7.1% ± 1.4 at 6M (n = 66)<br>Interviewed patients: 6.8% ± 0.9 |
| Glavas et al., 2024 [23] | Diabetes self-care | DSMQ | Moderate effect size, not significant |
| Roca et al., 2021 [30] | HbA1c, depressive symptoms, medication adherence | HbA1c, PHQ-9, MPR | ↓ HbA1c ($p = 0.02$)<br>↓ PHQ-9 ($p = 0.002$)<br>MPR ≥ 100% in several pts |
| Kannampallil et al., 2023 [24] | Neural activation | fMRI | No significant changes |

Abbreviations: HbA1c, Glycosylated Hemoglobin; DSMQ, Diabetes Self-Management Questionnaire; PHQ-9, Patient Health Questionnaire-9; MPR, Medication Possession Ratio; fMRI, Functional Magnetic Resonance Imaging.

### 3.3.3. Quality of Life

Three studies assessed quality of life using standardized tools such as the EQ-5D-5L, WEBWMS, and custom surveys. Glavas et al. (2024) found no significant differences in overall QoL scores but noted slight improvements in the intervention group's visual analog scale (VAS) ratings (79.2 ± 19.1 to 79.6 ± 21.7). Smith et al. (2023) reported that 80% of participants with intellectual disabilities felt more independent after using voice assistants, even though no significant improvements were observed in well-being scores as measured by WEBWMS. Kannampallil et al. [24] evaluated changes in positive and negative affect as proxies for quality of life. The Positive Affect Score showed a slight increase in the intervention group (from 25.21 ± 6.26 to +4.83 ± 7.79), compared to the control group (+2.43 ± 7.89), but with a negligible effect size (Cohen's d = 0.1). Negative Affect Scores decreased identically in both groups (−9.07 ± 7.58 in the intervention group and −9.07 ± 5.56 in the control group, Cohen's d = 0.1). No significant changes were observed in worry levels as measured by the Penn State Worry Questionnaire (PSWQ), with a reduction in the intervention group (−3.95 ± 11.01) and no change in the control group (0.0 ± 10.95), yielding a Cohen's d of 0.0 (Table 7)

**Table 7.** Quality of life (QoL) outcomes.

| Study | QoL Measure | Measurement Tool | Key Findings |
|---|---|---|---|
| Glavas et al., 2024 [23] | General QoL | EQ-5D-5L, VAS | No significant changes<br>Slight increase in ↑ VAS score: IG: 79.2 → 79.6, CG: 70.6 → 72.9 |
| Smith et al., 2023 [31] | Well-being, independence | WEBWMS, custom survey | 80% felt more independent<br>No significant change in WEBWMS |
| Kannampallil et al., 2023 [24] | Emotional well-being | PA, NA Scores | ↑ Increase in PA: +4.83 (IG) vs. +2.43 (CG), Cohen's d = 0.1<br>↓ Decrease in NA: −9.07 both groups (Cohen's d = 0.1) |

Abbreviations: QoL, Quality of Life; EQ-5D-5L, EuroQol-5 Dimensions-5 Levels; VAS, Visual Analog Scale; WEBWMS, Warwick–Edinburgh Mental Well-Being Scale; PA, Positive Affect; NA, Negative Affect; IG, Intervention Group; CG, Control Group.

#### 3.3.4. Usability

Six studies evaluated the usability of digital and voice-assisted technologies, providing insights into user experiences and challenges. Usability was generally rated positively, with System Usability Scale (SUS) scores ranging from 70.4 to 92, indicating good to excellent usability.

The "Vitória" virtual assistant for diabetes management [26] received SUS scores of 76.59 from end users and 70.2 from experts, highlighting its simplicity and ease of use; similarly, the "Laura" app [27] was found helpful by 86% of users, with a moderate user engagement (participants interacted with the app 18–36 times over the study period). In contrast, the "Medly" voice app for heart failure management [28] achieved an SUS score of 92/100 with 75% of users that prefer it over traditional methods, but 25% expressed privacy concerns, highlighting the need for better data management.

Amazon Alexa paired with the "Buddy Link" software [23] scored 70.4 on the SUS, reflecting good usability overall; nonetheless, some users faced challenges with specific interface elements, underscoring the variability in user experiences. Among individuals with intellectual disabilities, voice assistants like Amazon Echo and Google Home [31] were rated as easy to use by 73% of participants; however, 41% required frequent assistance, and 25% experienced frustration due to speech recognition issues. Despite these difficulties, 79% of users enjoyed using the devices and continued to engage with them. Among these, a virtual assistant for medication and reminder management [30] demonstrated consistent engagement, with 74.4% of reminders answered and 69% of users planning continued use, despite occasional comprehension issues (2.6%). Retention was high (77%), and older adults particularly appreciated its ease of use, reinforcing the importance of accessibility in digital health solutions (Table 8).

#### 3.3.5. Acceptability and Readiness

Four studies assessed the acceptability and readiness to adopt digital and voice-assisted technologies, highlighting overall positive perceptions and areas for improvement.

Baptista et al. [27] explored user satisfaction with the "Laura" app for diabetes management. The study found that 86% of participants considered the app helpful and friendly, and 73% expressed trust in the virtual assistant. However, some users experienced frustration due to mismatched verbal and nonverbal cues, which limited the overall user experience.

**Table 8.** Usability outcomes.

| Study | Usability Measure | Measurement Tool | Key Findings |
|---|---|---|---|
| Balsa et al., 2019 [26] | Usability | SUS | SUS: 76.59/100 (end-users), 70.2/100 (experts) Feedback: UI issues (small buttons, dialogue repetitions) |
| Baptista et al., 2020 [27] | User feedback | Survey | 86% found helpful, but with issues: monotone voice, gesture mismatch |
| Barbaric et al., 2022 [28] | Usability | SUS | SUS: 92/100 75% preferred VA over smartphone |
| Glavas et al., 2024 [23] | Usability | SUS | SUS: 70.4/100, high variability (SD = 16.9) |
| Roca et al., 2021 [30] | Usability | Acceptance and real use of the virtual assistant. | Daily interactions: 2.7/day (88.5% numeric-based); 74.4% of reminders answered; 77% retention (23% uninstalled); 69% planned continued use. Older adults noted ease of use despite occasional challenges. |
| Smith et al., 2023 [31] | Usability | Ease of Use: Likert-scale survey and staff observations. Challenges: Open-ended feedback and frustration ratings. | A total of 73% easy to use, 79% enjoy to use, 41% needed assistance, 25% had frustration (speech recognition issues). |

Abbreviations: SUS, System Usability Scale; UI, User Interface; VA, Virtual Assistant.

Kowalska et al. [29] investigated readiness for telemedicine and voice technology in cardiovascular patients. The study reported high readiness rates, with 83.9% of participants open to telemedicine and 66.7% willing to use voice technology. This readiness was particularly pronounced among individuals who had faced barriers to healthcare access and was influenced by factors such as higher education levels, urban residence, and strong family support.

Smith et al. [31] focused on individuals with intellectual disabilities using voice assistants like Amazon Echo and Google Home. The study revealed that 79% of participants enjoyed using the devices despite occasional frustration with speech intelligibility. However, 41% required frequent assistance, underscoring the importance of adequate training and support to maximize usability and satisfaction.

Barbaric et al. [28] evaluated the acceptability of the "Medly" app for heart failure management, with 75% of users preferring it over traditional methods (Table 9).

**Table 9.** Acceptability and readiness outcomes.

| Study | Acceptability/Readiness Measure | Measurement Tool | Key Findings |
|---|---|---|---|
| Baptista et al., 2020 [27] | Acceptability | Survey | 86% helpful, 85% competent, 73% trust VA |
| Kowalska et al., 2020 [29] | Readiness | Survey | 83.9% open to telemedicine, 66.7% willing to use VA |
| Smith et al., 2023 [31] | Acceptability and Readiness | Pre-intervention survey (Likert-scale) for readiness; user satisfaction survey (Likert-scale) on enjoyment for acceptability | 79% enjoyed VA use, 41% needed assistance |
| Barbaric et al., 2022 [28] | Acceptability | Survey | 75% preferred Medly VA over phone |

Abbreviations: VA, Virtual Assistant.

#### 3.3.6. Adherence

Adherence, defined as the level of engagement with voice assistants, was reported in only one study. Smith et al. [31] provided data showing that 57 out of 63 participants actively used the devices, while 6 did not engage with any features. Music was the most frequently used feature (~90%), followed by reminders and weather updates (~40%). Perseverance in using the devices was high, with 79% of participants continuing to use the voice assistants despite challenges such as intelligibility issues or phrasing commands.

Overall, the reviewed interventions demonstrated promising outcomes in usability, behavioral engagement, adherence, and clinical metrics, but challenges such as user training, privacy concerns, and occasional frustration with interfaces were identified, emphasizing the need for iterative design improvements and tailored implementation strategies (Table 10).

**Table 10.** Adherence outcomes.

| Study | Adherence Measure | Measurement Tool | Key Findings |
|---|---|---|---|
| Smith et al., 2023 [31] | Engagement with VA, feature utilization, perseverance | Self-reported usage and engagement data | A total of 57/63 participants actively used the devices;<br>6/63 did not engage with any features;<br>Music was the most used feature (~90%);<br>Reminders and weather updates were used by ~40%;<br>79% continued using VA despite challenges. |

Abbreviations: VA, Virtual Assistant.

## 4. Discussion

This systematic review highlights the potential and challenges of using voice VAs in managing NCDs, emphasizing their role in supporting behavioral engagement, clinical outcomes, and usability, while pointing out the need for improvements in accessibility, privacy, and personalization [32]. An initial aim of this review was to compare the effectiveness of VAs with other types of conversational agents (CAs) in NCD management. However, the current literature lacks studies that directly perform such comparisons and investigating this aspect in future research could provide valuable insights into user preferences and inform strategies to enhance adherence to these technologies. As noted in recent reviews [33,34], for example, incorporating anthropomorphic and context-aware features in conversational agents may strengthen relational outcomes and foster greater user adherence. Investigating these aspects further could guide the development of more tailored and effective interventions.

Furthermore, an important aspect of VA implementation in healthcare is their specific functionalities and regulatory approval status. The applications included in this review demonstrate a range of approaches to NCD management, from symptom tracking and behavior change [23,24,26] coaching to medication reminders [26,30] and clinician alerts [26,28]. For example, Amazon Alexa and Echo [23,29,35] integrates with wearable devices and mobile health apps to provide personalized lifestyle tracking and health coaching, making it a flexible tool for managing diabetes and obesity and cardiovascular disease. Similarly, Medly Voice Assistant [28] is specifically tailored for heart failure management, enabling remote symptom tracking, daily patient feedback, and clinician alerts when deterioration is detected. Other applications, such as Vitória and Laura [26,27], focus on diabetes self-management, offering medication reminders, dietary coaching, and emotional support through conversational artificial intelligence. In addition, the Signal-based virtual assistant studied by Roca et al. [30] is designed to enhance medication adherence in patients with type 2 diabetes and depressive disorder by providing structured reminders and enabling clinician monitoring through a secure messaging platform (Table 11).

**Table 11.** Comparative overview of voice assistant applications.

| Application | Disease | Key Features | AI Capabilities | User Interaction | FDA/MDR CE Approval |
|---|---|---|---|---|---|
| Amazon Alexa, Amazon Echo | Diabetes, Obesity, CVD | Personalized coaching, medication reminders, lifestyle tracking | Natural Language Processing (NLP), integration with wearables | Voice-based | Not specified |
| Medly | CVD | Symptom tracking, clinician alerts, remote monitoring | AI-driven alerts, symptom analysis | Voice + app | Not specified |
| Vitória | Type 2 Diabetes | Medication adherence, dietary support, behavior change | Behavior Change Techniques (BCTs), patient feedback | Voice-based | Not specified |
| Laura | Type 2 Diabetes | Emotional support, diabetes education, self-management tools | Avatar-based interactions, NLP | Voice + text | Not specified |
| Lumen | Mental Health | Cognitive Behavioral Therapy (CBT)-based problem solving | AI-driven conversation, NLP-based coaching | Voice-based | Not specified |
| Signal Platform | Type 2 Diabetes, Depressive Disorder | Medication reminders, clinician monitoring, patient self-reporting | AI-assisted chatbot or call-based structured messaging | Text- or call-based | Not specified |

Abbreviations: AI, Artificial Intelligence; BCTs, Behavior Change Techniques; CA, Conversational Agent; CBT, Cognitive Behavioral Therapy; CE, Conformité Européenne; CVD, Cardiovascular Disease; FDA, Food and Drug Administration; MDR, Medical Device Regulation; NCD, Non-Communicable Disease; NLP, Natural Language Processing; SaMD, Software as a Medical Device; VA, Virtual Assistant.

A key aspect emerging from this systematic review is the lack of explicit mention of regulatory approvals, such as FDA or MDR CE certification, in the included studies. None of the analyzed voice assistants were reported to have undergone regulatory approval processes, raising concerns about their compliance with established medical device regulations. This omission suggests that many of these technologies may not yet meet the safety, efficacy, and data protection standards required for clinical use.

The absence of regulatory approval may be attributed to several factors. First, some of the voice assistants examined in this review are research prototypes or commercially available AI-driven tools that have been repurposed for healthcare applications rather than specifically designed as certified medical devices. Second, the regulatory classification of voice assistants in healthcare remains an evolving area, and many interventions may not yet fall under the category of Software as a Medical Device (SaMD), thus operating in a regulatory gray zone.

This is further supported by the limited number of studies available, with only eight included in this review, all involving a small patient population. Given the growing emphasis on regulatory compliance for Software as a Medical Device (SaMD), future research should investigate how voice assistants can meet FDA and MDR requirements and explore strategies to ensure their clinical safety and effectiveness.

Regarding clinical and behavioral outcomes, the reviewed studies showed modest improvements. For instance, Roca et al. [30] observed better glycemic control and reduced depressive symptoms using a VA intervention. These findings align with broader evidence, suggesting that personalized conversational agents can deliver behavior change strategies effectively, as noted by Anisha et al. [33], who highlighted their role in promoting self-management and behavioral modifications for NCDs. However, some interventions, such as Kannampallil et al. [24], reported limited clinical impact, emphasizing the importance of targeting intervention design to user needs. A promising opportunity for delivering tailored interventions lies in the integration of artificial intelligence that enhances personalization with more precise recommendations and interventions with a positive impact on clinical and behavioral outcomes [36].

User experience and usability are investigated in most of the studies included in this review, highlighting their critical importance when discussing virtual assistants. This focus underscores the central role that ease of use, interface design, and user satisfaction play in determining the effectiveness and adoption of these technologies. In the included studies, usability scores ranged from moderate to excellent [23,26–28], and participants frequently reported ease of use but highlighted challenges such as speech recognition errors [31] and interface complexities [26]. For elderly users, usability issues can pose significant barriers, particularly when dealing with complex systems that fail to account for age-related sensory or cognitive impairments [37]. Anisha et al. [33] also identified usability as a key determinant of success for conversational agents, particularly in populations with low health literacy, and Sawad et al. [38] highlighted that user satisfaction with CAs often stems from their ability to provide nonjudgmental, easily accessible support. However, some users found certain embodied agents annoying or difficult to engage with. Improved designs incorporating adaptive learning and anthropomorphic features may further enhance usability and user trust.

Finally, adherence to VA interventions was generally moderate. For instance, Smith et al. [31] reported active engagement from 90% of users, with perseverance levels high, despite challenges that underline the need for improved user-centric design, tailored support systems, and rigorous testing to enhance the effectiveness and adherence to such interventions in diverse populations.

### 4.1. Conclusions

This systematic review underscores the potential of VAs as an innovative tool in managing NCDs, offering diverse benefits across clinical, behavioral, and usability domains. While VAs demonstrate promise in promoting self-management, enhancing patient engagement, and improving usability scores, their impact on clinical and quality-of-life outcomes remains modest, reflecting variability in user experiences and intervention designs, also with privacy concerns, speech recognition errors, and accessibility challenges that limit widespread adoption. Future research should focus on including larger, diverse populations to improve the generalizability of findings and ensure underrepresented groups are adequately studied, such as those with low health literacy or limited technological access. Employing more rigorous study designs, such as multicenter RCTs, can provide stronger evidence for the effectiveness of VAs. The adoption of standardized and validated outcome measures across studies will enable better comparisons and synthesis of results.

### 4.2. Limitations and Research Gaps

This review underscores several limitations that need to be addressed to optimize the effectiveness and adoption of voice assistants in healthcare. First of all, many of the included studies involved small participant groups, which limits the generalizability of findings. Observational and pilot studies formed a significant portion of the reviewed literature, reducing the ability to draw robust causal conclusions; secondly, the studies measured diverse outcomes ranging from usability and adherence to clinical and behavioral improvements, making direct comparisons challenging, and also the lack of standardized metrics further complicates synthesizing results. Finally, the majority of studies focused on specific demographic groups, such as adults with diabetes or cardiovascular diseases. Vulnerable populations, including those with lower health literacy, limited access to technology, or residing in rural areas, were underrepresented.

**Author Contributions:** Conceptualization: A.B., A.C., G.C., L.G., M.G. (Marina Garofano), M.G. (Massimo Giordano), C.P., G.M., M.P.D.P., F.D.S., M.A., M.B., R.D.S., M.C., P.B. and P.R.; Methodology: A.B., M.G. (Marina Garofano) and M.G. (Massimo Giordano); Formal Analysis and Investigation: M.G. (Marina Garofano), M.G. (Massimo Giordano), F.D.S. and M.C.; Data Curation: F.D.S. and M.P.D.P.; Writing—Original Draft Preparation: A.B., M.G. (Marina Garofano) and M.G. (Massimo Giordano); Writing—Review and Editing: G.C., L.G., C.P., G.M., M.P.D.P., F.D.S., M.A., M.B., R.D.S., M.C., P.B. and P.R. All authors have read and agreed to the published version of the manuscript.

**Funding:** The project "TED: The intElligent Doctor at your home" (PRIN 2022), classified under the LS4 (Life Sciences) sector, is supported through funding identified by the Ministerial Code 2022F7C2TA and the CUP (Codice Unico di Progetto) D53D23014300006. This initiative is part of the PRIN (Progetti di Ricerca di Rilevante Interesse Nazionale) program, aimed at advancing innovative solutions in healthcare delivery by leveraging cutting-edge technologies and interdisciplinary research.

**Institutional Review Board Statement:** Not applicable.

**Informed Consent Statement:** Not applicable.

**Data Availability Statement:** All data are included in this study.

**Conflicts of Interest:** The authors declare no conflicts of interest.

## References

1. Piovani, D.; Nikolopoulos, G.K.; Bonovas, S. Non-Communicable Diseases: The Invisible Epidemic. *J. Clin. Med.* **2022**, *11*, 5939. [CrossRef] [PubMed]
2. Global burden of 369 diseases and injuries in 204 countries and territories, 1990–2019: A systematic analysis for the Global Burden of Disease Study 2019. *Lancet* **2020**, *396*, 1204–1222. [CrossRef] [PubMed]
3. Peters, R.; Ee, N.; Peters, J.; Beckett, N.; Booth, A.; Rockwood, K.; Anstey, K.J. Common risk factors for major noncommunicable disease, a systematic overview of reviews and commentary: The implied potential for targeted risk reduction. *Ther. Adv. Chronic Dis.* **2019**, *10*, 2040622319880392. [CrossRef]
4. WHO. *Noncommunicable Diseases Country Profiles*; WHO: Geneva, Switzerland, 2018.
5. Laranjo, L.; Dunn, A.G.; Tong, H.L.; Kocaballi, A.B.; Chen, J.; Bashir, R.; Surian, D.; Gallego, B.; Magrabi, F.; Lau, A.Y.S.; et al. Conversational agents in healthcare: A systematic review. *J. Am. Med. Inform. Assoc.* **2018**, *25*, 1248–1258. [CrossRef]
6. Milne-Ives, M.; de Cock, C.; Lim, E.; Shehadeh, M.H.; de Pennington, N.; Mole, G.; Normando, E.; Meinert, E. The Effectiveness of Artificial Intelligence Conversational Agents in Health Care: Systematic Review. *J. Med. Internet Res.* **2020**, *22*, e20346. [CrossRef]
7. Hoy, M.B. Alexa, Siri, Cortana, and More: An Introduction to Voice Assistants. *Med. Ref. Serv. Q.* **2018**, *37*, 81–88. [CrossRef]
8. Minder, B.; Wolf, P.; Baldauf, M.; Verma, S. Voice assistants in private households: A conceptual framework for future research in an interdisciplinary field. *Humanit. Soc. Sci. Commun.* **2023**, *10*, 173. [CrossRef]
9. Ahanin, E.; Sade, A.B.; Tat, H.H. Applications of Artificial Intelligence and Voice Assistant in Healthcare. *Int. J. Acad. Res. Bus. Soc. Sci.* **2022**, *12*, 2545–2554. [CrossRef]
10. Bérubé, C.; Kovacs, Z.F.; Fleisch, E.; Kowatsch, T. Reliability of Commercial Voice Assistants' Responses to Health-Related Questions in Noncommunicable Disease Management: Factorial Experiment Assessing Response Rate and Source of Information. *J. Med. Internet Res.* **2021**, *23*, e32161. [CrossRef]
11. Sezgin, E.; Huang, Y.; Ramtekkar, U.; Lin, S. Readiness for voice assistants to support healthcare delivery during a health crisis and pandemic. *NPJ Digit. Med.* **2020**, *3*, 122. [CrossRef]
12. Schachner, T.; Keller, R.; von Wangenheim, F. Artificial Intelligence-Based Conversational Agents for Chronic Conditions: Systematic Literature Review. *J. Med. Internet Res.* **2020**, *22*, e20701. [CrossRef] [PubMed]
13. Vaidyam, A.N.; Wisniewski, H.; Halamka, J.D.; Kashavan, M.S.; Torous, J.B. Chatbots and Conversational Agents in Mental Health: A Review of the Psychiatric Landscape. *Can. J. Psychiatry* **2019**, *64*, 456–464. [CrossRef] [PubMed]
14. Abd-Alrazaq, A.A.; Rababeh, A.; Alajlani, M.; Bewick, B.M.; Househ, M. Effectiveness and Safety of Using Chatbots to Improve Mental Health: Systematic Review and Meta-Analysis. *J. Med. Internet Res.* **2020**, *22*, e16021. [CrossRef] [PubMed]
15. Kocaballi, A.B.; Berkovsky, S.; Quiroz, J.C.; Laranjo, L.; Tong, H.L.; Rezazadegan, D.; Briatore, A.; Coiera, E. The Personalization of Conversational Agents in Health Care: Systematic Review. *J. Med. Internet Res.* **2019**, *21*, e15360. [CrossRef]
16. Guarnera, J.; Yuen, E.; Macpherson, H. The Impact of Loneliness and Social Isolation on Cognitive Aging: A Narrative Review. *J. Alzheimers Dis. Rep.* **2023**, *7*, 699–714. [CrossRef]

17. Vitlin-Stein, I.; Gitlow, L.; Fusco, B.; Pathammavong, S.; Rajotte, C. A survey of the assistive technology experience of older adults in Tompkins County, NY. *Disabil. Rehabil. Assist. Technol.* **2024**, *19*, 2991–2997. [CrossRef]
18. Marasinghe, K.M.; Chaurasia, A.; Adil, M.; Liu, Q.Y.; Nur, T.I.; Oremus, M. The impact of assistive devices on community-dwelling older adults and their informal caregivers: A systematic review. *BMC Geriatr.* **2022**, *22*, 897. [CrossRef]
19. Albarqi, M.N. Exploring the Effectiveness of Technology-Assisted Interventions for Promoting Independence in Elderly Patients: A Systematic Review. *Healthcare* **2024**, *12*, 2105. [CrossRef]
20. Page, M.J.; McKenzie, J.E.; Bossuyt, P.M.; Boutron, I.; Hoffmann, T.C.; Mulrow, C.D.; Shamseer, L.; Tetzlaff, J.M.; Akl, E.A.; Brennan, S.E.; et al. The PRISMA 2020 statement: An updated guideline for reporting systematic reviews. *BMJ* **2021**, *372*, n71. [CrossRef]
21. Schardt, C.; Adams, M.B.; Owens, T.; Keitz, S.; Fontelo, P. Utilization of the PICO framework to improve searching PubMed for clinical questions. *BMC Med. Inform. Decis. Mak.* **2007**, *7*, 16. [CrossRef]
22. Sterne, J.A.C.; Savović, J.; Page, M.J.; Elbers, R.G.; Blencowe, N.S.; Boutron, I.; Cates, C.J.; Cheng, H.Y.; Corbett, M.S.; Eldridge, S.M.; et al. RoB 2: A revised tool for assessing risk of bias in randomised trials. *BMJ* **2019**, *366*, l4898. [CrossRef] [PubMed]
23. Glavas, C.; Scott, D.; Sood, S.; George, E.S.; Daly, R.M.; Gvozdenko, E.; de Courten, B.; Jansons, P. Exploring the Feasibility of Digital Voice Assistants for Delivery of a Home-Based Exercise Intervention in Older Adults With Obesity and Type 2 Diabetes Mellitus: Randomized Controlled Trial. *JMIR Aging* **2024**, *7*, e53064. [CrossRef]
24. Kannampallil, T.; Ajilore, O.A.; Lv, N.; Smyth, J.M.; Wittels, N.E.; Ronneberg, C.R.; Kumar, V.; Xiao, L.; Dosala, S.; Barve, A.; et al. Correction: Effects of a virtual voice-based coach delivering problem-solving treatment on emotional distress and brain function: A pilot RCT in depression and anxiety. *Transl Psychiatry* **2023**, *13*, 242. [CrossRef] [PubMed]
25. Sterne, J.A.; Hernán, M.A.; Reeves, B.C.; Savović, J.; Berkman, N.D.; Viswanathan, M.; Henry, D.; Altman, D.G.; Ansari, M.T.; Boutron, I.; et al. ROBINS-I: A tool for assessing risk of bias in non-randomised studies of interventions. *BMJ* **2016**, *355*, i4919. [CrossRef]
26. Balsa, J.; Félix, I.; Cláudio, A.P.; Carmo, M.B.; Silva, I.C.E.; Guerreiro, A.; Guedes, M.; Henriques, A.; Guerreiro, M.P. Usability of an Intelligent Virtual Assistant for Promoting Behavior Change and Self-Care in Older People with Type 2 Diabetes. *J. Med. Syst.* **2020**, *44*, 130. [CrossRef]
27. Baptista, S.; Wadley, G.; Bird, D.; Oldenburg, B.; Speight, J. Acceptability of an Embodied Conversational Agent for Type 2 Diabetes Self-Management Education and Support via a Smartphone App: Mixed Methods Study. *JMIR Mhealth Uhealth* **2020**, *8*, e17038. [CrossRef]
28. Barbaric, A.; Munteanu, C.; Ross, H.; Cafazzo, J.A. Design of a Patient Voice App Experience for Heart Failure Management: Usability Study. *JMIR Form. Res.* **2022**, *6*, e41628. [CrossRef]
29. Kowalska, M.; Gładyś, A.; Kalańska-Łukasik, B.; Gruz-Kwapisz, M.; Wojakowski, W.; Jadczyk, T. Readiness for Voice Technology in Patients With Cardiovascular Diseases: Cross-Sectional Study. *J. Med. Internet Res.* **2020**, *22*, e20456. [CrossRef]
30. Roca, S.; Lozano, M.L.; García, J.; Alesanco, Á. Validation of a Virtual Assistant for Improving Medication Adherence in Patients with Comorbid Type 2 Diabetes Mellitus and Depressive Disorder. *Int. J. Environ. Res. Public. Health* **2021**, *18*, 12056. [CrossRef]
31. Smith, E.; Sumner, P.; Hedge, C.; Powell, G. Smart-speaker technology and intellectual disabilities: Agency and wellbeing. *Disabil. Rehabil. Assist. Technol.* **2023**, *18*, 432–442. [CrossRef]
32. Angelelli, M.; Catalano, C.; Hill, D.; Koshutanski, H.; Pascarelli, C.; Rafferty, J. A reference architecture proposal for secure data management in mobile health. In Proceedings of the 2022 7th International Conference on Smart and Sustainable Technologies (SpliTech), Split, Croatia, 5–8 July 2022; pp. 1–6.
33. Anisha, S.A.; Sen, A.; Bain, C. Evaluating the Potential and Pitfalls of AI-Powered Conversational Agents as Humanlike Virtual Health Carers in the Remote Management of Noncommunicable Diseases: Scoping Review. *J. Med. Internet Res.* **2024**, *26*, e56114. [CrossRef]
34. Griffin, A.C.; Xing, Z.; Khairat, S.; Wang, Y.; Bailey, S.; Arguello, J.; Chung, A.E. Conversational Agents for Chronic Disease Self-Management: A Systematic Review. *AMIA Annu. Symp. Proc.* **2020**, *2020*, 504–513. [PubMed]
35. Pighin, M.; Choi, Y.K. The Evaluation of Smart Speaker Skills for Chronic Disease Management of Older Adults. *Innov. Aging* **2021**, *5*, 689. [CrossRef]
36. Al Kuwaiti, A.; Nazer, K.; Al-Reedy, A.; Al-Shehri, S.; Al-Muhanna, A.; Subbarayalu, A.V.; Al Muhanna, D.; Al-Muhanna, F.A. A Review of the Role of Artificial Intelligence in Healthcare. *J. Pers. Med.* **2023**, *13*, 951. [CrossRef] [PubMed]
37. De Cola, M.C.; Maresca, G.; D'Aleo, G.; Carnazza, L.; Giliberto, S.; Maggio, M.G.; Bramanti, A.; Calabrò, R.S. Teleassistance for frail elderly people: A usability and customer satisfaction study. *Geriatr. Nurs.* **2020**, *41*, 463–467. [CrossRef]
38. Bin Sawad, A.; Narayan, B.; Alnefaie, A.; Maqbool, A.; McKie, I.; Smith, J.; Yuksel, B.; Puthal, D.; Prasad, M.; Kocaballi, A.B. A Systematic Review on Healthcare Artificial Intelligent Conversational Agents for Chronic Conditions. *Sensors* **2022**, *22*, 2625. [CrossRef]

healthcare

MDPI

*Systematic Review*

# Interactive Conversational Agents for Perinatal Health: A Mixed Methods Systematic Review

**Samira Amil [1,2], Sié-Mathieu-Aymar-Romaric Da [2], James Plaisimond [2], Geneviève Roch [2,3,4,5], Maxime Sasseville [2,3], Frédéric Bergeron [6] and Marie-Pierre Gagnon [2,3,4,*]**

1 Centre NUTRISS, Institut sur la Nutrition et les Aliments Fonctionnels (INAF), Québec, QC G1V 0A6, Canada; samira.amil.1@ulaval.ca
2 VITAM-Centre de Recherche en Santé Durable, Québec, QC G1V 0A6, Canada; sie-mathieu-aymar-romaric.da.1@ulaval.ca (S.-M.-A.-R.D.); james.plaisimond.1@ulaval.ca (J.P.); genevieve.roch@fsi.ulaval.ca (G.R.); maxime.sasseville@fsi.ulaval.ca (M.S.)
3 Faculté des Sciences Infirmières, Université Laval, Québec, QC G1V 0A6, Canada
4 Centre de Recherche du CHU de Québec, Université Laval, Québec, QC G1E 6W2, Canada
5 Centre de Recherche du CISSS de Chaudière-Appalaches, Lévis, QC G6V 3Z1, Canada
6 Bibliothèque-Direction des Services-Conseil, Université Laval, Québec, QC G1V 0A6, Canada; frederic.bergeron@bibl.ulaval.ca
* Correspondence: marie-pierre.gagnon@fsi.ulaval.ca

**Abstract: Background:** Interactive conversational agents (chatbots) simulate human conversation using natural language processing and artificial intelligence. They enable dynamic interactions and are used in various fields, including education and healthcare. **Objective:** This systematic review aims to identify and synthesize studies on chatbots for women and expectant parents in the preconception, pregnancy, and postnatal period through 12 months postpartum. **Methods:** We searched in six electronic bibliographic databases (MEDLINE (Ovid), CINAHL (EBSCO), Embase, Web of Science, Inspec, and IEEE Xplore) using a pre-defined search strategy. We included sources if they focused on women in the preconception period, pregnant women and their partners, mothers, and fathers/coparents of babies up to 12 months old. Two reviewers independently screened studies and all disagreements were resolved by a third reviewer. Two reviewers independently extracted and validated data from the included studies into a standardized form and conducted quality appraisal. **Results:** Twelve studies met the inclusion criteria. Seven were from the USA, with others from Brazil, South Korea, Singapore, and Japan. The studies reported high user satisfaction, improved health intentions and behaviors, increased knowledge, and better prevention of preconception risks. Chatbots also facilitated access to health information and interactions with health professionals. **Conclusion:** We provide an overview of interactive conversational agents used in the perinatal period and their applications. Digital interventions using interactive conversational agents have a positive impact on knowledge, behaviors, attitudes, and the use of health services. Interventions using interactive conversational agents may be more effective than those using methods such as individual or group face-to-face delivery.

**Keywords:** conversational agents; chatbots; systematic review; maternal health care; perinatal health care

## 1. Introduction

For many women, gender-related social and physiological inequalities significantly impede the attainment of an overall state of health and, by extension, their ability to achieve


https://doi.org/10.3390/healthcare13040363

their full potential as individuals. Women's health is thus a global priority [1]. Indeed, although women have a higher life expectancy (74.2 years) than men (69.8 years), they have a higher morbidity rate than men and have greater recourse to health and social services, particularly for their sexual, reproductive, and mental health needs throughout the preconception and perinatal periods [2].

The "preconception period" is most often defined as the three months prior to conception [3,4]. The "perinatal period" is defined as from conception to one year postpartum [5]. These life stages involve changes at the biological, psychological, social, and cognitive levels that could negatively impact the health of women and babies before, during, and after birth (perinatal health). It is thus essential to consider women's needs specific to these life stages in the provision of care and services [6].

To meet these needs, women are increasingly turning to websites, social media, and smartphone apps for information [7]. The internet remains the most widely used tool for finding information on perinatal topics [8], and is also used as a virtual space for sharing experiences and peer support [9].

Recent studies have begun to explore the landscape of chatbot technology in maternal health. For example, Kaneho et al. [10] conducted a survey of existing chatbots specifically designed for maternal healthcare, providing valuable insights into current offerings and their potential impact on perinatal health. The use of technology was amplified during the COVID-19 pandemic, when most households worldwide faced restrictions and social isolation, limiting expectant and new parents' access to help and support [11].

In recent years, considerable technological advances have allowed for the development of conversational agents (chatbots) capable of interacting with a human using artificial intelligence. Chatbots are software packages that interact with users through text or voice exchanges and generate speech through natural language processing [10,12,13]. With the development of increasingly powerful and connected devices, smartphone chatbots are now widely used by consumers for everyday tasks such as information retrieval [14].

Considering their growing capabilities, chatbots have the potential to play an increasingly key role in the health care field, assisting women and expectant parents in the perinatal period and making the pregnancy and childbirth experience positive, allowing women and their babies to reach their full potential for health and well-being [14–17]. Indeed, the perinatal period, from conception to one year postpartum, is a crucial time when future parents and parents need health-care follow-up and information on many topics, including maternal-fetal needs, the course of pregnancy and its complications, vitamin and mineral supplementation, delivery and associated risks, postpartum, postpartum contraception, breastfeeding, baby's diet and dietary diversification, psychomotor development of the baby, vaccination, psychological and social adjustment to parenthood, and infant care abilities. They usually turn to electronic sources to find answers to their questions, but the information found there is not always credible or is even contradictory [15,17]. It is thus important to explore this question: What is the effectiveness and acceptability of interactive conversational agents in supporting various aspects of perinatal health for expectant and recent parents?

To our knowledge, no systematic review of chatbots in perinatal health has been undertaken. Our objective was to systematically identify sources and synthesize the evidence on chatbot interventions to support women and expectant parents in preconceptions, pregnancy, and postpartum through 12 months postpartum.

To address our research question, we conducted a systematic review following the PRISMA guidelines. A comprehensive search strategy was applied across six databases, including studies published between 2000 and 2022 in multiple languages. Eligible studies evaluated the effectiveness and acceptability of conversational tools in perinatal health, based on pre-defined PICOS criteria.

The paper is organized as follows: the Materials and Methods section describes the study design, inclusion criteria, and data synthesis. The Results section presents the findings, supported by four key tables summarizing study characteristics (Table 1), primary outcomes (Table 2), secondary outcomes (Table 3), and quality ratings (Table 4). The Discussion section analyses the implications of these findings and highlights research gaps, while the Conclusion section highlights the contribution of the review to advancing digital health interventions in perinatal care.

**Table 1.** Characteristics of the included studies.

| Studies | Country | Topics Covered | Study Population | Study Participants | Name of Chatbot | Functionalities | Study Design |
|---|---|---|---|---|---|---|---|
| Barreto, 2021 [18] | Brazil | Child health promotion | Mothers of new-borns | 142 | GISSA Mother-Baby | Text | Cross-sectional research with mixed study |
| Bickmore, 2020 [19] | USA | Preconception care risks | Female, Black, or African American aged 18–34 years, not pregnant | 262 | Gabby | Text Voice Avatar | Experimental study: randomized clinical trial |
| Chinkam, 2021 [20] | USA | Mode of birth after cesarean | Women with a previous cesarean and their prenatal providers | 20 | – | Audio Text Voice Avatar | Qualitative study |
| Chung, 2021 [21] | Republic of Korea | Obstetric and mental health care | Men aged between 38 and 40 years and women aged from 27 to 43 years | 15 | Dr. Joy | Text Voice | Observational study: descriptive study |
| Edwards, 2013 [22] | USA | Intent to breastfeed, attitudes towards breastfeeding, breastfeeding self-efficacy, exclusive breastfeeding expectation | Primipara, pregnant in the third trimester with one fetus, 18 years of age or older | 15 | Tanya | Text Avatar | Experimental study: randomized clinical trial |
| Gardiner, 2017 [23] | USA | Lifestyle changes | Women, 18–50 years | 57 | Gabby | Audio Text Avatar | Mixed study |
| Gardiner, 2021 [24] | USA | Preconception health risks | African American or Black women, ages 18–34 years | 229 | Gabby | Text Avatar | Experimental study: randomized clinical trial |
| Jack, 2015 [25] | USA | Preconception health risks | African American or Black women, 18–34 years of age | 77 | Gabby | Audio Text Avatar | Experimental study: randomized clinical trial |
| Jack, 2020 [26] | USA | Preconception related risks | African American or Black women | 528 | Gabby | Text Voice Avatar | Experimental study: randomized clinical trial |
| Maeda, 2020 [27] | Japan | Fertility and preconception health | Women aged between 20 and 34 years | 927 | – | Text | Experimental study: randomized clinical trial |

**Table 1.** *Cont.*

| Studies | Country | Topics Covered | Study Population | Study Participants | Name of Chatbot | Functionalities | Study Design |
|---|---|---|---|---|---|---|---|
| Montenegro, 2022 [28] | Brazil | Preconception health | Pregnant women in the prenatal or postnatal stages | 20 | Maria | Text | Mixed study |
| Wong, 2021 [29] | Singapore | Stress, sleep, infant feeding | Parents (women) aged ≥21 years | 26 | ClaimIt | Text | Observational descriptive study: multi-stage |

**Table 2.** Primary outcomes.

| Studies | | Usability/ Feasibility | Preconception Risks | Knowledge | Breastfeeding |
|---|---|---|---|---|---|
| Barreto, 2021 [18] | | * | – | – | – |
| Bickmore, 2020 [19] | | * | – | – | – |
| Chung, 2021 [21] | | √ | – | – | – |
| Edwards, 2013 [22] | | – | – | – | √ |
| Gardiner, 2017 [23] | | √ | – | √ | – |
| Gardiner, 2021 [24] | At 6 months | – | √ | – | – |
| | At 12 months | – | 0 | – | – |
| Jack, 2015 [25] | At 6 months | – | √ | – | – |
| Jack, 2020 [26] | At 6 months | – | √ | – | – |
| | At 12 months | – | √ | – | – |
| Maeda, 2020 [27] | Intervention vs. control 1 (no chatbot) | – | – | √ | – |
| | Intervention vs. control 2 (PDF document on irrelevant topic) | – | – | – | – |
| Montenegro, 2022 [28] | | * | – | – | – |
| Wong, 2021 [29] | | * | – | – | – |

**Legend:** √: Significant positive effect; 0: not statistically significant; *: positive correlation with no significant effect; –: not evaluated.

**Table 3.** Other Outcomes.

| Studies | Antecedents | Healthy Behaviors | Health Status or Health Services Utilization |
|---|---|---|---|
| Barreto, 2021 [18] | N/A | – | – |
| Bickmore, 2020 [19] | • Chatbot usability at 6 and 12 months: 62.9% and 67.9% (non-statistically significant).<br>• Satisfaction with chatbot at 6 and 12 months: 80.0% and 85.7% (non-statistically significant). | – | – |
| Chinkam, 2021 [20] | • Feasibility/Acceptability: The chatbot could support provider and patient discussions and offer programmed consistency in preparatory information. | – | – |

**Table 3.** *Cont.*

| Studies | Antecedents | Healthy Behaviors | Health Status or Health Services Utilization |
|---|---|---|---|
| Chung, 2021 [21] | • Usefulness: Less than half (M (SD) = 4.87 (1.11)) of the participants find the chatbot useful.<br>• Ease of use: More than half of the participants (M (SD) = 5.34 (0.73)) find the chatbot easy to use.<br>• Ease of learning: More than half of the participants (M (SD) = 6.35 (0.71)) find the chatbot easy to learn.<br>• Satisfaction: Less than half of the participants (M (SD) = 4.90 (1.26)) are satisfied with the chatbot. | – | – |
| Edwards, 2013 [22] | • Breastfeeding/Self-Efficacy: Higher for intervention group (58.7) than control group (54.1); $p = 0.35$.<br>• Satisfaction with the chatbot: 5.7/7-point scale for both the prenatal visit and perinatal visit (SD = 1.38 and 1.37, respectively).<br>• Confidence with the chatbot: 5.9/6.7-point scale for the prenatal visit (SD = 1.1) and perinatal visit 6.7 (SD = 0.5).<br>• Attitudes toward breastfeeding: No significant differences between groups. | – | – |
| Gardiner, 2017 [23] | • No significant difference in food knowledge, food insecurity, and breakfast consumption between groups ($p = 0.15$, $p = 0.99$, and $p = 0.11$, respectively). | • Physical activity: 52% of women utilized suggestions from Gabby to increase physical activity compared to 49% of women who utilized information sheet. This difference is not statistically significant | – |
| Gardiner, 2020 [24] | • Total usage: 198 of the 240 women in the IG interacted at least once with the entire Gabby system.<br>• After 12 months:<br>- Median number of logins = 6.<br>- Median duration per session = 13.7 min.<br>• Stage of change (food choices subdomain):<br>- At 6 months: IG versus CG = 62.76% versus 49.17%, $p = 0.165$.<br>- At 12 months: IG versus CG = 73.33% versus 62.38%, $p = 0.401$. | – | – |

**Table 3.** *Cont.*

| Studies | Antecedents | Healthy Behaviors | Health Status or Health Services Utilization |
| --- | --- | --- | --- |
| Jack, 2020 [26] | • Progressing forward on the stage of change scale:<br>- At 6 months: IG versus CG = 42.1% (SD = 26.2) versus 35.5% (SD = 23.2); $p = 0.00012$.<br>- At 12 months: IG versus CG = 43.7% (SD = 27.1) versus 40.2% (SD = 5.4); $p = 0.071$.<br>• Regressing backward on the stage of change scale:<br>- At 6 months: IG versus CG = 18.9% (SD = 22.1) versus 22.3% (SD = 22.3); $p = 0.01$.<br>- At 12 months: IG versus CG = 18.1% (SD = 20.4) versus 20.4% (21.4); $p = 0.03$.<br>• Use of the system Gabby: 76/118 (64%) of respondents rated it easy to use.<br>• Trust: 75/110 (68%) respondents trusted Gabby (much or very much). | – | • Clinical visits at 12 months: IG versus CG (587 vs. 812; $p = 0.02$). |
| Jack, 2015 [25] | • Average session lasted: 18.6 (SD = 12.1) minutes.<br>• Average interaction time with Gabby during the study: 63.7 (SD = 70.4, range 2.8–286) minutes per woman. | – | – |
| Maeda, 2020 [27] | – | – | • Post-test state anxiety scores on the STAI (mean ± SD):<br>- IG: (43.2 ± 9.5), $p < 0.001$.<br>- CG 1: (47.5 ± 9.5) < CG 2: (46.2 ± 9.0), $p < 0.001$. |
| Montenegro, 2022 [28] | • Self-efficacy:<br>- Mean according to feeling intimidated by using the chatbot for pregnant women: (mean = 4.00).<br>- Mean for agreement on facilitating conditions: (avg = 3.07). | – | – |

**Table 3.** *Cont.*

| Studies | Antecedents | Healthy Behaviors | Health Status or Health Services Utilization |
|---|---|---|---|
| Wong, 2021 [29] | • Preterm and term groups: Scored between «neutral» and «satisfied» with the chatbot, respectively, 3.62 (SD = 0.96) and 4.0, (SD = 0.82).<br>• Length of interactions:<br>- Preterm group: Interaction was between «long» to «neutral» (mean = 2.92, SD = 1.19).<br>- Term group: Interaction was between «manageable» and «easily manageable» (mean = 4.31 SD = 0.48).<br>• Experience of technical issues when using the chatbot: 46% (6/13) of the preterm parents and 23% (3/13) of the term parents. | – | – |

**Legend:** IG: Intervention group; CG: control group.

**Table 4.** Quality assessment of included studies based on the Mixed Methods Appraisal Tool.

| Authors | Study Design | Quantitative RCT | Quantitative Descriptive | Mixed Methods | Qualitative |
|---|---|---|---|---|---|
| Barreto, 2021 [18] | Cross-sectional research with mixed study | | | (4/5) **** | |
| Bickmore, 2020 [19] | Experimental study: randomized clinical trial | (3/5) *** | | | |
| Chinkam, 2021 [20] | Qualitative study | | | | (5/5) ***** |
| Chung, 2021 [21] | Observational study: descriptive study | | (2/5) ** | | |
| Edwards, 2013 [22] | Experimental study: randomized clinical trial | (4/5) **** | | | |
| Gardiner, 2017 [23] | Mixed study | (2/5) ** | | | |
| Gardiner, 2020 [24] | Experimental study: randomized clinical trial | (2/5) ** | | | |
| Jack, 2015 [25] | Experimental study: randomized clinical trial | (4/5) **** | | | |
| Jack, 2020 [26] | Experimental study: randomized clinical trial | (5/5) ***** | | | |
| Maeda, 2020 [27] | Experimental study: randomized clinical trial | (5/5) ***** | | | |
| Montenegro, 2022 [28] | Mixed study | (3/5) *** | | | |
| Wong, 2021 [29] | Observational descriptive study: multi-stage | | (2/5) ** | | |

**Legend:** **: Two stars; ***: Three stars; ****: Four stars; *****: Five stars.

## 2. Materials and Methods

### *2.1. Overview*

We used the Preferred Reporting Items for Systematic Reviews and Meta-Analysis (PRISMA) guidelines to plan this review [30]. The protocol of this review was registered on the International Prospective Register of Systematic Reviews (PROSPERO) (CRD42023376991).

### 2.2. Eligibility Criteria

We followed the PICOS (Population, Intervention, Comparison, Outcome and Study) framework to design the eligibility criteria.

Population: We included all trials that involved women in the preconception period, pregnant women and their partners, and mothers and fathers/co-parents of babies up to 12 months of age.

Interventions: We included any intervention with a conversational agent that allows participants to interact bidirectionally, either by voice or chat, or a combination of both. We excluded any intervention with a conversational agent used only to collect information or developed for the training of health professionals or students.

Comparator: We considered all comparators, including no intervention, usual care, or any other type of intervention.

Outcomes: We considered all outcomes reported in the studies that are related to the effectiveness of interactive conversational agents in any area of perinatal health or well-being such as pregnancy-related information seeking, childbirth, breastfeeding, dietary diversification, health, and support resources.

We were also interested in the non-clinical metrics such as user engagement, duration of adherence and duration of individual interaction, user experience, and acceptability.

Setting: We included studies taking place in primary health care, hospitals, community settings, third-sector organizations, or any other setting.

All types of studies were included (qualitative, quantitative, and mixed methods) if they had health-related outcomes.

### 2.3. Search Strategy

In collaboration with a librarian (FB), we developed a search strategy in six electronic bibliographic databases (MEDLINE (Ovid), CINAHL (EBSCO), Embase, Web of Science, Inspec, and IEEE Xplore). The sensitivity of the search strategy was tested before starting the screening process with five key articles.

Search strings combined free terms and, when supported, controlled vocabulary. The reference lists of relevant articles were also screened to ensure that all eligible studies were captured. All studies published from January 2000 to July 2022 in English, French, Spanish, Portuguese, and Italian (languages understood by the reviewers) were considered regardless of the study design.

We excluded the following types of publications: editorial comment, opinion, informative review, conference abstract, commentary, systematic review, and protocol. Grey literature such as dissertations, theses, and conference proceedings were not included. (The search strategy is presented in Appendix A).

### 2.4. Data Collection

We used the online platform Covidence to conduct the review (Covidence systematic review software). We imported all references to the tool and most duplicates were automatically removed. Two reviewers independently assessed the title and abstract of each reference using the criteria. We then obtained the full text of included references, and two reviewers independently assessed the studies for final inclusion. Two reviewers appraised the quality the studies included with the Mixed Methods Appraisal Tool (MMAT) [31]. Any disagreement was resolved by a third reviewer.

### 2.5. Data Extraction

An extraction grid was used in Covidence for the abstraction of data from included studies. The following data were collected for each study: first author, year of publication, type of study, type of technology (chat, voice, or a combination of both), intervention components and characteristics, study duration (if applicable), participants and setting characteristics, and health outcomes and non-clinical outcomes (if applicable). Two reviewers extracted data independently, and in case of missing data, direct requests were made to the study authors to supply the information.

### 2.6. Data Synthesis

We conducted descriptive and thematic analyses and presented the results in the form of a structured narrative synthesis of the main technologies used in perinatal care by fields of application. We used a prespecified thematic analysis grid based on 3 main categories of outcomes: 1, Antecedents; 2, Healthy behaviors; 3, Health status or health services utilization. We also conducted a narrative synthesis of qualitative findings, and we summarized the strengths and weaknesses reported for each conversational agent.

## 3. Results

A total of 162 publications were retrieved, and 36 duplicates were removed manually. The remaining 126 publications were screened by independent reviewers using titles and abstracts. Thirty-six publications were screened in full text, among which thirteen were retained. Two publications related to the same study were considered jointly, resulting in twelve studies suitable for inclusion in this review (see Figure 1).

A PRISMA flowchart describes the identification of studies, the screening process, and the application of inclusion and exclusion criteria [32] (Figure 1).

The selected studies were conducted between 2013 and 2022 (see Table 1). Seven studies were conducted in the USA, two in Brazil, one in the Republic of Korea, one in Singapore, and one in Japan. These studies evaluated the use and effectiveness of chatbots in various aspects of perinatal health. Most studies focused on the preconception period, particularly fertility [27], preconception health [27,28], and preconceptional-related risks [19,24–26]. Other studies focused on childbirth, specifically the mode of birth after cesarean [20], stress [29], and parental mental health during the perinatal period [21]. Some studies focused on sleep and neonatal dietary diversification [29], and various breastfeeding-related behaviors, including intentions, attitudes, and self-efficacy [22]. Only one study focused on child health promotion [18], and another on lifestyle changes in women of childbearing age [23].

The study population was generally female and ranged in age from 18 to 50 years. Only two studies included men aged 38 to 40 years [21] or parents aged 21 years and older [29]. Interventions to promote breastfeeding, dietary diversification, and infant health were mainly aimed at young primiparous women (new mothers) or young parents. In the trials that focused on the mode of birth after cesarean, the authors included women who already had a cesarean. The number of participants recruited ranged from 15 to 927 participants. All the chatbots studied interacted with their users via text messages, four via text messages and voice, three via audio, and seven integrated avatars into their chatbots.

Of the 12 studies included in our systematic review, 50% were randomized clinical trials (6/12), 25% were mixed methods studies (3/12), 17% (2/12) were observational descriptive studies (two or more phases), and only one study (0.9%) had a qualitative research design.

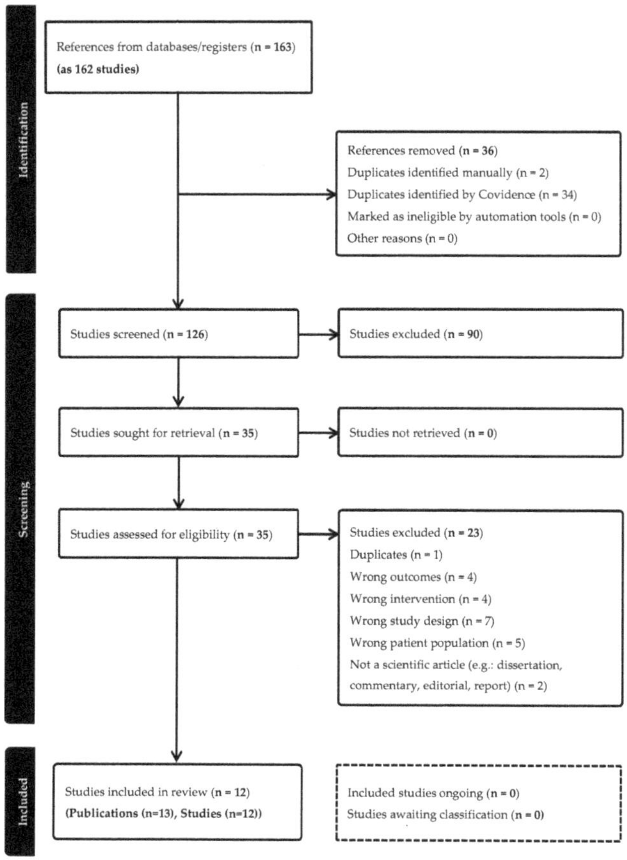


**Figure 1.** PRISMA flow diagram for inclusion of reviews.

### 3.1. Primary Outcomes Measured

The present review brings together heterogeneous studies with specific objectives and therefore different but complementary results, as shown in Table 2, which summarizes the main findings by topic.

Of the twelve included studies, six [18,19,21,23,28,29] assessed chatbot usability; three [23,25,26] preconception risks defined as health and nutrition risk factors that can have an impact on maternal and child health before conception; two studies [23,27] assessed knowledge; and one [22] breastfeeding. To assess usability, Barreto et al. [18] measured newborn mothers' user experience and satisfaction with the chatbot. The results indicate that women's level of agreement with the simplicity, good quality of information, clarity of content, usefulness, and overall satisfaction with the chatbot, was over 90%. In Wong's study [29], the usability assessment showed that parents found the chatbot easy to use (mean = 4.08, SD = 0.74; 1 = very difficult, 5 = very easy) and that they were satisfied (mean = 3.81, SD = 0.90; 1 = very dissatisfied, 5 = very satisfied).

Bickmore et al. [19] evaluated the acceptance, usability, and use of a chatbot to screen women for preconception care risks and treat them via an animated web-based virtual health advisor. Differences between younger (18–25 years old) and older (26–34 years old) in relation to chatbot acceptance and utilization were explored. No significant differences were found between the two age groups for either of these parameters. Chung et al. [21] evaluated a chatbot based on a question-and-answer knowledge database for obstetric and mental health care for perinatal women and their partners. The results indicate that, apart from ease of learning, total usability and the other three sub-factors (usefulness, ease of use, and satisfaction) had significant positive associations with each other.

In Montenegro's study [28], the usability assessment showed that the most significant and positive construct was related to chatbot performance expectations (mean = 4.61, SD = 0.74), while the construct with the least positive influence on pregnant women was facilitating conditions (mean = 3.30, SD = 1.24). From these results, it emerges that pregnant women believe that interaction with the chatbot has educated them and that their physician would approve their use [28].

Edwards et al. [22] looked at the evaluation of an animated, interactive computer agent designed to provide breastfeeding information and support mothers interested in breastfeeding. The results show that mothers who used the chatbot were more likely to breastfeed exclusively after being exposed to the chatbot ($p < 0.05$) [22].

Gardiner et al. [23] assessed the feasibility of using a chatbot to teach lifestyle modifications to urban women of childbearing age. In this regard, the results showed that after one month, among women randomized to the chatbot, alcohol consumption to reduce stress significantly decreased ($p = 0.03$) and daily fruit consumption increased by an average of two servings compared with the control ($p = 0.04$) [23]. Regarding knowledge assessment, this study compared food knowledge before and after the intervention, and the results were not statistically significant between the two study groups [23].

Maeda et al. [27] assessed the impact of a chatbot on fertility knowledge and the results indicate that fertility knowledge improved over time in the intervention group (chatbot) (+9.1 points, $p < 0.001$), control group 1 (+14.9 points, $p < 0.001$), and control group 2 (+1.1 points, $p = 0.24$). Preconception risk assessment was carried out in the studies by Gardiner et al. [24], and Jack et al. [25,26]. The results showed that the use of a chatbot for preconception risk assessment had a statistically significant positive effect between intervention and control groups at 6 months [24], as well as at 6 and 12 months [26]. However, the use of the chatbot had no statistically significant effect between groups at 12 months [24]. The results of Chinkam's study [20] are not included in Table 2, as it is a qualitative study with a small sample size (12 women). The findings of this study showed that women with previous cesarean sections and antenatal care providers viewed positively the use of an Embodied Conversational Agent (ECA) to support shared decision-making about the mode of delivery after a previous cesarean section. Participants commented that although the ECA might seem somewhat "robotic", it could provide easy access to information for patients and complement consultation with care providers. It was suggested that improvements be made to the visual appeal of the ECA, and that the role and timing of decision tools using ECA technology be clarified to improve the shared decision-making process [20].

### 3.2. Other Outcomes Measured

We carried out an additional analysis by secondary outcomes, which we categorized into three categories (Antecedents, Healthy Behaviors, and Health status or health services utilization). By antecedents, we mean outcomes related to usability (usefulness, ease of learning, feasibility, acceptability, engagement, trust, and satisfaction) as well as outcomes related to knowledge, attitude, and behavioral intention. As presented in Table 3, some authors evaluated the experience of using the technology [29] and usability [23,26,29], while others assessed participant engagement with the chatbot by measuring the number of interactions with the chatbot, the number of logins [29], and the duration of each session [29]. Other outcomes documented were the impact of chatbot interactions on improving levels of nutrition knowledge and adoption of dietary habits [23], knowledge related to food insecurity, and attitudes towards breastfeeding, confidence in breastfeeding, and intention to breastfeed exclusively [22]. Chung et al. [21] focused on the ease of learning with the chatbot. For their part, Jack et al. [26] and Gardiner et al. [24] were interested in demonstrating how the chatbot can help its users navigate the behavior-change process through the stages of change and achieving a sense of self-efficacy [22,28]. Other outcomes assessed included feasibility and acceptability [20], trust [26], and satisfaction [19,21,22]. Details are provided in Table 3. Based on the results of our review, user experience and the satisfaction of new mothers with the chatbot reports showed that women's level of agreement with the simplicity, good quality of information, clarity of content, usefulness, and overall satisfaction with the chatbot, was over 90% [18]. The Gabby system was also reported as usable for delivering lifestyle modifications and as easy to use and navigate [23].

Participants engaging with the chatbot demonstrated higher satisfaction levels in comparison to those utilizing patient education sheets, and they also expressed a willingness to recommend the system to others. Nguyen et al. [33] and Suharwardy et al. [34] pointed in the same direction by highlighting the high user satisfaction and usability of health chatbots, particularly among postpartum women seeking breastfeeding support. Despite some technical issues, most users expressed overall satisfaction with the platform's usability and reported positive experiences with the chatbot interface. These findings underscore the importance of chatbots as an accessible, user-friendly resource for maternal health support, and offer promising potential for meeting user needs in this specific population.

### 3.3. Quality Assessment

We used the Mixed Methods Appraisal Tool (MMAT) to assess the quality of all included studies [31]. After this analysis, we found that four of the six included RCTs were of very good to excellent quality (4 or 5 stars). The other RCTs were of average quality (from 2 to 3 stars). The most common methodological limitations for RCTs were: (1) lack of certainty that participants would adhere to the interventions, or outcome data are not complete, or information about the blinding of evaluators is not provided, or there was no blinding.

The three mixed-method studies were from average (2 stars) to very good (4 stars) quality, and the quality of the descriptive observational studies was average (2 stars). The most common methodological limitations were: (1) divergences and inconsistencies between quantitative and qualitative results that are not adequately addressed; (2) lack of adherence to the quality criteria of each tradition of the methods involved; (3) lack of adequate rationale for using a mixed methods design to address the research question. The only qualitative study included in the review was of excellent quality (5 stars). (see Table 4).

## 4. Discussion

### 4.1. Main Findings

In the rapidly evolving landscape of digital health interventions, chatbots have emerged as promising tools for supporting women's health. This systematic review aimed to identify and evaluate studies on chatbots designed to support women and expectant parents throughout the reproductive journey, from preconception to 12 months postpartum. Our review revealed the efficacy of chatbots in delivering perinatal care and promoting healthy lifestyles. Studies consistently demonstrated the feasibility of providing advice on physical activity, nutrition, mindfulness, and stress management through user-friendly chatbots. These digital tools, developed using text-mining techniques and contextual usability testing, proved particularly valuable in supporting women's health across diverse urban settings.

The effectiveness of chatbots aligns with previous findings on mobile phone-based interventions during pregnancy [35]. Both approaches have shown positive impacts on maternal behaviors, contributing to improved maternal- and fetal health outcomes. Specifically, these digital interventions have been associated with increased self-reported physical activity, higher rates of smoking cessation, improved dietary habits including increased fruit, vegetable, and folic acid intake, and reduced alcohol consumption among pregnant women.

The majority of studies in our review reported high feasibility and user acceptance of chatbot interventions which is consistent with the literature. These digital tools have been successfully implemented across various health domains, including mental health support for young adults [36], HIV testing and pre-exposure prophylaxis promotion [37], and COVID-19 guidance for pregnant and breastfeeding women [38]. Notably, users expressed high satisfaction with both web-based and app-based chatbots, underscoring their versatility and broad appeal [39].

Our findings extend beyond chatbots to encompass broader internet-based prenatal interventions. These digital tools have demonstrated positive impacts on various aspects of maternal health, including satisfaction, parent–child bonding, breastfeeding efficacy, social support, and overall quality of life [40,41]. While these results suggest that chatbot interventions could be an effective strategy for supporting perinatal women's health and well-being, we caution that careful consideration is needed when addressing anxiety in this population.

Recent research on perinatal women's engagement with digital emotional well-being interventions [42] has highlighted the critical role of usability. Our review corroborates these findings, emphasizing the importance of user experience and ease of interaction in digital health tools. By prioritizing usability as a primary outcome, researchers and developers can create more effective and engaging interventions that better address the unique needs of women during the perinatal period.

Our review underscores the potential of chatbots as effective tools for promoting healthy behaviors and engaging women in managing their well-being. The implementation of chatbots has shown a significant impact on user engagement, particularly in reducing stress-related alcohol consumption and increasing daily fruit intake. Users have reported a greater utilization of stress management techniques, with many acknowledging that they have adopted the chatbot's suggestions to help improve their stress levels. This indicates that chatbots not only provide valuable information but also encourage positive behavioral changes, making them a promising resource for enhancing health outcomes among women in urban settings.

These findings are further corroborated and expanded upon by a recent systematic review and meta-analysis of AI chatbot interventions in women's health [41,43]. This comprehensive analysis has illuminated the significant potential of these technologies to enhance healthcare outcomes across a broader spectrum of women's health issues. Chatbots have shown considerable promise in delivering health education, supporting mental health, managing chronic diseases, and providing targeted interventions for reproductive health and prenatal education. Notably, these interventions have been effective in improving both physical and mental health outcomes, particularly in reducing anxiety, underscoring the value of integrating AI chatbots into healthcare strategies for women.

The importance of leveraging digital technologies for preconceptional care was further emphasized by studies highlighting the role of chatbots in providing essential preconception information. These digital tools offer comprehensive support throughout the reproductive journey, empowering users to make informed health decisions and encouraging proactive health behaviors. Several studies in our review addressed preconception care risks both directly and indirectly. For instance, the Gabby system demonstrated effectiveness in delivering healthy lifestyle recommendations and addressing preconceptional risks among diverse populations, including African American and Black women [23–25]. Other studies focused on developing chatbots for perinatal care and parental support [21,29], indirectly contributing to preconceptional care through the promotion of maternal and infant health. For example, "Dina" a chatbot developed to inform and empower pregnant women with gestational diabetes mellitus promotes stable blood glucose and thereby prevent the development of adverse outcomes for the mother and the fetus [44]. In the same vein, "Wysa" is an AI-based emotionally intelligent mobile app aiming to build mental resilience and promote mental well-being in women with a self-reported maternal event, and its evaluation showed significant reductions in depressive symptoms [43].

However, it is important to recognize that equitable access to digital technologies is not guaranteed for all populations [45]. Disparities related to digital literacy, access to connected devices, and high-quality internet connections can limit adoption. These challenges are particularly pronounced in low-resource settings or among vulnerable groups such as migrants and refugees, or neurodiverse individuals [46–48]. Future research is needed to explore these issues and ensure that digital solutions are accessible and inclusive for all users.

In conclusion, our review reveals the multifaceted benefits of chatbots in improving health outcomes and enhancing user engagement across various stages of reproductive and maternal health. From preconception care to postpartum support and breastfeeding guidance, chatbots serve as valuable tools for disseminating knowledge and promoting proactive health behaviors. Their ability to provide anonymous, non-judgmental interactions makes them particularly effective in addressing sensitive health issues. As digital health continues to evolve, chatbots represent a promising avenue for delivering personalized, accessible, and effective support to women throughout their reproductive journey.

### 4.2. Strengths

This systematic review is underpinned by several methodological strengths that enhance its reliability and comprehensiveness. To ensure transparency and reproducibility, we pre-registered the study protocol with the International Prospective Register of Systematic Reviews (PROSPERO) and adhered strictly to the PRISMA guidelines throughout the review process, minimizing potential bias in our findings.

Our search strategy, developed and implemented by an experienced librarian, was both robust and comprehensive. We conducted searches in six databases, supplemented by hand searches to identify additional relevant studies. Notably, our literature search included five languages (English, French, Spanish, Portuguese, and Italian), allowing for a broad and inclusive review of the published literature on the topic.

To further reduce the risk of bias, two independent reviewers performed study selection and data extraction, with a consensus process for conflict resolution. This approach ensured agreement on the included studies and increased the reliability of our data synthesis. We used the Mixed Methods Appraisal Tool (MMAT) to critically appraise the methodological quality of the included studies, providing a standardized assessment of study rigor across our sample.

A key strength of our review is its comprehensive scope, covering the entire perinatal period from preconception through pregnancy and up to 12 months postpartum. This broad temporal range provides a holistic portrait of chatbot use across critical periods of maternal and infant life, allowing for a comprehensive understanding of their use and impact.

Together, these methodological strengths enhance the validity and reliability of our findings and provide a solid foundation for understanding the current state of chatbot use in perinatal care. By adhering to these rigorous standards, we aim to provide a trustworthy and comprehensive synthesis of the available evidence that can inform future research, clinical practice, and policy decisions in the area of digital health interventions for maternal and infant care.

*4.3. Limitations*

Despite our rigorous methodology, this systematic review has some limitations that should be considered when interpreting its results. The primary limitation was the limited number and heterogeneity of the included studies, which precluded the ability to perform a meta-analysis. This limitation hinders our ability to quantify the effect size of chatbot interventions on specific outcomes in perinatal care.

The paucity of qualitative studies in our sample, with only one such study included, limits our ability to provide a more nuanced, in-depth synthesis of user experiences and perspectives on chatbot interventions. This gap in qualitative data highlights the need for more diverse research approaches in this area

Although our initial protocol included plans to search the grey literature, we ultimately decided to focus solely on peer-reviewed publications. This decision was made due to time constraints and the desire to ensure a high level of scientific rigor in our included studies. While this approach may have resulted in the exclusion of some relevant unpublished data, it allowed us to focus on evidence that has undergone rigorous peer review. We acknowledge that this departure from our original protocol may limit the comprehensiveness of our findings. Future reviews on this topic may benefit from including grey literature to capture a broader range of evidence on chatbot interventions in perinatal care.

Another limitation is the lack of data collection on the source of funding (private versus government) of the included studies. This information could provide important context for understanding the goals and focus of different interventions. For example, funding sources may influence whether an intervention targets a specific phase of the perinatal period (e.g., pregnancy) rather than the entire continuum, due to budgetary constraints or alignment with specific program goals.

In addition, our review did not include an analysis stratified by country income level. Such an analysis could have provided insights into how economic factors may influence the outcomes of maternal and child health interventions using chatbots, potentially revealing important differences or trends across economic contexts.

These limitations highlight areas for improvement in future research and reviews in this area. They underscore the need for more diverse and comprehensive studies of chatbot interventions in perinatal care, including more qualitative research, consideration of funding sources, and analysis of economic factors that may influence intervention outcomes.

*4.4. Future Research Prospects*

This systematic review highlights several key areas for future research in chatbot interventions for perinatal care. There is a notable lack of studies that include male partners and both parents in perinatal health interventions. Given the positive impact of male support on maternal and newborn health, it is crucial to develop chatbot interventions that engage fathers and assess their influence on health outcomes.

Additionally, the variability in defining the perinatal period calls for a standardized definition to enhance consistency across research. This will help clarify how different definitions affect intervention design and outcomes.

The preconception period also requires more attention, as it significantly impacts fetal development. Future studies should focus on designing chatbot interventions for this phase and exploring their long-term effects on maternal and child health.

Longitudinal research is essential to understand the sustained impacts of chatbot interventions, tracking participants from preconception through to postpartum. Finally, culturally adapting chatbot interventions for diverse populations will ensure their effectiveness across various contexts.

The chatbots included in our review are primarily second-generation systems, which predate the integration of large language models (LLMs). These earlier systems represent a significant shift from first-generation chatbots, limited to predetermined question-and-answer scripts. Second-generation chatbots incorporate more advanced rule-based logic and can simulate more dynamic interactions, but their capabilities are still constrained compared to recent LLM-powered systems. The latest generation of conversational agents powered by LLMs—such as ChatGPT—have revolutionized human–computer interactions by enabling more realistic and context-aware dialogue [49].

Therefore, our review serves as a critical baseline assessment of these second-generation chatbots, allowing for the identification of their limitations and potential. The rapid progress in perinatal care conversational agents calls for future research to evaluate the impact of advanced AI technologies on maternal and infant health outcomes. Additionally, studies should explore how LLM-powered tools affect user engagement, access to care, and digital inclusion across diverse populations, especially considering disparities in healthcare access [50–52].

## 5. Conclusions

Research on interventions using digital technologies is booming, but the use of interactive conversational agents in the perinatal period is still in its infancy, with a limited number of studies that are highly heterogeneous. Our analysis shows that digital interventions using interactive conversational agents have a positive impact on several aspects of perinatal health, including knowledge, behaviors, attitudes, and the use of health services. These interventions appear to be more effective than traditional methods, highlighting the transformative potential of chatbots in perinatal care.

As we look to the future, chatbots represent a paradigm shift in how we deliver perinatal health support. Their ability to provide personalized, accessible, and timely information has the potential to revolutionize prenatal education, increase maternal and paternal engagement in health behaviors, and ultimately improve outcomes for mothers, fathers, and infants. By providing continuous, nonjudgmental support, chatbots can address critical gaps in care, particularly in underserved areas or for sensitive topics that individuals may be reluctant to discuss with healthcare providers.

However, realizing this potential requires overcoming current challenges. Innovative strategies are needed to increase engagement, reduce attrition, and engage partners at all stages of the perinatal period. In addition, integrating behavior-change theories and techniques into chatbot design is critical to optimizing their effectiveness, particularly in preconception interventions.

As we continue to refine and expand the use of chatbots in perinatal care, we are on the cusp of a digital revolution in maternal and child health. By harnessing the power of artificial intelligence and personalized digital support, we have the opportunity to create a future where every parent and child benefits from accessible, high-quality perinatal care, ultimately leading to healthier families and communities worldwide.

**Author Contributions:** All authors have participated sufficiently in the article to take public responsibility for the content. M.-P.G. and M.S. developed the study protocol. F.B. developed the search strategy. Search terms were agreed upon by all authors of the study. S.A., S.-M.-A.-R.D., J.P., G.R., M.-P.G. and M.S. screened the articles. S.A., S.-M.-A.-R.D. and J.P. conducted data extraction and quality assessment. Conflicts were resolved by S.A. and M.-P.G. S.A. wrote the first draft of the paper.

G.R., M.-P.G., M.S., F.B., S.-M.-A.-R.D. and J.P. revised the paper. All authors have read and agreed to the published version of the manuscript.

**Funding:** This project was funded by a Research Development Grant from the Faculty of Nursing Sciences, Université Laval (project #: SAR-2022-2023).

**Institutional Review Board Statement:** Not applicable.

**Informed Consent Statement:** Not applicable.

**Data Availability Statement:** The extracted data have been transposed into the results tables and the search strategy is provided in Appendix A. The data extraction grid can be shared upon reasonable request to the corresponding author. The corresponding author can be contacted for further information.

**Acknowledgments:** We would like to thank the Faculty of Nursing Sciences (Université Laval) for their support. We would also like to thank Érika Corona, who was part of the initial project team.

**Conflicts of Interest:** The authors declare no conflicts of interest.

## Appendix A

### Databases Search Strategy

Medline (OVID)
Date of the search: 09 November 2022

| Database Limit: Limit Results to Publications Date Between 23 July 2021 and 9 November 2022 | Search Strategy | Results |
|---|---|---|
| 1 | ("chat bot?" or chatterbot? or chatbot? or medbot? or "chatter bot?" or smart bot? or smartbot?).ti,ab,kw,kf | 574 |
| 2 | (Conversational adj2 (host or coach or avatar or advisor or "Artificial Intelligence" or interface or avatar or agent? or system or computer or humanoid or character or bot? or AI)).ti,ab,kw,kf | 475 |
| 3 | ((virtual or intelligent or chat or computer or AI or "artificial intelligence" or relational or embodied) adj2 agent?).ti,ab,kw,kf | 1022 |
| 4 | ((Conversational OR Virtual OR Voice OR "Artificial Intelligence" OR Digital) adj2 assistan*).ti,ab,kw,kf | 1528 |
| 5 | 1 or 2 or 3 or 4 | 3186 |
| 6 | Exp perinatal Care/OR Perinatology/OR exp "Infant, Newborn"/ OR Pregnant Women/OR Pregnancy/OR Obstetrics/ | 1451583 |
| 7 | newborn?.ti,ab,kw,kf OR Neonat*.ti,ab,kw,kf OR Pregnan*.ti,ab,kw,kf OR Perinat*.ti,ab,kw,kf OR Matern*.ti,ab,kw,kf OR Postpartum.ti,ab,kw,kf OR Postnatal.ti,ab,kw,kf OR Childbirth?.ti,ab,kw,kf OR Obstetric?.ti,ab,kw,kf OR "post natal".ti,ab,kw,kf | 1268687 |
| 8 | 6 or 7 | 1907674 |
| 9 | 5 AND 8 | 77 |
| 10 | limit 9 to ed = 20210723-20221109 | 8 |

Embase (Embase.com)
(accessed on 09 November 2022).
Database limit: limit results to publications date between 23 July 2021 and 09 November 2022

| # | Search Strategy | Results |
| --- | --- | --- |
| 1 | ("chat bot$" OR chatterbot$ OR chatbot$ OR medbot$ OR "chatter bot$" OR "smart bot$" OR smartbot$):ti,ab,kw | 576 |
| 2 | (Conversational NEAR/2 (host OR coach OR avatar OR advisor OR "Artificial Intelligence" OR interface OR avatar OR agent$ OR system OR computer OR humanoid OR character OR bot$ OR AI)):ti,ab,kw | 419 |
| 3 | ((virtual OR intelligent OR chat OR computer OR AI OR "artificial intelligence" OR relational OR embodied) NEAR/2 agent$):ti,ab,kw | 1054 |
| 4 | ((Conversational OR Virtual OR Voice OR "Artificial Intelligence" OR Digital) NEAR/2 assistan*):ti,ab,kw | 1841 |
| 5 | #1 OR #2 OR #3 OR #4 | 3566 |
| 6 | 'perinatal care'/exp OR 'newborn'/de OR 'pregnant woman'/de OR 'obstetric procedure'/de OR 'postnatal care'/exp OR 'pregnancy'/de OR 'hildbirth'/de OR 'perinatology'/de OR 'puerperium'/de | 1,481,462 |
| 7 | newborn$:ti,ab,kw OR Neonat*:ti,ab,kw OR Pregnan*:ti,ab,kw OR Perinat*:ti,ab,kw OR Matern*:ti,ab,kw OR Postpartum:ti,ab,kw OR Postnatal:ti,ab,kw OR Childbirth$:ti,ab,kw OR Obstetric$:ti,ab,kw OR "post natal":ti,ab,kw OR puerperium:ti,ab,kw | 1,633,076 |
| 8 | #6 OR #7 | 2,168,193 |
| 9 | #5 AND #8 | 98 |
| 10 | #9 AND [23-07-2021]/sd | 16 |

CINAHL
Date of the search: 09 November 2022
Database limit: limit results to publications date between 23 July 2021 and 09 November 2022

| # | Search Strategy | Results |
| --- | --- | --- |
| 1 | TI ("chat bot?" OR chatterbot? OR chatbot? OR medbot? OR "chatter bot?" OR smart bot? OR smartbot?) OR AB ("chat bot?" OR chatterbot? OR chatbot? OR medbot? OR "chatter bot?" OR smart bot? OR smartbot?) | 306 |
| 2 | TI (Conversational N2 (host OR coach OR avatar OR advisor OR "Artificial Intelligence" OR interface OR avatar OR agent? OR system OR computer OR humanoid OR character OR bot? OR AI)) OR AB (Conversational N2 (host OR coach OR avatar OR advisor OR "Artificial Intelligence" OR interface OR avatar OR agent? OR system OR computer OR humanoid OR character OR bot? OR AI)) | 194 |
| 3 | TI ((virtual OR intelligent OR chat OR computer OR AI OR "artificial intelligence" OR relational OR embodied) N2 agent?) OR AB ((virtual OR intelligent OR chat OR computer OR AI OR "artificial intelligence" OR relational OR embodied) N2 agent?) | 306 |
| 4 | TI ((Conversational OR Virtual OR Voice OR "Artificial Intelligence" OR Digital) N2 assistan*) OR AB ((Conversational OR Virtual OR Voice OR "Artificial Intelligence" OR Digital) N2 assistan*) | 981 |

| # | Search Strategy | Results |
|---|---|---|
| 5 | S1 OR S2 OR S3 OR S4 | 1637 |
| 6 | MH "Perinatal Care" OR MH "Maternal-Child Care" OR MH Perinatology OR MH "Expectant Mothers" OR MH "Infant, Newborn+" OR MH "Postnatal Care" OR MH "Prepregnancy Care" OR MH "Obstetric Care" OR MH "Childbirth" OR MH" Postnatal Period" OR MH Puerperium OR MH Pregnancy | 367,369 |
| 7 | TI newborn# OR AB newborn# OR TI Neonat* OR AB Neonat* OR TI Pregnan* OR AB Pregnan* OR TI Perinat* OR AB Perinat* OR TI Matern* OR AB Matern* TI newborn# OR AB newborn# OR TI Neonat* OR AB Neonat* OR TI Pregnan* OR AB Pregnan* OR TI Perinat* OR AB Perinat* OR TI Matern* OR AB Matern* | 307,158 |
| 8 | S6 OR S7 | 471,873 |
| 9 | S5 AND S8 | 36 |
| 10 | S9 AND DT 20210723-20221109 | 2 |

Web of Science
Date of the search: 09 November 2022
Database limit: database limit publications date between 23 July 2021and 09 November 2022 has been applied

| # | Search Strategy | Results |
|---|---|---|
| 1 | TS = ("chat bot$" OR chatterbot$ OR chatbot$ OR medbot$ OR "chatter bot$" OR smart bot$ OR smartbot$) | 7667 |
| 2 | TS = (Conversational NEAR/2 (host OR coach OR avatar OR advisor OR "Artificial Intelligence" OR interface OR avatar OR agent$ OR system OR computer OR humanoid OR character OR bot$ OR AI)) | 940 |
| 3 | TS = ((virtual OR intelligent OR chat OR computer OR AI OR "artificial intelligence" OR relational OR embodied) NEAR/2 agent$) | 1389 |
| 4 | TS = ((Conversational OR Virtual OR Voice OR "Artificial Intelligence" OR Digital) NEAR/2 assistan*) | 949 |
| 5 | #1 OR #2 OR #3 OR #4 | 10,146 |
| 6 | TS = (newborn$ OR Neonat* OR Pregnan* OR Perinat* OR Matern* OR Postpartum OR Postnatal OR Childbirth$ OR Obstetric$ OR "post natal" OR puerperium) | 91,419 |
| 7 | #5 AND #6 | 39 |

Inspec (Engineering Village)
Date of the search: 09 November 2022
Database limit: database limit publications date between 23 July 2021 and 09 November 2022 has been applied

| # | Search Strategy | Results |
|---|---|---|
| 1 | chatbots WN CV | 527 |
| 2 | "chat bot*" WN TI OR chatterbot* WN TI OR chatbot* WN TI OR medbot* WN TI OR "chatter bot*" WN TI OR smart bot* WN TI OR smartbot* WN TI OR "chat bot*" WN AU OR chatterbot* WN AU OR chatbot* WN AU OR medbot* WN AU OR "chatter bot*" WN AU OR smart bot* WN AU OR smartbot* WN AU | 591 |

| # | Search Strategy | Results |
|---|---|---|
| 3 | (Conversational NEAR/2 host) WN TI OR (Conversational NEAR/2 coach) WN TI OR (Conversational NEAR/2 avatar) WN TI OR (Conversational NEAR/2 advisor) WN TI OR (Conversational NEAR/2 Intelligence) WN TI OR (Conversational NEAR/2 interface) WN TI OR (Conversational NEAR/2 avatar) WN TI OR (Conversational NEAR/2 agent*) WN TI OR (Conversational NEAR/2 system) WN TI OR (Conversational NEAR/2 computer) WN TI OR (Conversational NEAR/2 humanoid) WN TI OR (Conversational NEAR/2 character) WN TI OR (Conversational NEAR/2 bot*) WN TI OR (Conversational NEAR/2 AI) WN TI OR (Conversational NEAR/2 host) WN AU OR (Conversational NEAR/2 coach) WN AU OR (Conversational NEAR/2 avatar) WN AU OR (Conversational NEAR/2 advisor) WN AU OR (Conversational NEAR/2 Intelligence) WN AU OR (Conversational NEAR/2 interface) WN AU OR (Conversational NEAR/2 avatar) WN AU OR (Conversational NEAR/2 agent*) WN AU OR (Conversational NEAR/2 system) WN AU OR (Conversational NEAR/2 computer) WN AU OR (Conversational NEAR/2 humanoid) WN AU OR (Conversational NEAR/2 character) WN AU OR (Conversational NEAR/2 bot*) WN AU OR (Conversational NEAR/2 AI) WN AU | 224 |
| 4 | (virtual NEAR/2 agent) WN TI OR (intelligent NEAR/2 agent) WN TI OR (chat NEAR/2 agent) WN TI OR (computer NEAR/2 agent) WN TI OR (AI NEAR/2 agent) WN TI OR ("artificial intelligence" NEAR/2 agent) WN TI OR (relational NEAR/2 agent) WN TI OR (embodied NEAR/2 agent) WN TI OR (virtual NEAR/2 agent) WN AU OR (intelligent NEAR/2 agent) WN AU OR (chat NEAR/2 agent) WN AU OR (computer NEAR/2 agent) WN AU OR (AI NEAR/2 agent) WN AU OR ("artificial intelligence" NEAR/2 agent) WN AU OR (relational NEAR/2 agent) WN AU OR (embodied NEAR/2 agent) WN AU | 115 |
| 5 | (Conversational NEAR/2 assistan*) WN TI OR (Virtual NEAR/2 assistan*) WN TI OR (Voice NEAR/2 assistan*) WN TI OR ("Artificial Intelligence" NEAR/2 assistan*) WN TI OR (Digital NEAR/2 assistan*) WN TI OR (Conversational NEAR/2 assistan*) WN AB OR (Virtual NEAR/2 assistan*) WN TI OR (Voice NEAR/2 assistan*) WN AB OR ("Artificial Intelligence" NEAR/2 assistan*) WN AB OR (Digital NEAR/2 assistan*) WN AB | 1402 |
| 6 | #1 OR #2 OR #3 OR #4 OR #5 | 2386 |
| 7 | newborn* WN TI OR newborn* WN AB OR Neonat* WN TI OR Neonat* WN AB OR Pregnan* WN TI OR Pregnan* WN AB OR Perinat* WN TI OR Perinat* WN AB OR Matern* WN TI OR Matern* WN AB OR Postpartum WN TI OR Postpartum WN AB OR Postnatal WN TI OR Postnatal WN AB OR Childbirth* WN TI OR Childbirth* WN AB OR Obstetric* WN TI OR Obstetric* WN AB OR "post natal" WN TI OR "post natal" WN AB OR puerperium WN TI OR puerperium WN AB | 16,208 |
| 8 | #6 AND #7 | 5 |

IEEE Xplore
Date of the search: 09 November 2022
Database limit: limit results to publications date between 23 July 2021 and 09 November 2022

| # | Search Strategy | Results |
|---|---|---|
| 1 | "All Metadata":chatbot AND (Pregnant OR pregnancy OR perinatal) | 3 |

Google Scholar (https://harzing.com/resources/publish-or-perish) (accessed on 9 November 2022).
Database limits: only up to the 20 first results per string have been considered; publications between 2021 and 2022 limit has been applied; citations and patents options have been removed

| # | Search | # Results Screened |
| --- | --- | --- |
| 1 | "Conversational agent" AND (Pregnant OR pregnancy OR perinatal) | 20 |
| 2 | Conversational AND assistant AND (Pregnant OR pregnancy OR perinatal) | 20 |
| 3 | chatbot AND (Pregnant OR pregnancy OR perinatal) | 20 |
| 4 | chatbots AND (Pregnant OR pregnancy OR perinatal) | 20 |
| | Total number of results | 80 |

## References


1. Coen, S.; Banister, E. *What a Difference Sex and Gender Make: A Gender, Sex and Health Research Casebook*; CIHR Institute of Gender and Health: Canada, 2012. [CrossRef]
2. World Health Organization (WHO). Women's Health. Fact Sheets. Available online: https://www.who.int/fr/news-room/fact-sheets/detail/women-s-health (accessed on 13 February 2023).
3. Potter, R.G.; Parker, M.P. Predicting the time required to conceive. *Popul. Stud.* **1964**, *18*, 99–116. [CrossRef]
4. Gnoth, C.; Godehardt, D.; Godehardt, E.; Frank-Herrmann, P.; Freundl, G. Time to pregnancy: Results of the German prospective study and impact on the management of infertility. *Hum. Reprod.* **2003**, *18*, 1959–1966. [CrossRef] [PubMed]
5. Garcia, E.R.; Yim, I.S. A systematic review of concepts related to women's empowerment in the perinatal period and their associations with perinatal depressive symptoms and premature birth. *BMC Pregnancy Childbirth* **2017**, *17*, 347. [CrossRef] [PubMed]
6. BC Reproductive Mental Health Program; Williams, J. Best Practice Guidelines for Mental Health Disorders in the Perinatal Period. 2014. Available online: http://www.bcwomens.ca/Professional-Resources-site/Documents/Best%20Practice%20Guidelines%20for%20Mental%20Health%20Disorders%20in%20the%20Perinatal%20Period%20(2014).pdf (accessed on 15 January 2023).
7. Wallwiener, S.; Müller, M.; Doster, A.; Laserer, W.; Reck, C.; Pauluschke-Fröhlich, J.; Brucker, S.Y.; Wallwiener, C.W.; Wallwiener, M. Pregnancy eHealth and mHealth: User proportions and characteristics of pregnant women using Web-based information sources—A cross-sectional study. *Arch. Gynecol. Obstet.* **2016**, *294*, 937–944. [CrossRef]
8. Fabrizio, B.; Maria Rosaria, G.; Silvio, B.; De Elisabetta, V.; de Chiara, W.; Giuseppe La, T.; Lamberto, M.; Gabriele, M.; Tullia, T.; Maria Valeria, T.; et al. Pregnancy e-health: A multicenter Italian cross-sectional study on internet use and decision-making among pregnant women. *J. Epidemiol. Community Health* **2013**, *67*, 1013. [CrossRef]
9. Johnson, S.A. 'Intimate mothering publics': Comparing face-to-face support groups and Internet use for women seeking information and advice in the transition to first-time motherhood. *Cult. Health Sex.* **2015**, *17*, 237–251. [CrossRef]
10. Kaneho, A.E.A.; Zrira, N.; Bokonda, P.L.; Ouazzani-Touhami, K. A Survey on Existing Chatbots for Pregnant Women's Healthcare. In Proceedings of the 2022 IEEE 3rd International Conference on Electronics, Control, Optimization and Computer Science (ICECOCS), Fez, Morocco, 1–2 December 2022; pp. 1–6.
11. Aziz, A.; Zork, N.; Aubey, J.J.; Baptiste, C.D.; D'Alton, M.E.; Emeruwa, U.N.; Fuchs, K.M.; Goffman, D.; Gyamfi-Bannerman, C.; Haythe, J.H.; et al. Telehealth for High-Risk Pregnancies in the Setting of the COVID-19 Pandemic. *Am. J. Perinatol.* **2020**, *37*, 800–808. [CrossRef]
12. Stone, P.; Brooks, R.; Brynjolfsson, E.; Calo, R.; Etzioni, O.; Hager, G.; Hirschberg, J.; Kalyanakrishnan, S.; Kamar, E.; Kraus, S. Artificial intelligence and life in 2030: The one hundred year study on artificial intelligence. *arXiv* **2022**, arXiv:2211.06318.
13. McTear, M.F. Spoken dialogue technology: Enabling the conversational user interface. *ACM Comput. Surv. (CSUR)* **2002**, *34*, 90–169. [CrossRef]
14. Laranjo, L.; Dunn, A.G.; Tong, H.L.; Kocaballi, A.B.; Chen, J.; Bashir, R.; Surian, D.; Gallego, B.; Magrabi, F.; Lau, A.Y.S.; et al. Conversational agents in healthcare: A systematic review. *J. Am. Med. Inform. Assoc. JAMIA* **2018**, *25*, 1248–1258. [CrossRef]
15. Chung, K.; Cho, H.Y.; Kim, Y.R.; Jhung, K.; Koo, H.S.; Park, J.Y. Medical Help-Seeking Strategies for Perinatal Women With Obstetric and Mental Health Problems and Changes in Medical Decision Making Based on Online Health Information: Path Analysis. *J. Med. Internet Res.* **2020**, *22*, e14095. [CrossRef] [PubMed]
16. Hämeen-Anttila, K.; Jyrkkä, J.; Enlund, H.; Nordeng, H.; Lupattelli, A.; Kokki, E. Medicines information needs during pregnancy: A multinational comparison. *BMJ Open* **2013**, *3*, e002594. [CrossRef] [PubMed]
17. Hämeen-Anttila, K.; Nordeng, H.; Kokki, E.; Jyrkkä, J.; Lupattelli, A.; Vainio, K.; Enlund, H. Multiple information sources and consequences of conflicting information about medicine use during pregnancy: A multinational Internet-based survey. *J. Med. Internet Res.* **2014**, *16*, e60. [CrossRef]
18. Barreto, I.C.d.H.C.; Barros, N.B.S.; Theophilo, R.L.; Viana, V.F.; Silveira, F.R.d.V.; Souza, O.d.; Sousa, F.J.G.d.; Oliveira, A.M.B.d.; Andrade, L.O.M.d. Development and evaluation of the GISSA Mother-Baby ChatBot application in promoting child health. *Ciência Saúde Coletiva* **2021**, *26*, 1679–1690. [CrossRef]

19. Bickmore, T.; Zhang, Z.; Reichert, M.; Julce, C.; Jack, B. Promotion of preconception care among adolescents and young adults by conversational agent. *J. Adolesc. Health* **2020**, *67*, S45–S51. [CrossRef]
20. Chinkam, S.; Steer-Massaro, C.; Herbey, I.; Zhang, Z.; Bickmore, T.; Shorten, A. The Perspectives of Women and Their Health-Care Providers Regarding Using an ECA to Support Mode of Birth Decisions. *J. Perinat. Educ.* **2021**, *30*, 135–144. [CrossRef]
21. Chung, K.; Cho, H.; Park, J. A Chatbot for Perinatal Women's and Partners' Obstetric and Mental Health Care: Development and Usability Evaluation Study. *JMIR Med. Inform.* **2021**, *9*, e18607. [CrossRef]
22. Edwards, R.A.; Bickmore, T.; Jenkins, L.; Foley, M.; Manjourides, J. Use of an interactive computer agent to support breastfeeding. *Matern. Child Health J.* **2013**, *17*, 1961–1968. [CrossRef]
23. Gardiner, P.M.; McCue, K.D.; Negash, L.M.; Cheng, T.; White, L.F.; Yinusa-Nyahkoon, L.; Jack, B.W.; Bickmore, T.W. Engaging women with an embodied conversational agent to deliver mindfulness and lifestyle recommendations: A feasibility randomized control trial. *Patient Educ. Couns.* **2017**, *100*, 1720–1729. [CrossRef]
24. Gardiner, P.; Bickmore, T.; Yinusa-Nyahkoon, L.; Reichert, M.; Julce, C.; Sidduri, N.; Martin-Howard, J.; Woodhams, E.; Aryan, J.; Zhang, Z. Using health information technology to engage African American women on nutrition and supplement use during the preconception period. *Front. Endocrinol.* **2021**, *11*, 571705. [CrossRef]
25. Jack, B.; Bickmore, T.; Hempstead, M.; Yinusa-Nyahkoon, L.; Sadikova, E.; Mitchell, S.; Gardiner, P.; Adigun, F.; Penti, B.; Schulman, D.; et al. Reducing Preconception Risks Among African American Women with Conversational Agent Technology. *J. Am. Board Fam. Med.* **2015**, *28*, 441–451. [CrossRef]
26. Jack, B.W.; Bickmore, T.; Yinusa-Nyahkoon, L.; Reichert, M.; Julce, C.; Sidduri, N.; Martin-Howard, J.; Zhang, Z.; Woodhams, E.; Fernandez, J. Improving the health of young African American women in the preconception period using health information technology: A randomised controlled trial. *Lancet Digit. Health* **2020**, *2*, e475–e485. [CrossRef]
27. Maeda, E.; Miyata, A.; Boivin, J.; Nomura, K.; Kumazawa, Y.; Shirasawa, H.; Saito, H.; Terada, Y. Promoting fertility awareness and preconception health using a chatbot: A randomized controlled trial. *Reprod. Biomed. Online* **2020**, *41*, 1133–1143. [CrossRef] [PubMed]
28. Montenegro, J.L.Z.; da Costa, C.A.; Janssen, L.P. Evaluating the use of chatbot during pregnancy: A usability study. *Healthc. Anal.* **2022**, *2*, 100072. [CrossRef]
29. Wong, J.; Foussat, A.C.; Ting, S.; Acerbi, E.; van Elburg, R.M.; Chien, C.M. A chatbot to engage parents of preterm and term infants on parental stress, parental sleep, and infant feeding: Usability and feasibility study. *JMIR Pediatr. Parent.* **2021**, *4*, e30169. [CrossRef] [PubMed]
30. Moher, D.; Shamseer, L.; Clarke, M.; Ghersi, D.; Liberati, A.; Petticrew, M.; Shekelle, P.; Stewart, L.A.; Group, P.-P. Preferred reporting items for systematic review and meta-analysis protocols (PRISMA-P) 2015 statement. *Syst. Rev.* **2015**, *4*, 1. [CrossRef] [PubMed]
31. Hong, Q.N.; Fàbregues, S.; Bartlett, G.; Boardman, F.; Cargo, M.; Dagenais, P.; Gagnon, M.-P.; Griffiths, F.; Nicolau, B.; O'Cathain, A.; et al. The Mixed Methods Appraisal Tool (MMAT) version 2018 for information professionals and researchers. *Educ. Inf.* **2018**, *34*, 285–291. [CrossRef]
32. Page, M.J.; McKenzie, J.E.; Bossuyt, P.M.; Boutron, I.; Hoffmann, T.C.; Mulrow, C.D.; Shamseer, L.; Tetzlaff, J.M.; Akl, E.A.; Brennan, S.E.; et al. The PRISMA 2020 statement: An updated guideline for reporting systematic reviews. *Syst. Rev.* **2021**, *10*, 89. [CrossRef]
33. Nguyen, Q.C.; Aparicio, E.M.; Jasczynski, M.; Doig, A.C.; Yue, X.; Mane, H.; Srikanth, N.; Gutierrez, F.X.M.; Delcid, N.; He, X. Rosie, a Health Education Question-and-Answer Chatbot for New Mothers: Randomized Pilot Study. *JMIR Form. Res.* **2024**, *8*, e51361. [CrossRef]
34. Suharwardy, S.; Ramachandran, M.; Leonard, S.A.; Gunaseelan, A.; Lyell, D.J.; Darcy, A.; Robinson, A.; Judy, A. Feasibility and impact of a mental health chatbot on postpartum mental health: A randomized controlled trial. *AJOG Glob. Rep.* **2023**, *3*, 100165. [CrossRef]
35. Hussain, T.; Smith, P.; Yee, L.M. Mobile Phone–Based Behavioral Interventions in Pregnancy to Promote Maternal and Fetal Health in High-Income Countries: Systematic Review. *JMIR Mhealth Uhealth* **2020**, *8*, e15111. [CrossRef] [PubMed]
36. Koulouri, T.; Macredie, R.D.; Olakitan, D. Chatbots to Support Young Adults' Mental Health: An Exploratory Study of Acceptability. *ACM Trans. Interact. Intell. Syst.* **2022**, *12*, 11. [CrossRef]
37. Cheah, M.H.; Gan, Y.N.; Altice, F.L.; Wickersham, J.A.; Shrestha, R.; Salleh, N.A.M.; Ng, K.S.; Azwa, I.; Balakrishnan, V.; Kamarulzaman, A.; et al. Testing the Feasibility and Acceptability of Using an Artificial Intelligence Chatbot to Promote HIV Testing and Pre-Exposure Prophylaxis in Malaysia: Mixed Methods Study. *JMIR Hum. Factors* **2024**, *11*, e52055. [CrossRef] [PubMed]
38. El Ayadi, A.M.; Singh, P.; Duggal, M.; Kumar, V.; Kaur, J.; Sharma, P.; Vosburg, K.B.; Diamond-Smith, N.G. Feasibility and acceptability of Saheli, a WhatsApp Chatbot, on COVID-19 vaccination among pregnant and breastfeeding women in rural North India. *BMJ Innov.* **2023**, *9*, 195. [CrossRef]

39. Martínez-Borba, V.; Suso-Ribera, C.; Osma, J. Usability, acceptability, and feasibility of two technology-based devices for mental health screening in perinatal care: A Comparison of web versus app. In *Pervasive Computing Paradigms for Mental Health: 9th International Conference, MindCare 2019, Buenos Aires, Argentina, April 23–24, 2019, Proceedings 9*; Springer: Cham, Switzerland, 2019.
40. Chae, J.; Kim, H.K. Internet-based prenatal interventions for maternal health among pregnant women: A systematic review and meta-analysis. *Child. Youth Serv. Rev.* **2021**, *127*, 106079. [CrossRef]
41. Kim, H.K. The Effects of Artificial Intelligence Chatbots on Women's Health: A Systematic Review and Meta-Analysis. *Healthcare* **2024**, *12*, 534. [CrossRef]
42. Davis, J.A.; Ohan, J.L.; Gregory, S.; Kottampally, K.; Silva, D.; Prescott, S.L.; Finlay-Jones, A.L. Perinatal Women's Perspectives of, and Engagement in, Digital Emotional Well-Being Training: Mixed Methods Study. *J. Med. Internet Res.* **2023**, *25*, e46852. [CrossRef]
43. Inkster, B.; Kadaba, M.; Subramanian, V. Understanding the impact of an AI-enabled conversational agent mobile app on users' mental health and wellbeing with a self-reported maternal event: A mixed method real-world data mHealth study. *Front. Glob. Women's Health* **2023**, *4*, 1084302. [CrossRef]
44. Sagstad, M.H.; Morken, N.-H.; Lund, A.; Dingsør, L.J.; Nilsen, A.B.V.; Sorbye, L.M. Quantitative User Data From a Chatbot Developed for Women With Gestational Diabetes Mellitus: Observational Study. *JMIR Form. Res.* **2022**, *6*, e28091. [CrossRef]
45. Shaw, J.; Abejirinde, I.-O.O.; Agarwal, P.; Shahid, S.; Martin, D. Digital health and equitable access to care. *PLoS Digit. Health* **2024**, *3*, e0000573. [CrossRef]
46. Badr, J.; Motulsky, A.; Denis, J.-L. Digital health technologies and inequalities: A scoping review of potential impacts and policy recommendations. *Health Policy* **2024**, *146*, 105122. [CrossRef] [PubMed]
47. Reddy, P.; Sharma, B.; Chaudhary, K. Digital literacy: A review of literature. *Int. J. Technoethics (IJT)* **2020**, *11*, 65–94. [CrossRef]
48. Robinson, L.; Cotten, S.R.; Ono, H.; Quan-Haase, A.; Mesch, G.; Chen, W.; Schulz, J.; Hale, T.M.; Stern, M.J. Digital inequalities and why they matter. *Inf. Commun. Soc.* **2015**, *18*, 569–582. [CrossRef]
49. Singh, S.U.; Namin, A.S. A survey on chatbots and large language models: Testing and evaluation techniques. *Nat. Lang. Process. J.* **2025**, *10*, 100128. [CrossRef]
50. Bachmann, M.; Duta, I.; Mazey, E.; Cooke, W.; Vatish, M.; Davis Jones, G. Exploring the capabilities of ChatGPT in women's health: Obstetrics and gynaecology. *npj Womens Health* **2024**, *2*, 26. [CrossRef]
51. Mennickent, D.; Rodríguez, A.; Opazo, M.C.; Riedel, C.A.; Castro, E.; Eriz-Salinas, A.; Appel-Rubio, J.; Aguayo, C.; Damiano, A.E.; Guzmán-Gutiérrez, E.; et al. Machine learning applied in maternal and fetal health: A narrative review focused on pregnancy diseases and complications. *Front. Endocrinol.* **2023**, *14*, 1130139. [CrossRef]
52. Kwok, W.H.; Zhang, Y.; Wang, G. Artificial intelligence in perinatal mental health research: A scoping review. *Comput. Biol. Med.* **2024**, 108685. [CrossRef]

healthcare MDPI

*Systematic Review*

# Effects of Digital Psychotherapy on Suicide: A Systematic Review and Meta-Analysis

**Jinseok Oh, Jonggab Ho, Sanghee Lee and Jin-Hyuck Park ***

Special Child Education Research Institute, University of Soonchunhyang, Asan 31538, Republic of Korea; oh486255@naver.com (J.O.); hodori1988@sch.ac.kr (J.H.); sanglh@sch.ac.kr (S.L.)
* Correspondence: roophy@naver.com

**Abstract:** Previous studies reported that digital psychotherapy was a clinically beneficial intervention for suicide ideation. However, the effects of digital psychotherapy on other aspects of suicide beyond ideation remain unclear. Therefore, this study investigated the effects of digital psychotherapy on suicide and depression. Articles were identified by searching Cochrane, Google Scholar, Medline, PubMed, Web of Science, and PsycINFO in line with the PRISMA statement, yielding nine randomized controlled trials. The difference between conditions regarding suicide and depression in the effect size of the individual article was calculated using Hedges' $g$. Most digital psychotherapy interventions were based on cognitive behavioral therapy and delivered via apps or the web for at least six weeks. Suicide outcomes primarily focused on suicide ideation. The findings showed digital psychotherapy achieved a significantly larger effect size for suicide ($g = 0.488$, $p < 0.001$) and depression ($g = 0.316$, $p < 0.001$), compared to controls. Specifically, digital psychotherapy showed a significant effect on both suicide ideation ($g = 0.478$, $p < 0.001$) and other suicidal variables ($g = 0.330$, $p < 0.001$). These results suggest the effectiveness of digital psychotherapy in reducing suicide and depression compared to traditional face-to-face therapy. Future research should consider a wider range of outcomes and examine the long-term effectiveness of digital psychotherapy to better understand its effects on suicide prevention.

**Keywords:** suicide; psychotherapy; digital psychotherapy; depression; meta-analysis

## 1. Introduction

Suicide is the most severe consequence of mental health issues, impacting not only individuals but also their families and friends, both directly and indirectly [1]. According to the World Health Organization's 2019 Suicide Worldwide data, over 700,000 people die by suicide annually, highlighting troubling increases in global suicide rates [2]. These statistics underscore the urgent need for enhanced mental health care to prevent suicide.

Notably, the COVID-19 pandemic has further exacerbated the global demand for mental health care. However, the existing supply of mental health services has struggled to meet this increased demand, prompting many individuals to seek alternative solutions, such as digital mental health services. Advances in information and communication technology have driven the growth of the digital health market, offering new avenues for mental health care [3,4]. Digital mental health services encompass a wide range of offerings, including suicide prevention, mental health promotion, and treatment for drug and alcohol addiction, all delivered through digital platforms such as websites and mobile applications [4].

Digital mental health services offer several advantages: they are not limited by geographic location and can make mental health knowledge more accessible, thereby reducing barriers to care and encouraging wider uptake [4,5]. Consequently, digital psychotherapy has been increasingly applied to various clinical populations with mental health issues. Specifically, digital psychotherapy has proven beneficial for suicide prevention, particularly for individuals with suicidal ideation, for whom face-to-face treatment may pose significant barriers [6].

A prior meta-analysis on digital psychotherapy for suicide prevention included 16 randomized controlled trials to evaluate its efficacy [7]. Among these, 10 studies focused directly on suicide, while six addressed depressive symptoms. The interventions, primarily based on cognitive behavioral therapy or dialectical therapy, were delivered via web or mobile applications. The number of sessions ranged from 4 to more than 10, with the main outcome measures including suicidal ideation and depression. The findings indicated that digital psychotherapy significantly reduced both suicidal ideation and depression compared to waitlist or placebo control groups. Another recent meta-analysis reviewed nine randomized controlled trials of digital psychotherapy for suicide prevention [1]. Of these, three trials were guided by clinical teams and six were self-guided, all utilizing cognitive behavioral therapy. The interventions were delivered via web or mobile applications, with sessions ranging from 2 to 10. The main outcome measures included depression, anxiety, and hopelessness. The findings demonstrated that digital psychotherapy significantly outperformed waitlist or conventional care control groups in reducing depression. Taken together, these studies suggest that digital psychotherapy could be effective in preventing suicide and improving mental health.

However, previous meta-analyses have primarily focused on suicidal ideation and depression, overlooking other critical suicidal variables such as suicide risk, behavior, or severity [1,7]. In the process leading to suicide, not only suicide ideation but also suicide planning and execution are important. Consequently, it is crucial to investigate other suicidal variables alongside suicide ideation. Therefore, this study aimed to conduct a systematic review and meta-analysis of randomized controlled trials to investigate the effects of digital psychotherapy on a broader range of suicidal variables.

## 2. Materials and Methods

This systematic review and meta-analysis followed the Preferred Reporting Items for Systematic Reviews and Meta-Analyses Statement (PRISMA).

### 2.1. Search Strategy

A literature search was completed in April 2024. This search focused on articles published from 2014 to 10 April 2024 to exclude outdated methods. Six databases were searched (Cochrane, Google Scholar, Medline, PubMed, Web of Science, and PsycINFO) in accordance with a previous meta-analysis [7]. The search terms were "suicide" or "suicidal" or "self-injurious behavior" and "psychotherapy" or "therapy" and "web" or "internet" or "online" or "mobile" or "smartphone" or "phone" or "app" or "mhealth" and "randomise*" or "randomize*". This study was registered with PROSPERO (ID: CRD42024537058)

### 2.2. Eligibility Criteria

The eligibility criteria for this study were as follows:

1. Study design: randomized controlled trials (RCTs).
2. Population: no restrictions were placed on population.
3. Intervention: (a) interventions related to suicide prevention; (b) interventions that were digitally delivered (web or app); (c) interventions that delivered theory-based therapeutic content (e.g., cognitive behavioral therapy or dialectical behavioral therapy); (d) interventions that were directed toward subjects.
4. Control: controls received treatment-as-usual or minimal attention (e.g., psychoeducation) or were on a waitlist.
5. Outcomes: (a) primary outcomes were pre- and post-test measures of suicidal thoughts and behaviors, and (b) secondary outcomes included the symptoms of depression.
6. Language: studies written in English or Korean.
7. Full-text articles.

### 2.3. Article Selection

The article search and selection processes reviewed the titles and abstracts of the searched articles following a database search. Then two independent authors finalized the article selection based on the eligibility criteria. Disagreements between the authors were resolved through consultation with a third author.

### 2.4. Risk of Bias and Methodological Quality

To investigate the risk of bias in the selected studies, the Risk of Bias Assessment tool for randomized trials with the Review Manager (RevMan) program (version 5.4.1, The Cochrane Collaboration, 2020) was utilized. The risk of bias was determined by selection bias, allocation, detection bias, performance bias, attrition bias, and reporting bias. Three levels of bias (low, unclear, and high) were assigned. The methodological quality of the selected studies was assessed by the PEDro scale. Two authors independently assessed the risk of bias and methodological quality, resolving discrepancies through discussion with a third author.

### 2.5. Data Extraction and Statistical Analysis

Data extraction from the selected studies was performed by two independent authors. Extracted data included: population characteristics, features of digital psychotherapy, control conditions, and primary and secondary outcomes. All data were coded using means, standard deviations, *p*-values, and t-values for both experimental and control groups at pre-test and post-test.

Statistical analysis was conducted using Comprehensive Meta-Analysis 2.0 (Biostat, Englewood, NJ, USA). Heterogeneity was considered acceptable when $I^2 < 50\%$. For $I^2$ values less than 50%, a fixed-effects model was used. Pooled effect sizes were analyzed using Hedges' g with 95% confidence intervals (CI). Hedges' $g$ adjusts for intervention differences between experimental and control groups (where Hedges' $g < 0.3$ indicates a small effect, $0.3 \leq g < 0.6$ indicates a moderate effect size, and $g \geq 0.6$ indicates a large effect size). Mean, standard deviation, and sample size were utilized for result calculations and analyses.

The pooled effect sizes and directions of the selected articles were visually represented using a forest plot. Statistical heterogeneity was assessed by $I^2$. Egger's regression test was employed to evaluate publication bias, with a *p*-value above 0.05 indicating no publication bias [8]. Sensitivity analysis, conducted through Hedges' $g$, verified the robustness of results across varying conditions, excluding studies with outlier results.

## 3. Results

### 3.1. Study Selection

A total of 394 studies were identified in the initial literature review. Among them, 256 duplicate articles were excluded. The titles and abstracts of the remaining 138 articles were reviewed for preliminary screening. Out of these, nine articles that met the inclusion criteria were finally selected (Figure 1).

### 3.2. Characteristics of the Included Studies

A total of 1779 subjects were included (intervention: n = 887, mean group size: n = 98.5, control: n = 892, mean group size: n = 99.1), with ages ranging from 14.8 to 47.46 years (Table 1). The subjects in the included studies were adolescents, adults, or veterans with suicide ideation in the past month. The educational levels of the subjects were not reported uniformly, leading to disparities in reporting.

Most interventions in the study utilized cognitive behavioral therapy (CBT), dialectical behavioral therapy (DBT), or a combination of treatments. Specifically, there were eight CBT-based interventions: Frame-IT program, ibobly program, LEAP, Virtual Hope Box (VHB), LifeApp'tite, Think Life, Online Self-Help for Suicidal Thought, and Living with Deadly Thought (LwDT). Additionally, two interventions were DBT-based: iDBT-ST and

LwDT (Living with Deadly Thought) combined with CBT. Regarding delivery methods, the majority of interventions (66.7%) were web-based, while three were app-based. This indicates a preference for web-based programs over app-based ones in the studies.

The intervention periods ranged mostly from at least 6 weeks to 12 weeks, with some studies extending up to 4 months. Various assessment tools were used to evaluate suicide and depression outcomes, including the Beck Scale for Suicide Ideation (BSS), Suicidal Ideation Attributes Scale (SIDAS), Suicidal Ideation Questionnaire (SIQ), Depressive Symptom Inventory-Suicidality Subscale (DIS-SS), Suicide Status Form (SSF), Columbia Suicide Severity Rating Scale (C-SSRS), and Scale for Suicidal Ideation (SSI). The majority of studies focused on assessing suicide ideation, with eight out of nine studies using these measures. Only one study each utilized assessments for evaluating suicide risk (SSF) and suicide severity and suicide behavior (C-SSRS).

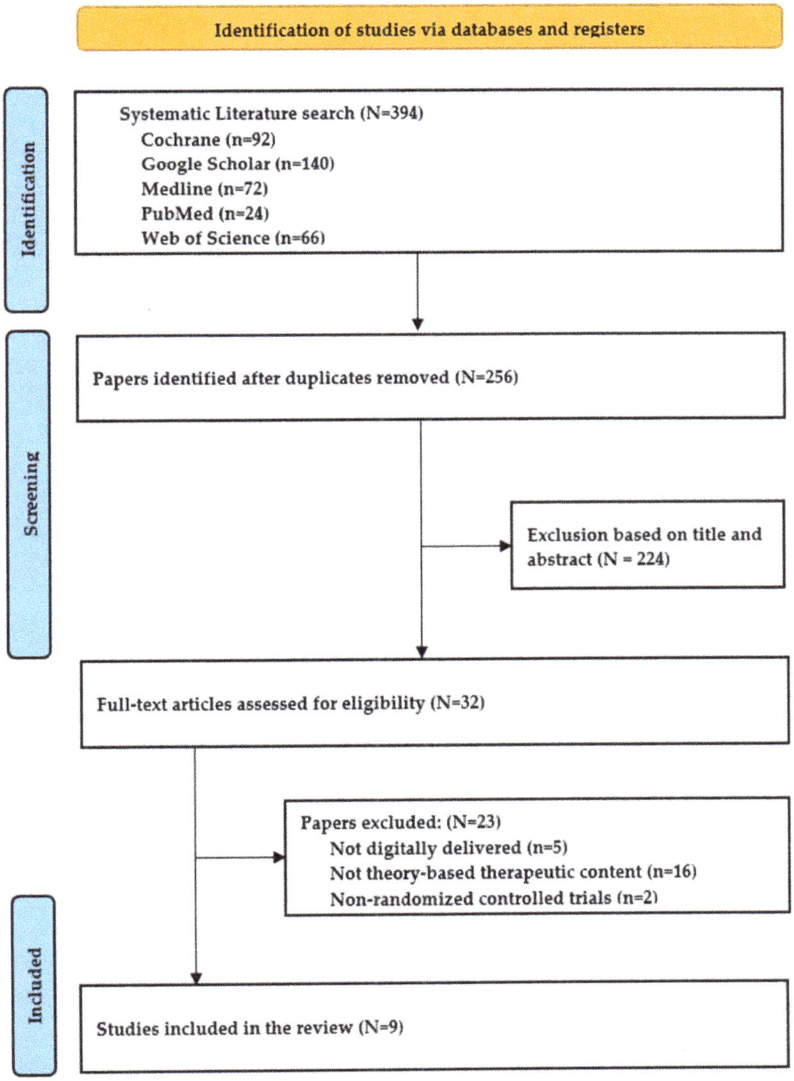


**Figure 1.** PRISMA Flow chart of the study selection process.

**Table 1.** Characteristics of studies included in meta-analysis.

| Reference | Study Design | Participants | Intervention | Duration | Outcomes | PEDro-Scale |
|---|---|---|---|---|---|---|
| Denneson et al., 2019 [9] | RCT | Veterans N = 117 (EG = 58, CG = 59) | App-based CBT Virtual Hope Box(VHB) | 12 weeks | (Suicide) BSS | 7 |
| De Jaegere et al., 2019 [10] | RCT | Adults N = 724 (EG = 365, CG = 359) | Web-based CBT, DBT, and Mindfulness Think Life | 12 weeks | (Suicide) BSS/SIDAS (Depression) BDI-II | 6 |
| Hill & Pettit 2019 [11] | RCT | Adolescents N = 80 (EG = 31, CG = 30) | Web-based CBT LEAP | 6 weeks | (Suicide) BSS (Depression) RADS-2 | 7 |
| O'Toole, Arendt, and Pedersen, 2019 [12] | RCT | Adults N = 129 (EG = 60, CG = 69) | App-based CBT LifeApp'tite | 4 months | (Suicide) SSF (Depression) MDI | 7 |
| Van Spijker et al., 2018. [13] | RCT | Adults N = 323 (EG = 160, CG = 163) | Web-based CBT, DBT, and Mindfulness LwDT | 6 weeks | (Suicide) C-SSRS/SIDAS (Depression) CES-D | 9 |
| Wilks et al., 2018 [14] | RCT | Adults N = 59 (EG = 30, CG = 29) | Web-based DBT Idbt-ST | 8 weeks | (Suicide) SSI | 7 |
| Hetrick et al., 2017 [15] | RCT | Adolescents N = 50 (EG = 26, CG = 24) | Web-based CBT Reframe-IT | 10 weeks | (Suicide) SIQ (Depression) RADS-2/CDRS-R | 8 |
| Tighe et al., 2017 [16] | RCT | Youth N = 62 (EG = 31, CG = 30) | App-based CBT ibobbly | 6 weeks | (Suicide) DIS-SS (Depression) PHQ-9 | 6 |
| Van Spijke, Straten, & Kerkhof, 2014 [17] | RCT | Adults N = 236 (EG = 116, CG = 120) | Web-based CBT, DBT, and Mindfulness Online Self-Help for Suicidal Thoughts | 18 weeks | (Suicide) BSS (Depression) BDI-II | 7 |

Note: EG = experiment group; CG = control group; CBT = cognitive behavior therapy; DBT = dialectical behavior therapy; BSS = Beck Scale for Suicide Ideation; RADS-2 = Reynolds Adolescent Depression Scale-2; SIDAS = Suicidal Ideation Attributes Scale; BDI-II = Beck Depression Inventory-second edition; SSF = Suicide Status Form; MDI = Major Depression Inventory; C-SSRS = Columbia Suicide Severity Rating Scale; CES-D = Centre for Epidemiological Studies Depression Scale; SSI = Scale for Suicidal Ideation; SIQ = Suicidal Ideation Questionnaire; CDRS-R = Children Depression Rating Scale Revised; DSI-SS = Depressive Symptom Inventory-Suicidality Subscale; PHQ-9 = Patient Health Questionnaire.

For depression assessment, tools such as the Children Depression Rating Scale Revised (CDRS-R), Reynolds Adolescent Depression Scale-2 (RADS-2), Patient Health Questionnaire-9 (PHQ-9), Major Depression Inventory (MDI), and Beck Depression Inventory (BDI) were employed.

The mean PEDro score was 7.1 out of 10, with all nine studies rated low for random sequence generation and incomplete outcome data (Figure 2). However, most of the included studies showed unclear or high risk in blinding of participants and personnel, blinding of outcome assessment, and selective reporting (Figure 2).

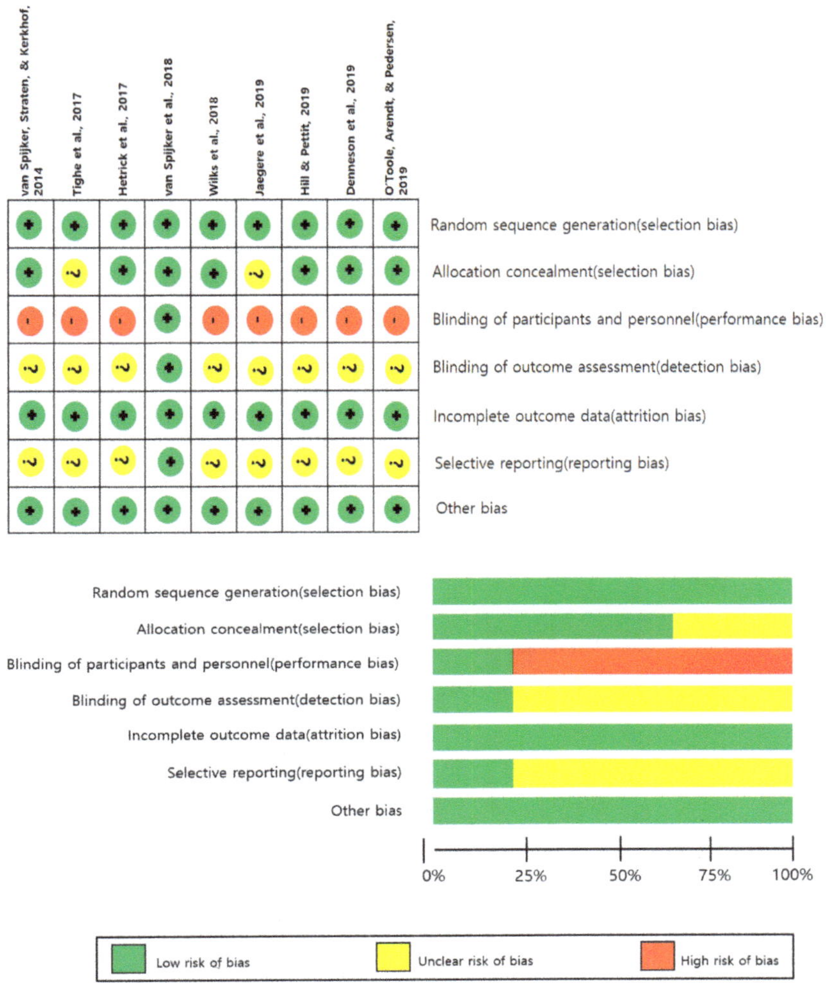


**Figure 2.** Summary of the risk of bias in the included studies in this meta-analysis. Overall, the risk of bias in the included studies is low. Green with plus mark indicates a low risk of bias, yellow with question mark indicates unclear bias, and red with minus mark indicates a high risk of bias. Van Spijker et al. (2014) [17]; Tighe et al. (2017) [16]; Hetrick et al. (2017) [15]; Van Spijker et al. (2018) [13]; Wilks et al. (2018) [14]; De Jaegere (2019) [10]; Hill et al. (2019) [11]; Denneson et al. (2019) [9]; O'Toole et al. (2019) [12].

### 3.3. *Effect Size of Digital Psychotherapy*

#### 3.3.1. Effect on Suicide

The analysis revealed significant heterogeneity across the included studies regarding the effect of digital psychotherapy on suicide ($I^2 = 88.73\%$, $p < 0.001$). Therefore, a random-effects model was used to determine effect sizes. The pooled effect size was found to be moderate and statistically significant (k = 11, $g = 0.488$, 95% CI = 0.224–0.752, $p < 0.001$) when compared to control groups (Table 2). Additionally, Egger's test indicated no significant publication bias (Egger's intercept = 1.40, $p = 0.52$).

**Table 2.** The summary of the pooled effect size on outcomes.

| | Overall Suicide | Suicide Ideation | Other Suicidal Variables | Depression |
|---|---|---|---|---|
| Hedge's *g* (95% CI) | 0.488 *** (0.224–0.752) | 0.478 *** (0.379–0.578) | 0.330 *** (0.182–0.477) | 0.316 *** (0.207–0.426) |
| $I^2$ | 88.73% | 88.02% | 92.90% | 12.64% |
| Egger's intercept | 1.40 | 0.81 | 6.01 | −0.06 |

Note: *** $p < 0.001$; CI = confidence interval.

Sub-group analyses were conducted for each pooled effect size, distinguishing between suicide ideation and other suicidal variables. Significant heterogeneity was observed across the sub-grouped studies (suicide ideation: $I^2 = 88.02\%$, $p < 0.001$; other suicidal variables: $I^2 = 92.90\%$, $p < 0.001$). A random-effects model revealed that the pooled effect size on suicide ideation (k = 8, $g = 0.478$, 95% CI = 0.379–0.578, $p < 0.01$) and other suicidal variables (k = 2, $g = 0.330$, 95% CI = 0.182–0.477, $p < 0.001$) was moderate and statistically significant (Figure 3). Additionally, Egger's test indicated no significant publication bias (suicide ideation: Egger's intercept = 0.81, $p = 0.73$; other suicidal variables: Egger's intercept = 6.01, $p = 0.65$).

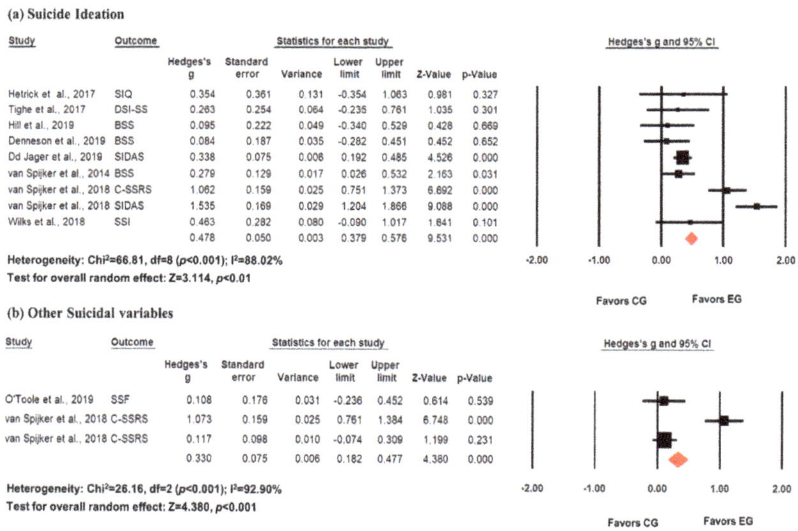


**Figure 3.** Forest plot for a meta-analysis of the effect of digital psychotherapy on (**a**) suicide and (**b**) other suicidal variables (suicide behavior, risk, and severity). The pooled effect size of digital psychotherapy on suicide and other suicidal variables was moderate and statistically significant. Van Spijker et al. (2018) [13]; Van Spijker et al. (2014) [17]; Tighe et al. (2017) [16]; De Jaegere (2019) [10]; Hetrick et al. (2017) [15]; Hill et al. (2019) [11]; Wilks et al. (2018) [14]; Denneson et al. (2019) [9]; O'Toole et al. (2019) [12].

### 3.3.2. Effect on Depression

Regarding the effect of digital psychotherapy on depression, the included studies showed no significant heterogeneity ($I^2 = 12.64\%$, $p = 0.333$). Therefore, a fixed-effect model was utilized. The pooled effect size was moderate and statistically significant (k = 6, $g = 0.316$, 95% CI = 0.207–0.426, $p < 0.001$) compared to control groups (Figure 4, Table 2). Egger's test also indicated no significant publication bias (Egger's intercept = −0.06, $p = 0.94$).

| Study | Outcome | Statistics for each study | | | | | | |
|---|---|---|---|---|---|---|---|---|
| | | Hedges's g | Standard error | Variance | Lower limit | Upper limit | Z-Value | p-Value |
| Hetrick et al., 2017 | CDRS | 0.438 | 0.363 | 0.132 | -0.273 | 1.149 | 1.206 | 0.228 |
| Hetrick et al., 2017 | RADS | 0.449 | 0.363 | 0.132 | -0.263 | 1.161 | 1.237 | 0.216 |
| Tighe et al., 2017 | PHQ-9 | 0.725 | 0.261 | 0.068 | 0.213 | 1.237 | 2.774 | 0.006 |
| Hill et al., 2019 | RADS | 0.095 | 0.222 | 0.049 | -0.340 | 0.529 | 0.427 | 0.669 |
| O'Toole et al., 2019 | MDI | 0.068 | 0.176 | 0.031 | -0.276 | 0.412 | 0.386 | 0.699 |
| Dd Jager et al., 2019 | BDI | 0.375 | 0.075 | 0.006 | 0.228 | 0.522 | 5.004 | 0.000 |
| van Spijker et al., 2014 | BDI | 0.219 | 0.129 | 0.017 | -0.034 | 0.472 | 1.700 | 0.089 |
| | | 0.316 | 0.056 | 0.003 | 0.207 | 0.426 | 5.663 | 0.000 |

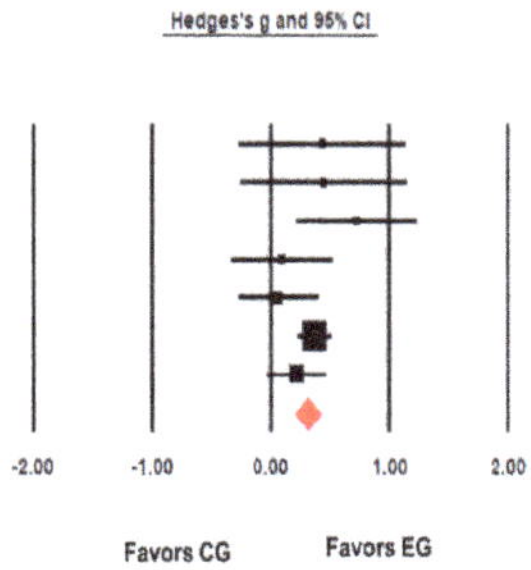


Heterogeneity: $Chi^2=6.868$, $df=6$ ($p=.333$); $I^2=12.64\%$

Test for overall fixed effect: $Z=5.663$, $p<0.001$

**Figure 4.** Forest plot for meta-analysis of the effect of digital psychotherapy on depression. The pooled effect size of digital psychotherapy on depression was moderate and statistically significant. Van Spijker et al. (2014) [17]; Tighe et al. (2017) [16]; De Jaegere (2019) [10]; Hetrick et al. (2017) [15]; Hill et al. (2019) [11]; O'Toole et al. (2019) [12].

## 4. Discussion

### 4.1. Overall Results

This study is a systematic review and meta-analysis investigating the effects of digital psychotherapy on suicide and depression. The findings indicate that digital psychotherapy was more effective than control conditions in preventing suicide and alleviating depression. The effect sizes ranged from small to moderate with statistical significance, which is consistent with findings from previous systematic reviews and meta-analyses [1,18,19].

### 4.2. Characteristics of Digital Psychotherapy

The digital psychotherapy utilized in the included studies primarily employed CBT, a widely recognized intervention for addressing suicide-related behaviors in young individuals. CBT for suicide prevention targets suicidal thoughts and behaviors through several core modules [1,2]. Firstly, it includes strategies for developing skills to identify and distance oneself from thoughts, feelings, and behaviors associated with suicide. Secondly, it focuses on managing emotions and behaviors using relaxation techniques. Thirdly, it emphasizes problem-solving and cognitive restructuring. Previous research has consistently shown that CBT, particularly when tailored for suicide prevention, effectively reduces suicidal thoughts, decreases the frequency of suicide attempts, alleviates symptoms of depression, hopelessness, and anxiety, and enhances problem-solving skills, which aligns with the findings of our study [1–4]. In addition to CBT, DBT was utilized in four of the included studies. DBT is another well-established intervention for treating adolescent depression and is specifically designed for high-risk groups prone to suicide, characterized by emotional dysregulation and behavioral dysfunction [20]. Studies applying DBT have demonstrated its effectiveness in reducing behaviors associated with emotional dysregulation [20,21], which is consistent with our study's findings. Previous meta-analyses suggest that DBT may have greater efficacy than CBT in some contexts of suicide prevention. Furthermore, acceptance and commitment therapy, therapeutic evaluative conditioning, and mixed-component approaches have also shown effectiveness in addressing suicide-related issues [18]. In our study, three of the included studies incorporated these alternative approaches alongside CBT, highlighting the need to further explore their efficacy. However, due to the limited number of studies applying these treatments in a manner conducive to comparison with CBT, our analysis did not permit a definitive assessment of their relative effectiveness.

### 4.3. Suicide and Depression Outcomes

To evaluate the effects of digital psychotherapy, the studies included assessments for suicidal variables and depression. Most assessments focused heavily on suicide ideation, indicating that digital psychotherapy primarily targeted reducing suicidal thoughts. Only a few studies included assessments of suicide risk and severity, suggesting that digital psychotherapy addressed more than just ideation. Additionally, we observed differences in how depression assessments were utilized compared to assessments for suicidal variables.

### 4.4. Effectiveness of Digital Psychotherapy

Previous studies have shown that transitioning face-to-face treatment to a digital format positively impacts the reduction of suicidal ideation and depression. as well as lowering suicide risk and improving overall mental health [18]. In another meta-analysis, the effectiveness of digital psychotherapy was assessed by distinguishing between studies that directly targeted suicide prevention and those that indirectly addressed suicide-related factors. The findings indicated that direct interventions for suicide-related issues were more effective in reducing suicidal ideation [7]. Consistent with our findings, previous meta-analyses consistently demonstrate that digital psychotherapy effectively prevents suicide and reduces depression, particularly when directly targeting suicide prevention [7,18].

### 4.5. Comparison with Previous Literature

Unfortunately, previous meta-analyses have only focused on the effect of digital psychotherapy on suicide ideation, without encompassing other aspects of suicide risk or severity. Indeed, most previous studies did not consider suicidal severity, possibly due to the perception that digital psychotherapy can only be applied to individuals with low suicidal severity [21]. In contrast, the significance of this study lies in its analysis of the effects of digital psychotherapy by including not only suicidal ideation but also suicide risk and severity as outcomes. Suicidal ideation is crucially important in predicting suicide. However, in the progression from suicidal ideation to actual suicide planning and execution, there are also various factors related to suicidal risk and severity [10,16,17]. Therefore, to effectively prevent suicide, it is essential to consider not only suicidal ideation but also diverse variables like suicidal risk and severity, comprehensively examining the entire process of suicide. Our study uniquely addresses this gap by holistically analyzing the entire spectrum of suicide, thus providing a more nuanced understanding of the potential of digital psychotherapy in suicide prevention.

### 4.6. Significance of Digital Platform

In this study, digital psychotherapy was delivered via a web- or app-based program, which is more accessible compared to traditional face-to-face approaches. Digital psychotherapy reduces social stigma and has been found effective in treating depression and anxiety in adolescents, offering a cost-effective approach [22]. Furthermore, the internet is easily accessible to individuals experiencing suicidal thoughts and holds the potential to prevent these thoughts from escalating into suicidal behavior or suicide attempts [23]. Therefore, in settings where face-to-face psychotherapy is limited, digital psychotherapy could be an alternative. Specifically, web-based digital psychotherapy is cost-effective and ensures anonymity and confidentiality. Additionally, compared to face-to-face approaches, web-based digital psychotherapy could offer the advantage of providing service by periodically checking client information in addition to real-time services [10,11,14,15,17]. On the other hand, app-based programs follow a similar approach to web-based programs but offer the added benefit of being more accessible on mobile devices, which are easier to carry and use compared to computers [9,12,16]. However, the proportion of web-based digital psychotherapy was higher in the included studies. This suggests that despite the increased number of smartphone users compared to the past, a significant number of people still access the internet via computers. Furthermore, while the differences are not substantial, it is hypothesized that this could be due to the higher development costs associated with app-based digital psychotherapy.

### 4.7. Clinical Implication

In this meta-analysis, we aimed to overcome the limitations of previous meta-analyses by analyzing the effects of suicidal variables without restricting them to suicide ideation.

However, most of the included studies primarily assessed suicide ideation, which limits our ability to demonstrate significant differences from prior studies. Nevertheless, our study is significant as it confirmed that digital psychotherapy targeting suicide risk and severity did not differ significantly in content from digital psychotherapy focusing solely on suicide ideation [1,7]. Furthermore, the effect size of digital psychotherapy remained significant even when these additional variables were included. Therefore, this study suggests that effective suicide prevention requires a comprehensive examination of the entire suicide process, considering not only suicide ideation but also various variables such as suicide risk and severity. Consequently, the clinical implication of this study is that digital psychotherapy should be implemented from early interventions aimed at preventing suicide ideation to later interventions designed to mitigate suicide risk and severity, utilizing content based on multiple theories.

### *4.8. Limitation*

Although this study analyzed the effects of digital psychotherapy by broadly including suicidal variables, unlike previous meta-analyses, it has several limitations. Firstly, since considerable heterogeneity was observed in the findings related to suicide, its interpretation requires caution. Secondly, while the included studies were selected with careful consideration of various suicidal variables, they did not analyze variables encompassing the entire suicide process, such as suicide plans and attempts. Future studies should expand their scope to include variables that cover the complete trajectory of suicide. Thirdly, digital psychotherapy was proposed as an alternative to face-to-face therapy, but its comparative effectiveness was not conclusively demonstrated. However, given that digital psychotherapy primarily differs in delivery methods, it is anticipated that effectiveness may not significantly differ. Fourthly, this study did not assess the long-term effects of digital psychotherapy. By focusing solely on immediate post-intervention effects, it is limited in its ability to determine the duration of treatment effects. Therefore, future research should adopt a broader perspective by considering a wider range of variables and examining the long-term impacts of both face-to-face and digital psychotherapy to better understand the effects of digital psychotherapy across the entire spectrum of suicide prevention. In addition, since the number of studies on other theories is relatively small compared to CBT, further validation of its effectiveness is necessary in the future.

## 5. Conclusions

This study explored the effects of digital psychotherapy on suicide and depression. The findings demonstrate that digital psychotherapy is more beneficial to prevent suicide and ameliorate depression. These findings suggest that digital psychotherapy could be an alternative option when face-to-face psychotherapy is not available. Future research should consider a broader range of suicide variables and examine the long-term impact of digital psychotherapy to better understand its effects on suicide prevention.

**Author Contributions:** Conceptualization, J.O. and J.-H.P.; methodology, J.O. and J.H.; software, J.O. and J.-H.P.; formal analysis, J.O., J.H. and J.-H.P.; investigation, J.O. and J.H.; resources, S.L.; data curation, J.O., J.H. and J.-H.P.; writing—original draft preparation, J.O. and J.H.; writing—review and editing, J.-H.P.; visualization, J.O. and J.-H.P.; supervision, S.L. and J.-H.P.; project administration, J.-H.P.; funding acquisition, S.L. All authors have read and agreed to the published version of the manuscript.

**Funding:** This research was supported by the Soonchunhyang University Research Fund, the Ministry of Education of the Republic of Korea, and the National Research Foundation of Korea (NRF-2023S1A5C2A03099545).

**Institutional Review Board Statement:** Not applicable.

**Informed Consent Statement:** Not applicable.

**Data Availability Statement:** Data sharing is not applicable; no new data were created or analyzed in this study.

**Conflicts of Interest:** The authors declare no conflicts of interest.

## References

1. Sander, L.B.; Beisemann, M.; Doebler, P.; Micklitz, H.M.; Kerkhof, A.; Cuijpers, P.; Batterham, P.; Calear, A.; Christensen, H.; Jaegere, E.D.; et al. The effects of internet-based cognitive Behavioral therapy for suicidal ideation or behaviors on depression, anxiety, and hopelessness in individuals with suicidal ideation: Systematic review and Meta-analysis of individual participant data. *J. Med. Internet Res.* **2023**, *25*, e46771. [CrossRef] [PubMed]
2. World Health Organization. Suicide Worldwide in 2019: Global Health Estimates. 2021. Available online: https://www.who.int/publications/i/item/9789240026643 (accessed on 17 June 2024).
3. Büscher, R.; Beisemann, M.; Doebler, P.; Micklitz, H.M.; Kerkhof, A.; Cuijpers, P.; Batterham, P.J.; Calear, A.L.; Christensen, H.; De Jaegere, E.; et al. Digital cognitive–behavioural therapy to reduce suicidal ideation and behaviours: A systematic review and meta-analysis of individual participant data. *BMJ Ment. Health* **2022**, *25*, e8–e17. [CrossRef] [PubMed]
4. Marshall, J.M.; Dunstan, D.A.; Bartik, W. The role of digital mental health resources to treat trauma symptoms in Australia during COVID-19. *Psychol. Trauma* **2020**, *12*, S269–S271. [CrossRef] [PubMed]
5. Büscher, R.; Torok, M.; Terhorst, Y.; Sander, L. Internet-based cognitive behavioral therapy to reduce suicidal ideation: A systematic review and meta-analysis. *JAMA Netw. Open* **2020**, *3*, e203933. [CrossRef] [PubMed]
6. Reily, N.M.; Tang, S.; Batterham, P.J.; Aadam, B.; Draper, B.; Shand, F.; Han, J.; Nicholas, A.; Christensen, H. Help-seeking and barriers to service use amongst men with past-year suicidal ideation and not in contact with mental health services. *Arch. Suicide Res.* **2024**, *28*, 482–498. [CrossRef] [PubMed]
7. Torok, M.; Han, J.; Baker, S.; Werner-Seidler, A.; Wong, I.; Larsen, M.E.; Christensen, H. Suicide prevention using self-guided digital interventions: A systematic review and meta-analysis of randomised controlled trials. *Lancet Digit. Health* **2020**, *2*, e25–e36. [CrossRef] [PubMed]
8. Cooper, H. *Research Synthesis and Meta-Analysis: A Step-by-Step Approach*, 5th ed.; Sage Publications: Newbury Park, CA, USA, 2015; pp. 239–249.
9. Denneson, L.M.; Smolenski, D.J.; Bauer, B.W.; Dobscha, S.K.; Bush, N.E. The mediating role of coping self-efficacy in hope box use and suicidal ideation severity. *Arch. Suicide Res.* **2019**, *23*, 234–246. [CrossRef] [PubMed]
10. De Jaegere, E.; van Landschoot, R.; Van Heeringen, K.; van Spijker, B.A.; Kerkhof, A.J.; Mokkenstorm, J.K.; Portzky, G. The online treatment of suicidal ideation: A randomised controlled trial of an unguided web-based intervention. *Behav. Res. Ther.* **2019**, *119*, 103406. [CrossRef] [PubMed]
11. Hill, R.M.; Pettit, J.W. Pilot randomized controlled trial of LEAP: A selective preventive intervention to reduce adolescents' perceived burdensomeness. *J. Clin. Child Adolesc. Psychol.* **2019**, *48*, S45–S56. [CrossRef] [PubMed]
12. O'Toole, M.S.; Arendt, M.B.; Pedersen, C.M. Testing an app-assisted treatment for suicide prevention in a randomized controlled trial: Effects on suicide risk and depression. *Behav. Ther.* **2019**, *50*, 421–429. [CrossRef] [PubMed]
13. Van Spijker, B.A.; Werner-Seidler, A.; Batterham, P.J.; Mackinnon, A.; Calear, A.L.; Gosling, J.A.; Reynolds, J.; Kerkhof, A.J.; Solomon, D.; Shand, F.; et al. Effectiveness of a web-based self-help program for suicidal thinking in an Australian community sample: Randomized controlled trial. *J. Med. Internet Res.* **2018**, *20*, e15. [CrossRef] [PubMed]
14. Wilks, C.R.; Lungu, A.; Ang, S.Y.; Matsumiya, B.; Yin, Q.; Linehan, M.M. A randomized controlled trial of an Internet delivered dialectical behavior therapy skills training for suicidal and heavy episodic drinkers. *J. Affect. Disord.* **2018**, *232*, 219–228. [CrossRef] [PubMed]
15. Hetrick, S.E.; Yuen, H.P.; Bailey, E.; Cox, G.R.; Templer, K.; Rice, S.M.; Bendall, S.; Robinson, J. Internet-based cognitive behavioural therapy for young people with suicide-related behaviour (Reframe-IT): A randomised controlled trial. *BMJ Ment. Health* **2017**, *20*, 76–82. [CrossRef] [PubMed]
16. Tighe, J.; Shand, F.; Ridani, R.; Mackinnon, A.; De La Mata, N.; Christensen, H. Ibobbly mobile health intervention for suicide prevention in Australian Indigenous youth: A pilot randomised controlled trial. *BMJ Open* **2017**, *7*, e013518. [CrossRef] [PubMed]
17. Van Spijker, B.A.; van Straten, A.; Kerkhof, A.J. Effectiveness of online self-help for suicidal thoughts: Results of a randomised controlled trial. *PLoS ONE* **2014**, *9*, e90118. [CrossRef] [PubMed]
18. Malakouti, S.K.; Rasouli, N.; Rezaeian, M.; Nojomi, M.; Ghanbari, B.; Mohammadi, A.S. Effectiveness of self-help mobile telephone applications (apps) for suicide prevention: A systematic review. *Med. J. Islam. Repub. Iran* **2020**, *34*, 85. [CrossRef] [PubMed]
19. Chen, M.; Chan, K.L. Effectiveness of digital health interventions on unintentional injury, violence, and suicide: Meta-analysis. *Trauma Violence Abus.* **2022**, *23*, 605–619. [CrossRef] [PubMed]
20. Linehan, M.M.; Korslund, K.E.; Harned, M.S.; Gallop, R.J.; Lungu, A.; Neacsiu, A.D.; McDavid, J.; Comtois, K.A.; Murray-Gregory, A.M. Dialectical behavior therapy for high suicide risk in individuals with borderline personality disorder: A randomized clinical trial and component analysis. *JAMA Psychiatry* **2015**, *72*, 475–482. [CrossRef] [PubMed]

21. Valentine, S.E.; Bankoff, S.M.; Poulin, R.M.; Reidler, E.B.; Pantalone, D.W. The use of dialectical behavior therapy skills training as stand-alone treatment: A systematic review of the treatment outcome literature. *J. Clin. Psychol.* **2015**, *71*, 1–20. [CrossRef] [PubMed]
22. Andrews, G.; Cuijpers, P.; Craske, M.G.; McEvoy, P.; Titov, N. Computer therapy for the anxiety and depressive disorders is effective, acceptable and practical health care: A meta-analysis. *PLoS ONE* **2010**, *5*, e13196. [CrossRef] [PubMed]
23. Andersson, G.; Cuijpers, P.; Carlbring, P.; Riper, H.; Hedman, E. Guided Internet-based vs. face-to-face cognitive behavior therapy for psychiatric and somatic disorders: A systematic review and meta-analysis. *World Psychiatry* **2014**, *13*, 288–295. [CrossRef] [PubMed]

healthcare

MDPI

Systematic Review

# Detection of Arrhythmias Using Smartwatches—A Systematic Literature Review

**Bence Bogár [1,*], Dániel Pető [1], Dávid Sipos [2], Gábor Füredi [1], Antónia Keszthelyi [3], József Betlehem [1] and Attila András Pandur [1]**

[1] Department of Oxyology and Emergency Care, Pedagogy of Health and Nursing Sciences, Institute of Emergency Care, Faculty of Health Sciences, University of Pécs, 7624 Pécs, Hungary; daniel.peto@etk.pte.hu (D.P.); gabor.furedi@etk.pte.hu (G.F.); betlehem@etk.pte.hu (J.B.); attila.pandur@etk.pte.hu (A.A.P.)

[2] Department of Medical Imaging, Faculty of Health Sciences, University of Pécs, 7400 Kaposvár, Hungary; david.sipos@etk.pte.hu

[3] Human Patient Simulation Center for Health Sciences, Faculty of Health Sciences, University of Pécs, 7624 Pécs, Hungary; keszthelyi.antonia@pte.hu

* Correspondence: bence.bogar@etk.pte.hu; Tel.: +36-308-804-565

**Abstract:** Smartwatches represent one of the most widely adopted technological innovations among wearable devices. Their evolution has equipped them with an increasing array of features, including the capability to record an electrocardiogram. This functionality allows users to detect potential arrhythmias, enabling prompt intervention or monitoring of existing arrhythmias, such as atrial fibrillation. In our research, we aimed to compile case reports, case series, and cohort studies from the Web of Science, PubMed, Scopus, and Embase databases published until 1 August 2023. The search employed keywords such as "Smart Watch", "Apple Watch", "Samsung Gear", "Samsung Galaxy Watch", "Google Pixel Watch", "Fitbit", "Huawei Watch", "Withings", "Garmin", "Atrial Fibrillation", "Supraventricular Tachycardia", "Cardiac Arrhythmia", "Ventricular Tachycardia", "Atrioventricular Nodal Reentrant Tachycardia", "Atrioventricular Reentrant Tachycardia", "Heart Block", "Atrial Flutter", "Ectopic Atrial Tachycardia", and "Bradyarrhythmia." We obtained a total of 758 results, from which we selected 57 articles, including 33 case reports and case series, as well as 24 cohort studies. Most of the scientific works focused on atrial fibrillation, which is often detected using Apple Watches. Nevertheless, we also included articles investigating arrhythmias with the potential for circulatory collapse without immediate intervention. This systematic literature review provides a comprehensive overview of the current state of research on arrhythmia detection using smartwatches. Through further research, it may be possible to develop a care protocol that integrates arrhythmias recorded by smartwatches, allowing for timely access to appropriate medical care for patients. Additionally, continuous monitoring of existing arrhythmias using smartwatches could facilitate the assessment of the effectiveness of prescribed therapies.

**Keywords:** arrhythmia; atrial fibrillation; smartwatch

## 1. Introduction

Among the challenges encountered in emergency departments, cardiovascular disorders stand out as the most common and severe conditions, contributing significantly to global morbidity and mortality [1]. Globally, cardiovascular diseases are recognized as a leading cause of death, accounting for an estimated 17.9 million lives annually, constituting approximately 45% of all deaths [2,3]. In Europe, over 1.4 million premature deaths occur annually due to cardiovascular diseases in individuals under the age of 75 [3]. Common cardiovascular conditions include myocardial infarction, stroke, heart failure, cardiac arrhythmias, and heart valve issues [4].

Among cardiac arrhythmias, atrial fibrillation (AF) is the most prevalent, affecting 8.8 million individuals aged 55 and older in Europe in 2010. Projections indicate that this number will increase to more than double to 17.9 million by 2060 [5]. However, various other arrhythmias may develop, posing potential threats to patients' lives, including sinus tachycardia, atrial flutter, supraventricular tachycardia, ventricular fibrillation, ventricular tachycardia, sinus arrest, sick sinus syndrome, or atrioventricular blocks [6]. Arrhythmias are associated with 15–20% of all deaths, particularly sudden cardiac death, emphasizing the need for heightened attention to these conditions [7].

Fortunately, advancements in technology have introduced wearable smart devices, such as smartwatches, capable of assisting in the detection and management of cardiac arrhythmias and various health conditions [8,9]. Wearable smart devices have become one of the fastest-growing sectors in the technology industry, with major tech companies like Apple (Apple Watch), Google (Fitbit), and Samsung (Galaxy) developing smartwatches capable of monitoring biometric data, including heart rhythm, pulse rate, oxygen saturation, blood pressure, and sleep pattern [10]. Some devices utilizing photoplethysmography (PPG) can register patients' electrocardiography (ECG) within a 30-s interval, playing a crucial role in monitoring AF [11–13].

Beyond detecting AF, smartwatches can prove valuable in identifying other ECG abnormalities, such as bradyarrhythmias, tachyarrhythmias, or deviations indicative of ischemia [14]. With their current capabilities, smartwatches can provide excellent support for healthcare professionals in recognizing and managing various ECG abnormalities [8]. In our current research, we systematically aim to compile literature that specifically focuses on the registration of ECG abnormalities via smartwatches, particularly those relating to arrhythmias.

## 2. Methods

Our systematic literature review gathered available case reports, case series, and cohort studies. The literature review was conducted following the 2020 PRISMA (Preferred Reporting Items for Systematic Reviews and Meta-Analyses) guidelines, utilizing the PRISMA 2020 Checklist for the article's preparation [15].

### 2.1. Procedure for Literature Search

The search encompassed four databases: Web of Science, PubMed, Scopus, and Embase. Specifically, we sought articles and research focusing on the detection or monitoring of arrhythmias and other ECG abnormalities utilizing smartwatches. The systematic literature review included scientific works published from 1 January 2019 to 1 August 2023.

During the research, we utilized the following keywords: "smart watch" OR "smartwatch" OR "smart watches" OR "smartwatches" AND "Apple Watch" OR "Samsung Gear" OR "Samsung Galaxy Watch" OR "Google Pixel Watch" OR "Fitbit" OR "Huawei Watch" OR "Withings" OR "Garmin" AND "Atrial Fibrillation" OR "Supraventricular Tachycardia" OR "Cardiac Arrhythmia" OR "Ventricular Tachycardia" OR "Atrioventricular Nodal Reentrant Tachycardia" OR "Atrioventricular Reentrant Tachycardia" OR "Heart Block" OR "Atrial Flutter" OR "Ectopic Atrial Tachycardia" OR "Bradyarrhythmia". We experimented with various combinations of keywords and utilized Boolean operators to refine the search results. These searches were complemented with keywords and MeSH terms to broaden the scope of the findings. Additionally, we examined the bibliography of the selected literature to identify further relevant articles for inclusion.

Initially, we filtered articles based on titles and abstracts. Subsequently, we selected scientific works that were written in English or German and identified arrhythmias or other ECG abnormalities using smartwatches. We excluded conference abstracts, editorials, letters, guidelines, literature reviews, and meta-analyses from this systematic literature review. Studies issued by tech companies that manufacture smartwatches were also excluded.

### 2.2. Quality Assessment

Using the Newcastle-Ottawa Scale, we assessed the methodological quality and appropriateness of all case reports, case series, and cohort studies [16,17].

### 2.3. Data Organization

From the selected articles, we organized data by author(s), place of origin, publication year, study type, detected arrhythmia(s)/ECG deviation(s), sample size, average age of participants, and the smartwatches employed.

## 3. Results

We included a total of 57 articles in our research. Among the scientific works, there were 33 case reports or case series, and in addition, we selected 24 cohort studies where various arrhythmias and ECG abnormalities were recorded (Figure 1).

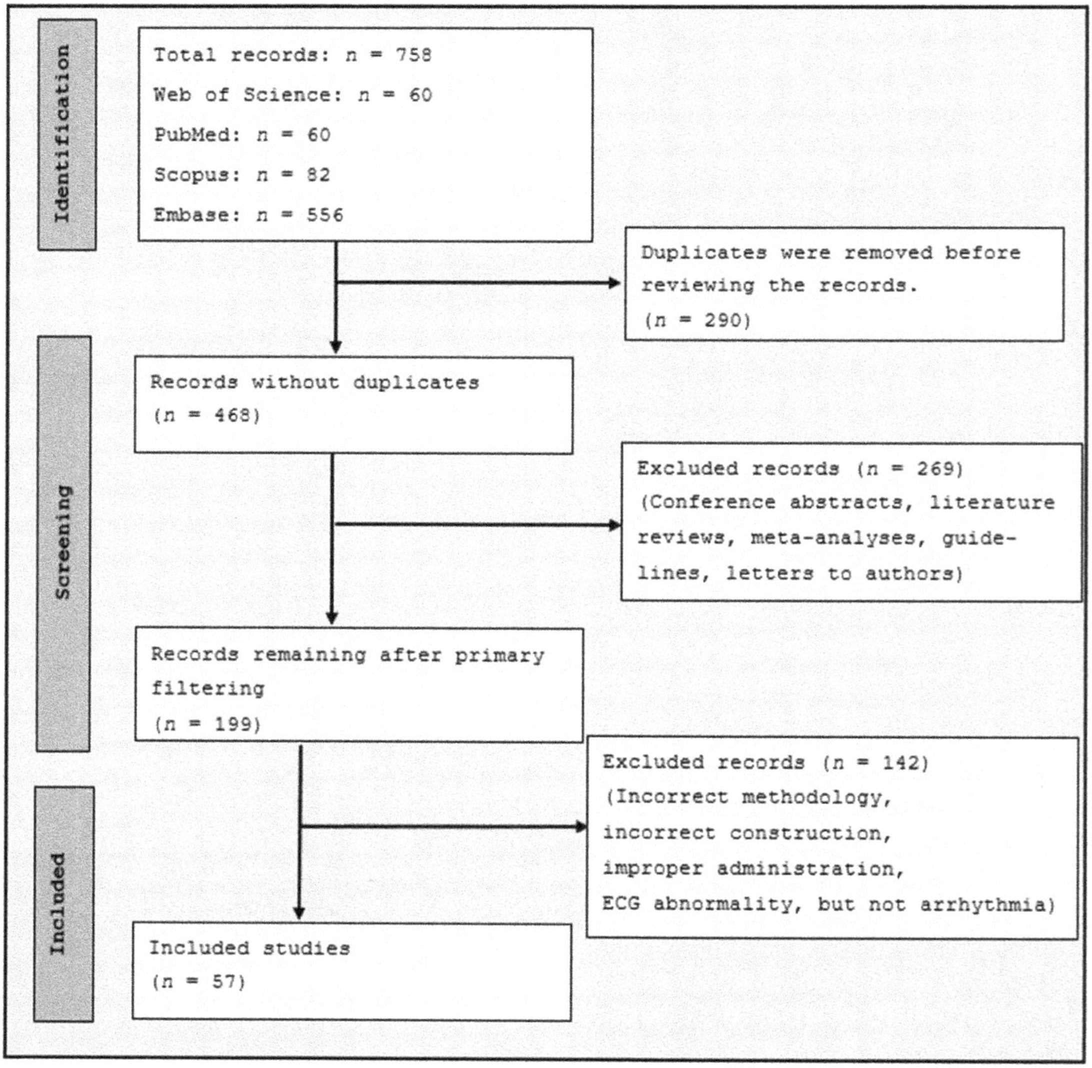


**Figure 1.** PRISMA Flow Diagram.

### 3.1. Case Reports

We selected 33 articles from case reports and case series detailing events involving a total of 44 patients. Most of the reports come from the United States ($n$ = 12). In the selected articles, the youngest subject was 10 days old, and the oldest was 72 years old. In most cases ($n$ = 30), the Apple Watch was used, while Samsung Galaxy Fit was used for arrhythmia registration in one patient. The smartwatch type was not precisely specified in two articles. Atrial fibrillation was recorded in 6 patient cases, and atrial flutter (AFL) was observed in 3 patients. The most frequently recorded arrhythmia was supraventricular tachycardia (SVT) (including atrioventricular re-entry tachycardia (AVRT) and atrioventricular nodal re-entry tachycardia (AVNRT), occurring a total of 13 times. Ventricular tachycardia (VT) was recorded in 7 patients. Third-degree atrioventricular (AV) block occurred 5 times. Other arrhythmias or ECG abnormalities (sinus bradycardia, sinus tachycardia, sick sinus syndrome (SSS)/tachycardia-bradycardia syndrome, Wolff–Parkinson–White (WPW) syndrome, bigeminy, ST-segment elevation/depression, ventricular fibrillation (VF) was described once each. (Table 1: Summary table of case descriptions).

**Table 1.** Summary table of case descriptions.

| Authors | Country | Year | Arrhythmia Type/ECG Abnormality | Number of Patients | Age | Smartwatch Type |
|---|---|---|---|---|---|---|
| Sanchez et al. [18] | USA | 2022 | Sinus bradycardia | 1 | 32 | NA |
| Kasai et al. [19] | Japan | 2021 | AVNRT, AVRT | 1 | 52 | Apple Watch |
| Ocher et al. [20] | USA | 2023 | VT | 1 | 36 | Apple Watch |
| Hawrysko et al. [21] | Poland | 2022 | AVNRT | 1 | 35 | Apple Watch |
| Al-Sudani et al. [22] | USA | 2023 | Third-degree AV block | 1 | 44 | Apple Watch |
| Siddeek et al. [23] | USA | 2020 | AVNRT | 1 | 16 | Apple Watch |
| Wu et al. [24] | Taiwan | 2022 | SVT | 3 | 59, 60, 48 | Apple Watch |
| Leroux et al. [25] | France | 2021 | Sinus tachycardia, SVT, Third-degree AV block | 3 | 10 days, 4 months, 16 months | Apple Watch |
| Kassam et al. [26] | Tanzania | 2021 | AVRT | 1 | 42 | Apple Watch |
| Ringwald et al. [27] | Switzerland | 2020 | VT | 1 | 45 | Apple Watch |
| Goldstein and Wells [28] | South Africa | 2019 | AFL | 1 | 56 | Apple Watch |
| Bedi et al. [29] | USA | 2023 | AF | 1 | 25 | NA |
| Bogossian et al. [30] | Germany | 2020 | AVNRT | 1 | 65 | Apple Watch |
| Gu et al. [31] | Canada | 2022 | VT | 1 | 64 | Apple Watch |
| Burke et al. [32] | USA | 2020 | VT | 2 | 60, 63 | Apple Watch |
| Jeong [33] | South Korea | 2022 | AVNRT | 1 | 23 | Apple Watch |
| Ahmed et al. [34] | USA | 2020 | AFL | 1 | 54 | Apple Watch |
| Yeo et al. [35] | Singapore | 2021 | SVT with aberrant conduction | 1 | NA | Apple Watch |
| Russo et al. [36] | Italy | 2023 | "Narrow-wide-narrow" QRS tachycardia | 1 | NA | Apple Watch |
| Glöckner et al. [37] | Germany | 2022 | NSVT, ST-segment elevation | 1 | 44 | Apple Watch |
| Leroux et al. [38] | France | 2022 | SVT, WPW syndrome, Third-degree AV block | 6 | 5, 6, 7, 9, 11, 13 | Apple Watch |
| Overbeek et al. [39] | USA | 2019 | Third-degree AV block | 1 | 60 | Apple Watch |

**Table 1.** *Cont.*

| Authors | Country | Year | Arrhythmia Type/ECG Abnormality | Number of Patients | Age | Smartwatch Type |
|---|---|---|---|---|---|---|
| Yerasi et al. [40] | USA | 2020 | Third-degree AV block | 1 | 68 | Apple Watch |
| Itoh [41] | Japan | 2022 | AF | 1 | 60 | Apple Watch |
| Mun et al. [42] | South Korea | 2021 | WPW syndrome | 1 | 26 | Samsung Galaxy Fit |
| Delinière et al. [43] | Switzerland | 2021 | ST-segment depression, VT | 1 | 45 | Apple Watch |
| Walker et al. [44] | USA | 2023 | AFL | 1 | 37 | Apple Watch |
| Weichert [45] | UK | 2019 | AF | 1 | 59 | Apple Watch |
| Samal et al. [46] | USA | 2020 | AF | 1 | 39 | Apple Watch |
| Jariwala and Jadhav [47] | India | 2021 | AF, SSS (tachycardia-bradycardia syndrome) | 2 | 72, 69 | Apple Watch |
| Pasli and Imamoglu [48] | Turkey | 2023 | Bigeminy | 1 | 41 | Apple Watch |
| Patel and Tarakji [49] | USA | 2021 | AF | 1 | 70 | Apple Watch |
| Provencio and Gil [50] | Spain | 2022 | ST-segment depression, PVCs, VF | 1 | 72 | Apple Watch |

NA = Not available.

### 3.2. Cohort Studies

Among the cohort studies, 24 articles met the inclusion criteria. Most of these studies originated from the United States ($n$ = 6). The cardiac arrhythmia investigated most often was atrial fibrillation, documented in a total of 1294 cases throughout the studies. Other arrhythmias included atrial flutter (77 cases), atrioventricular nodal reentrant tachycardia (64 cases), atrioventricular reentrant tachycardia (36 cases), (paroxysmal) supraventricular tachycardia (PSVT) or sinus tachycardia (27 cases), ventricular tachycardia (5 cases), and second- or third-degree atrioventricular block (49 cases). Sinus bradycardia was recorded in 27 cases.

The cohort studies showed that the smartwatch that was used the most for ECG recordings was the Apple Watch, which was employed in 4479 cases. Additionally, ECGs that used Samsung ($n$ = 978) were recorded 2743 times, Withings ($n$ = 942), Fitbit ($n$ = 360), Garmin ($n$ = 223), Acer ($n$ = 116), Huawei ($n$ = 100), and Polar ($n$ = 24) devices. (Table 2: Summary table of cohort studies).

**Table 2.** Summary table of cohort studies.

| Author(s) | Country | Year | Arrhythmia Type/ECG Abnormality | Number of Patients | Average Age | Smart-Watch Type(s) |
|---|---|---|---|---|---|---|
| Seshadri et al. [51] | USA | 2019 | AF | 50 | 61.4 ± 10.4 | Apple Watch |
| Hwang et al. [52] | South Korea | 2019 | PSVT | 51 | 44.4 ± 16.6 | Apple Watch, Samsung Galaxy Gear, Fitbit Charge |
| Ploux et al. [53] | France | 2022 | Sinus bradycardia, Second-, Third-degree AV block, AF, AFL/AT, ST-, T-wave changes, RBBB, LBBB, Pathological Q-wave | 260 | 66 ± 6 | Apple Watch |

**Table 2.** *Cont.*

| Author(s) | Country | Year | Arrhythmia Type/ECG Abnormality | Number of Patients | Average Age | Smart-Watch Type(s) |
|---|---|---|---|---|---|---|
| Sequeira et al. [54] | Canada | 2020 | AVNRT, AVRT | 52 | 52.3 ± 17.2 | Apple Watch, Fitbit Charge, Garmin Vivo-Smart, Polar A360 |
| Leroux et al. [55] | France | 2022 | BBB, AV block, WPW, SVT, Long-QT | 110 | 1 week–16 years | Apple Watch |
| Koshy et al. [56] | Australia | 2018 | AF, AFL | 102 | 68 ± 15 | Apple Watch, Fitbit Blaze |
| Abu-Alrub et al. [57] | France | 2022 | AF | 200 | 62 ± 7 | Apple Watch, Samsung Galaxy Watch, Withings Move |
| Han et al. [58] | USA | 2021 | AF | 35 | 50–91 | Samsung |
| Mannhart et al. [59] | Switzerland | 2023 | AF | 201 | 66.7 | Apple Watch, Samsung Galaxy Watch, Withings Scan-watch, Fitbit Sense, AliveCor Kardia-Mobile |
| Racine et al. [60] | Canada | 2022 | AF, AFL/AT, VT, SVT, sinus dysfunction, second-and third-degree AV block, ventricular ectopic beats, RBBB, LBBB | 734 | 66 | Apple Watch |
| Pengel et al. [61] | Netherlands | 2022 | AF | 222 | 40 ± 17 | Withings Scan-watch |
| Pepplinkhuizen et al. [62] | Netherlands | 2022 | AF | 74 | 67.1 ± 12.3 | Apple Watch |
| Rajakariar et al. [63] | Australia | 2020 | AF | 200 | 67 ± 16 | Apple Watch |
| Wasserlauf et al. [64] | USA | 2023 | AF | 30 | 65.4 ± 12.2 | Apple Watch |
| Chang et al. [65] | Taiwan | 2022 | AF | 200 | 66.1 ± 12.6 | Garmin |
| Wyatt et al. [66] | USA | 2020 | AF | 264 | 55 | Apple Watch |
| Badertscher et al. [67] | Switzerland | 2022 | AF | 319 | 67 | Withings Scan-watch |
| Ford et al. [68] | Australia | 2022 | AF | 125 | 76 ± 7 | Apple Watch |
| Lee et al. [69] | Canada | 2022 | AF | 200 | 65.6 ± 14.6 | Apple Watch |
| Roelle et al. [70] | USA | 2022 | SVT, Arrhythmia Syndrome, Syncope, Sinus arrest, Sinus tachycardia | 30 | 11.6 | Apple Watch |
| Liao et al. [71] | Taiwan | 2022 | AF | 116 | 59.6 ± 11.4 | Acer Leap Ware |
| Dörr et al. [72] | Germany | 2019 | Paroxysmal Fibrillation (PF) | 508 | 76.4 | Samsung |
| Liu et al. [73] | China | 2022 | Brady-arrhythmia, Mobitz I, Mobitz II, Third-degree AV block, LBBB, Tachy-arrhythmia, AF, AFL | 100 | 73.1 ± 7.6 | Huawei |
| Feldman et al. [74] | USA | 2022 | Paroxysmal Fibrillation (PF) | 1802 | 45.96 | Apple Watch |

Of the cohort studies, the first was conducted by Seshadri et al. They aimed to evaluate the precision of the Apple Watch during exercise of fifty patients with common cardiac arrhythmias like atrial fibrillation. They compared its accuracy against telemetry. The findings of this preliminary clinical investigation revealed a correlation coefficient of 0.7 between all Apple Watch readings and telemetry. Additionally, the Apple Watch exhibited greater accuracy in assessing heart rate among patients with atrial fibrillation compared to those without ($rc = 0.86$ for patients in AF, versus $rc = 0.64$ for patients not in AF) [51].

Hwang et al. conducted a study to evaluate the precision of three smartwatch models: the Apple Watch Series 2, the Samsung Galaxy Gear S3, and the Fitbit Charge 2. This research involved 51 patients with a history of paroxysmal supraventricular tachyarrhythmia (SVT) or paroxysmal palpitations. Patients were randomly assigned to wear two different devices. The initial heart rate measurements showed accuracies of 100%, 100%, and 94% for Apple, Samsung, and Fitbit, respectively. During induced SVT, in which heart rates ranged from 108 to 228 beats per minute, the accuracy was 100%, 90%, and 87% for Apple, Samsung, and Fitbit, respectively. While the devices demonstrated acceptable accuracy, it tended to decrease as heart rate increased and exhibited variations between the different models [52].

Ploux et al. evaluated the sensitivity and specificity of the Apple Watch Series 4 among 260 patients, both with and without a history of cardiovascular disease. Their findings indicate that the Apple Watch Series 4 can detect ECG abnormalities with a sensitivity of 91% and a specificity of 94% (95% CI) [53].

Sequeira et al. investigated the precision of four common wearable devices (Apple Watch, Fitbit Charge HR, Garmin VivoSmart HR, and Polar A360) in monitoring heart rate during episodes of paroxysmal supraventricular tachycardia (SVT). Their study involved 52 patients. The researchers concluded that all wearable devices showed inaccuracy for short-duration (<60 s) SVT episodes. Only the Apple Watch (23 out of 23) and Polar (19 out of 21) devices demonstrated an accuracy exceeding 90% for long-duration ($\geq$60 s) SVT episodes [54].

Leroux et al. evaluated the sensitivity and specificity of the Apple Watch in 110 children, ranging from 1 week to 16 years old, who had either normal ($n = 75$) or abnormal ($n = 35$) 12-lead ECGs. The smartwatch tracings showed a sensitivity of 84% and specificity of 100% in detecting abnormal ECG [55].

Koshy et al. assessed the accuracy of heart rate measurement using the Apple Watch Series 1 and Fitbit Blaze among patients diagnosed with atrial fibrillation (AF) and atrial flutter (AFL). The Apple Watch demonstrated accuracies of 86%, 100%, and 99% for AF, AFL, and both conditions, respectively, when compared to an ECG monitor. Similarly, the Fitbit showed accuracies of 87%, 99%, and 98% for AF, AFL, and both conditions, respectively, when compared to an ECG monitor [56].

Abu-Alrub et al. conducted a comparison of the diagnostic capabilities for detecting atrial fibrillation (AF) among three commercially available smartwatches. Their study involved 100 patients with AF and 100 patients with sinus rhythm. They found that the Apple Watch Series 5, the Samsung Galaxy Watch Active 3, and the Withings Move ECG exhibited sensitivities/specificities of 87%/86%, 88%/81%, and 78%/80%, respectively ($p < 0.05$) [57].

Han et al. developed an algorithm aimed at detecting atrial fibrillation using a Samsung Simband 2. Their study involved 35 participants. The sensitivity, specificity, positive predictive value, negative predictive value, and accuracy for subjects with atrial fibrillation were 92%, 96%, 85%, 98%, and 95%, respectively [58].

Mannhart et al. conducted a study to evaluate the accuracy of five smart devices in detecting atrial fibrillation compared to a physician-interpreted 12-lead electrocardiogram. They prospectively analyzed 201 patients, among whom 62 had atrial fibrillation. The sensitivity and specificity for atrial fibrillation detection were similar across devices: 85% and 75% for the Apple Watch 6, 85% and 75% for the Samsung Galaxy Watch 3, 58% and 75% for the Withings Scanwatch, 66% and 79% for the Fitbit Sense, and 79% and 69% for the AliveCor KardiaMobile, respectively. In terms of patient preference, the Apple Watch ranked highest (preferred by 39% of participants) [59].

Racine et al. wanted to evaluate the precision of the Apple Watch ECG in detecting atrial fibrillation (AF) among 734 patients, of whom 21% were diagnosed with AF and had various ECG abnormalities in their study. Upon excluding unclassified ECGs from the analysis, the sensitivity was found to be 88% (95% CI 82–93%), and specificity was 98% (95% CI 97–99%). However, when unclassified ECGs were considered as false results, the sensitivity and specificity for AF detection were 69% (95% CI 61–76%) and 81% (95% CI 76–84%), respectively [60].

Pengel et al. evaluated the diagnostic precision of various ECG-based devices in comparison to the standard 12-lead ECG in a cohort of 222 patients. Their study found that for atrial fibrillation (AF) detection, the Withings Scanwatch achieved 100% accuracy, sensitivity, and specificity. Additionally, only 5% of cases were deemed uninterpretable with this smartwatch. The Kardia 6L demonstrated 97% accuracy, 100% sensitivity, and 97% specificity, albeit with 31% of cases were uninterpretable [61].

Pepplinkhuizen et al. investigated the effectiveness of the Apple Watch (AW) ECG in detecting atrial fibrillation (AF) among patients scheduled for electrical cardioversion (ECV). Their study involved obtaining AW ECGs before and after ECV, with up to three attempts made in case of unclassified recordings. Sensitivity, specificity, and kappa coefficient were calculated for analysis. A total of 65 AF and 64 sinus rhythm measurements were recorded. The initial AW measurement showed a sensitivity of 93.5% and a specificity of 100% ($\kappa = 0.94$). Subsequent measurements yielded a sensitivity of 94.6% and specificity of 100% ($\kappa = 0.95$) for the second attempt and a sensitivity of 93% and specificity of 96.5% ($\kappa = 0.90$) for the third attempt [62].

Rajakariar et al. assessed the accuracy of using an Apple Watch with AliveCor KardiaBand (KB) for diagnosing atrial fibrillation (AF) in comparison to a 12-lead ECG. The KB, when paired with a smartwatch, provided an automated diagnosis of either AF or sinus rhythm. The sensitivity and specificity of KB were 94.4% and 81.9%, respectively, with a positive predictive value of 54.8% and a negative predictive value of 98.4%. The agreement between the diagnosis from the 12-lead ECG and KB was moderate, especially when including unclassified tracings ($\kappa = 0.60$, 95% CI 0.47 to 0.72) [63].

Wasserlauf et al. recruited thirty participants for their study, aiming to evaluate the precision of the Apple Watch in detecting atrial fibrillation. Their primary goal was to ascertain the accuracy of the irregular rhythm notification (IRN) among individuals previously diagnosed with non-permanent AF. The study found no instances of false positive IRN detections, achieving a sensitivity of 72%, a specificity of 100%, a PPV (Positive predictive value.) of 100%, and a NPV (Negative predictive value) of 90% [64].

Chang et al. examined the precision of the Garmin Forerunner 945 smartwatch in identifying atrial fibrillation (AF) in comparison to a Holter electrocardiogram. Their study involved 200 participants. The sensitivity, specificity, positive predictive value, and negative predictive value for AF detection among participants were 97.3%, 88.6%, 91.6%, and 96.3%, respectively. The accuracy of the Garmin smartwatch was reported at 93.5% [65].

Wyat et al. aimed to characterize the assessments of patients who seek medical attention after detecting an abnormal pulse using the Apple Watch. They conducted a retrospective analysis of patients evaluated for an abnormal pulse detected via the Apple Watch over a four-month period. Out of the 264 patients included in the study, clinical documentation explicitly noted an abnormal pulse alert in 41 patients (15.5%). Preexisting atrial fibrillation was identified in 58 patients (22.0%). Only 30 patients (11.4%) received a clinically actionable cardiovascular diagnosis of interest, with 6 out of 41 patients (15%) who received an explicit alert among them [66].

Badertscher et al. made a prospective observational study involving patients attending a cardiology service at a tertiary referral center. Their objective was to evaluate the diagnostic accuracy of the intelligent ECG feature of the Withings Scanwatch in detecting atrial fibrillation (AF) compared to a concurrently obtained cardiologist-interpreted 12-lead

ECG. In total, AF was diagnosed in 34 patients (11%). Among the ECG tracings analyzed by the algorithm, it demonstrated a sensitivity of 76% (95% CI 55–91%), a specificity of 99% (95% CI 97–100%), and a Kappa coefficient of 0.72 when compared to cardiologist-interpreted 12-lead ECGs [67].

Ford et al. conducted a comparative analysis between the Apple Watch Series 4 (AW) and the AliveCor KardiaBand (KB) for the detection of atrial fibrillation (AF) in a cohort of 125 patients. The results showed that AW automatically detected AF with an accuracy of 93%, a sensitivity of 50%, a specificity of 100%, a positive predictive value of 100%, and a negative predictive value of 92%. KB automatically detected AF with an accuracy of 94%, a sensitivity of 96%, a specificity of 93%, a positive predictive value of 84%, and a negative predictive value of 99% [68].

Lee et al. compared the Apple Watch Series 4 (AW) and KardiaMobile (KM), involving 200 participants in their study. The accuracy of rhythm detection for sinus rhythm was found to be 100% for AW and 99.03% for KM. In detecting atrial fibrillation, AW exhibited an accuracy of 90.48%, whereas KM achieved 100% accuracy. Regarding heart rate accuracy for sinus rhythm, KM showed 94.39% accuracy, while the AW photoplethysmography function had 90.65% accuracy, and the AW ECG function had 96.26% accuracy. For heart rate accuracy during atrial fibrillation, KM demonstrated 91.30% accuracy, while the AW photoplethysmography function showed 82.61% accuracy, and the AW ECG function exhibited 86.96% accuracy [69].

Roelle et al. assessed the effectiveness of digital health technologies in pediatric electrophysiology telehealth consultations. Providers evaluated the data quality from these devices using a post-visit usability survey. Regarding ECG devices, providers reported high-quality tracings from KardiaMobile (62%; 18/29), Apple Watch (93%; 28/30), and Coala monitor (86%; 24/28) [70].

Liao et al. evaluated the Acer Leap Ware smartwatch for its ability to detect atrial fibrillation (AF). Data were gathered from patients undergoing radiofrequency or cryotherapy ablation for AF. A total of 116 patients were enrolled, of which 76 had previously been diagnosed with paroxysmal AF and 40 with persistent AF. The overall accuracy of the smartwatch was summarized as 95.02%, with a sensitivity of 95.68% and specificity of 93.66% [71].

Dörr et al. utilized the photoplethysmography algorithm and discovered a sensitivity of 93.7% (95% CI: 89.8% to 96.4%), a specificity of 98.2% (95% CI: 95.8% to 99.4%), and an accuracy of 96.1% (95% CI: 94.0% to 97.5%) for detecting atrial fibrillation with a Samsung Gear Fit 2 [72].

Liu et al. employed a Huawei Watch GT 2 Pro ECG edition to identify arrhythmias in a cohort of 100 patients. Throughout their investigation, they recorded 52 instances of bradyarrhythmias, encompassing Mobitz I, Mobitz II, and third-degree atrioventricular block, as well as 16 occurrences of tachyarrhythmias, including atrial fibrillations and atrial flutters [73].

Feldman et al. aimed to provide real-world insights into the proportion of individuals who would potentially benefit from anticoagulation therapy if diagnosed with atrial fibrillation using data from wearable devices. This study utilized electronic health records (EHR) and Apple Watch data obtained from an observational cohort comprising 1802 patients. Utilizing this dataset, they estimated the number of high-risk patients eligible for anticoagulation based on their medical history, Apple Watch usage patterns, and atrial fibrillation (AF) risk determined by a validated model. Considering the characteristics of this cohort, they found that, on average, 0.25% ($n$ = 4.58, 95% CI, 2.0–8.0) of patients could be considered suitable candidates for initiating anticoagulation therapy due to AF detection through their Apple Watch [74].

## 4. Discussion

Numerous studies have explored the capability of various smartwatches, including Apple Watch Series 4®, Samsung Simband®, Samsung Galaxy Watch 3®, Huawei Watch GT

2 Pro®, Fitbit Sense 2®, Withings Scanwatch®, Garmin Venu 2®, Polar A360®, Acer Leap Ware®, and their subsequent generations, to detect both brady- and tachyarrhythmias. Additionally, there are non-invasive devices such as AliveCor KardiaMobile®, ATsens®, Polar H10®, or Coala Heart Monitor®, and invasive measurement methods, such as Implantable Loop Recorder or Implantable Cardiac Monitor, for continuous heart rhythm monitoring.

The systematic literature review aimed to collect articles on how smartwatches were utilized for detecting arrhythmias.

The case reports and case series highlight key demographic information such as the age range of patients, the geographic distribution of cases, and the prevalence of specific arrhythmias recorded. The inclusion of patients spanning from 10 days old to 72 years old emphasizes the broad applicability of smartwatch-based arrhythmia monitoring across different age groups. Most of the cases originated from the United States, suggesting a potential concentration of research and clinical use of smartwatches for cardiac monitoring in this region. Atrial fibrillation and supraventricular tachycardia were the most recorded types of arrhythmias. This reflects the known prevalence of these arrhythmias in clinical practice and presents the importance of early detection and monitoring, particularly in high-risk populations. The smartwatch model that is used most often is the Apple Watch, which suggests its popularity and reliability.

In the cohort studies, our focus was on understanding the effectiveness of smartwatches in arrhythmia detection. The most studied arrhythmia was atrial fibrillation, with Apple Watch being the predominant device used for its detection. Studies revealed that the Apple Watch, either standalone or supplemented with KardiaBand, demonstrated over 90% accuracy in AF detection [53,63,68,69]. Diagnostic sensitivity and specificity were also consistently around 90% [53,57,60,62–64,68]. Moreover, the Apple Watch proved effective in accurately determining heart rate, even during tachyarrhythmias [51,52,56]. Similar results were observed with smartwatches from other manufacturers, including Samsung, Withings, Fitbit, Garmin, Huawei, and Acer [52,56–58,61,65,67,71,72]. Apart from AF, these devices demonstrated capability in detecting various other arrhythmias, such as second- and third-degree atrioventricular block, atrial flutter, atrial tachycardia, supraventricular tachycardia, atrioventricular nodal reentrant tachycardia, atrioventricular reentrant tachycardia, or ventricular tachycardia [52–55,60,70,73]. In addition to having good accuracy, as well as high sensitivity and specificity, smartwatches can be used easily and conveniently, which is why the majority of research participants prefer smartwatches, above all the Apple Watch, over other ECG-capable devices [59,61,70]. Their wide applicability is also facilitated by the fact that they can be used not only for adults but also for children where necessary [55,70]. Despite the convenience and accuracy of smartwatches, they are still underutilized in clinical practice for prevention and therapy adjustment. This is despite potential benefits, such as aiding in initiating anticoagulant therapy in patients with detected atrial fibrillation [74]. It is important to acknowledge false-positive events, as smartwatches may incorrectly indicate arrhythmias, potentially contributing to the burden on the healthcare system [66].

## 5. Conclusions

Our systematic literature review presents a comprehensive overview of the utilization of smartwatches for monitoring cardiac arrhythmias, focusing on both case reports and cohort studies. Let us delve into some key points drawn from these findings:

1. Diversity in patient demographics and arrhythmias: The study encompassed a wide range of patients, spanning from a 1-week-old infant to a 91-year-old individual, showcasing the applicability of smartwatch technology across various age groups. Moreover, the diversity of recorded arrhythmias, including atrial fibrillation, atrial flutter, supraventricular tachycardia, ventricular tachycardia, and others, highlights the versatility of smartwatches in detecting different cardiac anomalies.
2. Prevalence of Apple Watch usage: The Apple Watch emerged as the most utilized and most reliable smartwatch for arrhythmia monitoring in both case reports and

cohort studies. This prevalence might be attributed to its widespread availability, user-friendly interface, and integration with healthcare systems.

3. Accuracy and precision across different studies: Several cohort studies evaluated the accuracy of smartwatch models in detecting cardiac arrhythmias. Findings varied across studies, with some reporting high sensitivity and specificity, particularly for atrial fibrillation detection, while others noted variations in accuracy depending on the smartwatch model and type of arrhythmia.
4. Comparison studies: Comparative studies, such as those assessing different smartwatch models or comparing smartwatch performance with standard ECG monitoring, provided valuable insights into the strengths and limitations of each device. These comparisons aid in guiding clinicians and patients in selecting the most suitable device for their specific monitoring needs.
5. Clinical implications: The study's findings have significant clinical implications, particularly in the early detection and management of cardiac arrhythmias. Smartwatches offer the potential for continuous monitoring outside clinical settings. It could be helpful for monitoring a patient in need or who underwent a major intervention, to improve the patient's outcome.
6. Challenges and future directions: Despite promising results, challenges such as accuracy during high heart rates and variability across different smartwatch models underscore the need for further research and technological advancements. Future studies may focus on enhancing the accuracy, reliability, and usability of smartwatch-based arrhythmia detection systems.

In summary, this study provides insights into the evolving role of smartwatches in cardiac arrhythmia monitoring. While advancements in wearable technology hold promise for revolutionizing healthcare delivery, continued research and validation are essential to optimize their clinical utility and ensure patient safety and efficacy.

**Author Contributions:** Conceptualization, A.A.P. and B.B.; methodology, D.P.; validation, D.S., G.F. and J.B.; formal analysis, B.B.; investigation, A.K.; resources, A.A.P. and J.B.; data curation, B.B.; writing—original draft preparation, B.B.; writing—review and editing, B.B.; supervision, A.A.P.; project administration, A.A.P. and J.B.; funding acquisition, A.A.P. All authors have read and agreed to the published version of the manuscript.

**Funding:** The project No. 2022-2.1.1-NL-2022-00012, "National Laboratory of Cooperative Technologies", was realized with the support provided by the Ministry of Culture and Innovation from the National Research, Development, and Innovation Fund, financed by the National Laboratories tender program.

**Institutional Review Board Statement:** Not applicable.

**Informed Consent Statement:** Not applicable.

**Data Availability Statement:** Not applicable.

**Conflicts of Interest:** The authors declare no conflict of interest.

## References

1. Shahzad, A. Systematic Approach to Acute Cardiovascular Emergencies. In *Essentials of Accident and Emergency Medicine*; 2018. Available online: https://www.intechopen.com/chapters/60421 (accessed on 2 April 2018).
2. WHO. World Health Organization/Health Topic/Cardiovascular Diseases. 2023. Available online: https://www.who.int/health-topics/cardiovascular-diseases#tab=tab_1 (accessed on 3 November 2023).
3. Townsend, N.; Wilson, L.; Bhatnagar, P.; Wickramasinghe, K.; Rayner, M.; Nichols, M. Cardiovascular disease in Europe: Epidemiological update 2016. *Eur. Heart J.* **2016**, *37*, 3232–3245. [CrossRef] [PubMed]
4. Benjamin, E.J.; Blaha, M.J.; Chiuve, S.E.; Cushman, M.; Das, S.R.; Deo, R.; Ferranti, S.D.; Floyd, J.; Fornage, M.; Gillespie, C. Heart Disease and Stroke *Statistics*—2017 Update: A Report from the American Heart Association. *Circulation* **2017**, *135*, e146–e603. [CrossRef] [PubMed]
5. Krijthe, B.P.; Kunst, A.; Benjamin, E.J.; Lip, G.Y.; Franco, O.H.; Hofman, A.; Witteman, J.C.; Stricker, B.H.; Herringa, J. Projections on the number of individuals with atrial fibrillation in the European Union, from 2000 to 2060. *Eur. Heart J.* **2013**, *34*, 2746–2751. [CrossRef]

6. NHLBI. National Heart, Lung, and Blood Institute. Available online: https://web.archive.org/web/20150607165144/http://www.nhlbi.nih.gov/health/health-topics/topics/arr/types. (accessed on 1 July 2023).
7. Srinivasan, N.T.; Schilling, R.J. Sudden Cardiac Death and Arrhythmias. *Arrhythmia Electrophysiol. Rev.* **2018**, *7*, 111–117. [CrossRef] [PubMed]
8. Garikapati, K.; Turnbull, S.; Bennett, R.G.; Campbell, T.G.; Kanawati, J.; Wong, M.S.; Thomas, S.P.; Chow, C.K.; Kumar, S. The Role of Contemporary Wearable and Handheld Devices in the Diagnosis and Management of Cardiac Arrhythmias. *Heart Lung Circ.* **2022**, *31*, 1432–1449. [CrossRef] [PubMed]
9. Xiao-Yong, C.; Bo-Xiong, Y.; Shuai, Z.; Jie, D.; Peng, S.; Lindi, G.L. Intelligent health management based on analysis of big data collected by wearable smart watch. *Cogn. Robot.* **2023**, *3*, 1–7. [CrossRef]
10. Lima, F.V.; Kadiyala, V.; Huang, A.; Agusala, K.; Cho, D.; Freeman, A.M.; Druz, R. At the Crossroads! Time to Start Taking Smartwatches Seriously. *Am. J. Cardiol.* **2022**, *179*, 96–101. [CrossRef]
11. Turakhia, M.P.; Desai, M.; Hedlin, H.; Rajmane, A.; Talati, N.; Ferris, T.; Desai, S.; Nag, D.; Patel, M.; Kowey, P.; et al. Rationale and design of a large-scale, app-based study to identify cardiac arrhythmias using a smartwatch: The Apple Heart Study. *Am. Heart J.* **2019**, *207*, 66–75. [CrossRef] [PubMed]
12. Lubitz, S.A.; Faranesh, A.Z.; Atlas, S.J.; McManus, D.D.; Singer, D.E.; Pagoto, S.; Pantelopoulos, A.; Foulkes, A.S. Rationale and design of a large population study to validate software for the assessment of atrial fibrillation from data acquired by a consumer tracker or smartwatch: The Fitbit heart study. *Am. Heart J.* **2021**, *238*, 16–26. [CrossRef]
13. Guo, Y.; Wang, H.; Zhang, H.; Liu, T.; Liang, Z.; Xia, Y.; Yan, L.; Xing, Y.; Shi, H.; Li, S.; et al. Mobile Photoplethysmographic Technology to Detect Atrial Fibrillation. *J. Am. Coll. Cardiol.* **2019**, *74*, 2365–2375. [CrossRef]
14. Caillol, T.; Strik, M.; Ramirez, D.F.; Abu-Alrub, S.; Marchand, H.; Buliard, S.; Welte, N.; Ploux, S.; Haïssaguerre, M.; Bordachar, P. Accuracy of a Smartwatch-Derived ECG for Diagnosing Bradyarrhythmias, Tachyarrhythmias, and Cardiac Ischemia. *Circ. Arrhythmia Electrophysiol.* **2021**, *14*, e009260. [CrossRef] [PubMed]
15. Page, M.J.; McKenzie, J.E.; Bossuyt, P.M.; Boutron, I.; Hoffmann, T.C.; Mulrow, C.D.; Shamseer, L.; Tetzlaff, J.M.; Akl, E.A.; Brennan, S.E.; et al. The PRISMA 2020 statement: An updated guideline for reporting systematic reviews. *Int. J. Surg.* **2021**, *88*, 105906. [CrossRef] [PubMed]
16. Murad, M.H.; Sultan, S.; Haffar, S.; Bazerbachi, F. Methodological quality and synthesis of case series and case reports. *BMJ Evid.-Based Med.* **2018**, *23*, 60–63. [CrossRef] [PubMed]
17. Stang, A. Critical evaluation of the Newcastle-Ottawa scale for the assessment of the quality of nonrandomized studies in meta-analyses. *Eur. J. Epidemiol.* **2010**, *25*, 603–605. [CrossRef] [PubMed]
18. Sanchez, A.C.; Chohan, M.; Olatunde, O.; White, C. A Rare Case of Ciprofloxacin-Induced Bradycardia Recognized by a Smartwatch. *J. Investig. Med. High Impact Case Rep.* **2022**, *10*, 1–3.
19. Kasai, Y.; Kasai, J.; Sekihuchi, Y.; Asano, S.; Fukunaga, H.; Nagase, T.; Nitta, J. Apple Watch® facilitates single-session catheter ablation of coexisting atrioventricular nodal reentrant tachycardia and atrioventricular reentrant tachycardia. *Clin. Case Rep.* **2021**, *9*, e04702. [CrossRef] [PubMed]
20. Ocher, R.; Shahid, M.; Sridharan, A.; Parikh, R.; Bradfield, J.S.; Vaseghi, M.; Shahandeh, N. Apple Watch Detected Ventricular Tachycardia in a Pregnant Patient. *J. Am. Coll. Cardiol.* **2023**, *81*, 3874. [CrossRef]
21. Hawryszko, M.; Sławiński, G.; Kozłowski, D.; Lewicka, E. Apple Watch-guided diagnosis of AVNRT in a pregnant woman—A case report and literature review. *Front. Cardiovasc. Med.* **2022**, *9*, 985421. [CrossRef] [PubMed]
22. Al-Sudani, H.; Motupalli, S.N.V.V.; Adekayode, C.; Boris, J.; Jacob, D. Asymptomatic Heart Block in Cardiac Sarcoidosis Identified by Apple Watch and Managed with icd. *J. Am. Coll. Cardiol.* **2023**, *81*, 2795. [CrossRef]
23. Siddeek, H.; Fisher, K.; McMakin, S.; Bass, J.L.; Cortez, D. AVNRT captured by Apple Watch Series 4: Can the Apple watch be used as an event monitor? *Ann. Noninvasive. Electrocardiol.* **2020**, *25*, e12742. [CrossRef]
24. Wu, S.-J.; Li, C.-H.; Lin, J.-C.; Weng, C.-J.; Lin, W.-W.; Hsieh, Y.-C. Detecting supraventricular tachycardia with smartwatches facilitates the decision for catheter ablation: A case series. *Pacing Clin. Electrophysiol.* **2022**, *45*, 157–159. [CrossRef] [PubMed]
25. Leroux, J.; Bordachar, P.; Strik, M.; Ramirez, D.F.; Ploux, S.; Chabaneix-Thomas, J.; Jalal, Z.; Thambo, J.-B. Recording an ECG With a Smartwatch in Newborns and Young Children: Feasibility and Perspectives. *Can. J. Cardiol.* **2021**, *37*, 1877–1879. [CrossRef] [PubMed]
26. Kassam, N.; Aziz, O.; Eghan, E.; Somji, S.; Mbithe, H.; Bapumia, M.; Mvungi, R.; Surani, S. Smart Watch Detection of Supraventricular Tachycardia (SVT): First Case from Tanzania. *Int. Med. Case Rep. J.* **2021**, *14*, 563–566. [CrossRef] [PubMed]
27. Ringwald, M.; Crich, A.; Beysard, N. Smart watch recording of ventricular tachycardia: Case study. *Am. J. Emerg. Med.* **2020**, *38*, 849.e3–849.e5. [CrossRef] [PubMed]
28. Goldstein, L.N.; Wells, M. Smart watch-detected tachycardia: A case of atrial flutter. *Oxf. Med. Case Rep.* **2019**, *2019*, 495–497. [CrossRef] [PubMed]
29. Bedi, A.; Al Masri, M.K.; Al Hennawi, H.; Qadir, S.; Ottman, P. The Integration of Artificial Intelligence into Patient Care: A Case of Atrial Fibrillation Caught by a Smartwatch. *Cureus* **2023**, *15*, e35941. [CrossRef] [PubMed]
30. Bogossian, H.; Iliodromitis, K.; Robl, S. Jump-Phänomen zur SVT-Induktion und die Korrelation mit der EKG-Dokumentation über die Apple Watch™. *Herzschr Elektrophys* **2020**, *31*, 426–429. [CrossRef] [PubMed]
31. Gu, K.; Marshall, K.; Robertson-Stovel, Q.; Zieroth, S. Polymorphic Ventricular Tachycardia Detected with a Smartwatch. *CJC Open* **2022**, *4*, 424–427. [CrossRef]

32. Burke, J.; Haigney, M.C.; Borne, R.; Krantz, M.J. Smartwatch detection of ventricular tachycardia: Case series. *Hear. Case Rep.* **2020**, *6*, 800–804. [CrossRef]
33. Jeong, H.K. Supraventricular Tachycardia Detected by Smart Watch. *Chonnam Med. J.* **2022**, *58*, 59–60. [CrossRef]
34. Ahmed, A.S.; Golden, K.M.; Foreman, J.R.; Padanilam, B.J. Using a smartwatch to identify the morphology of atrial flutter. *Hear. Case Rep.* **2020**, *6*, 808–809. [CrossRef] [PubMed]
35. Yeo, C.; Wang, Y.; Tan, V.H. Wide complex tachycardia captured on smartwatch. *Heart* **2021**, *107*, 626–684. [CrossRef]
36. Russo, V.; Ascrizzi, A.; Mauriello, A. "Narrow-Wide-Narrow" QRS Complex Tachycardia—Beware the Smartwatch Monsters. *JAMA Intern. Med.* **2023**, *183*, 726–727. [CrossRef]
37. Glöckner, D.; Zeus, T.; Kelm, M.; Makimoto, H. Recurrent nocturnal ST-T deviation and nonsustained ventricular tachycardias recorded with a smartwatch: A case report. *J. Cardiol. Cases* **2022**, *26*, 169–172. [CrossRef] [PubMed]
38. Leroux, J.; Strik, M.; Ramirez, D.F.; Ploux, S.; Sacristan, B.; Chabaneix-Thomas, J.; Jalal, Z.; Thambo, J.-B.; Bordachar, P. Using a smartwatch to record an electrocardiogram in the pediatric population. *J. Electrocardiol.* **2022**, *71*, 25–27. [CrossRef] [PubMed]
39. Overbeek, D.L.; Hogikyan, E.M.; Davis, M.; McGullicuddy, D.C. A unique case of bradycardia recognized by wearable technology as first presentation of complete heart block. *Am. J. Emerg. Med.* **2019**, *37*, 1989.e5–1989.e7. [CrossRef] [PubMed]
40. Yerasi, C.; O'Donoghue, S.; Satler, L.F.; Waksman, R. Apple Watch detecting high-grade block after transcatheter aortic valve implantation. *Eur. Heart J.* **2020**, *41*, 1096. [CrossRef] [PubMed]
41. Itoh, A. Apple Watch is useful in demonstrating coffee-triggered atrial fibrillation with a very short duration: A case report. *Eur. Heart J.* **2022**, *6*, ytac252. [CrossRef]
42. Mun, E.; Hong, J.; Kwon, S.; Lee, S.H.; Kim, W.; Lee, C. Digital health care and arrhythmia: A case of WPW syndrome in South Korea, 2020. *Ann. Occup. Environ. Med.* **2021**, *33*, e8. [CrossRef]
43. Deliniere, A.; Desgraz, B.; Herrera-Siklody, C.; Pascale, P.; Muller, O.; Pruvot, E. First case reported of a Prinzmetal vasospastic angina diagnosed with the help of a smartwatch. *EP Eur.* **2021**, *23*, 982. [CrossRef]
44. Walker, S.; Mallidi, J.R.; Gray, M.; Thakkar, A.B.; Song, E.J.; Hill, A.C.; Wisneski, A.D.; Phinney, L.; Quaye, E.; MacGregor, J.S. In the Nick of Time-Apple Watch Aids in Diagnosis of Chronic Type a Aortic Dissection. *J. Am. Coll. Cardiol.* **2023**, *81*, 3134. [CrossRef]
45. Weichert, I. 'My watch kept on alarming all night about my heart rate': Diagnosis of asymptomatic atrial fibrillation with fast ventricular response in a patient with a recent TIA as the result of a smartwatch alarm. *Oxf. Med. Case Rep.* **2019**, *2019*, omz014. [CrossRef] [PubMed]
46. Samal, S.; Singhania, N.; Bansal, S.; Sahoo, A. New-onset atrial fibrillation in a young patient detected by smartwatch. *Clin. Case Rep.* **2020**, *8*, 1331–1332. [CrossRef] [PubMed]
47. Jariwala, P.; Jadhav, K.P. Remote detection of arrhythmias using Apple watch: A useful wearable during COVID-19 pandemic. *IHJ Cardiovasc. Case Rep.* **2021**, *5*, 119–122. [CrossRef]
48. Pasli, S.; Imamoglu, M. Smart watch detected ventricular bigeminy during chest palpitations. *Am. J. Emerg. Med.* **2023**, *69*, 220.e1–220.e3. [CrossRef] [PubMed]
49. Patel, D.; Tarakji, K.G. Smartwatch diagnosis of atrial fibrillation in patient with embolic stroke of unknown source: A case report. *Cardiovasc. Digit. Health J.* **2021**, *2*, 84–87. [CrossRef] [PubMed]
50. Provencio, A.; Gil, M.Á.C. Smartwatch electrocardiogram records ST depression, premature ventricular complexes, and ventricular fibrillation. *Lancet* **2022**, *400*, e12. [CrossRef]
51. Seshadri, D.R.; Bittel, B.; Browsky, D.; Houghtaling, P.; Drummond, C.K.; Desai, M.; Gillinov, A.M. Accuracy of the Apple Watch 4 to Measure Heart Rate in Patients with Atrial Fibrillation. *IEEE J. Transl. Eng. Health Med.* **2020**, *8*, 1–4. [CrossRef] [PubMed]
52. Hwang, J.; Kim, J.; Choi, K.-J.; Cho, M.S.; Nam, G.-B.; Kim, Y.-H. Assessing Accuracy of Wrist-Worn Wearable Devices in Measurement of Paroxysmal Supraventricular Tachycardia Heart Rate. *Korean Circ. J.* **2019**, *49*, 437–445. [CrossRef]
53. Ploux, S.; Strik, M.; Caillol, T.; Ramirez, F.; Abu-Alrub, S.; Marchand, H.; Buliard, S.; Haïssaguerre, M.; Bordachar, P. Beyond the wrist: Using a smartwatch electrocardiogram to detect electrocardiographic abnormalities. *Arch. Cardiovasc. Dis.* **2022**, *115*, 29–36. [CrossRef]
54. Sequeira, N.; D'Shouza, D.; Angaran, P.; Aves, T.; Dorian, P. Common wearable devices demonstrate variable accuracy in measuring heart rate during supraventricular tachycardia. *HeartRhythm* **2020**, *17*, 854–859. [CrossRef] [PubMed]
55. Leroux, J.; Strik, M.; Ramirez, F.; Jalal, Z.; Thambo, J.-B.; Bordachar, P.; Racine, H.P.; Ploux, S.; Sacristan, B.; Chabaneix-Thomas, J. Feasibility and Diagnostic Value of Recording Smartwatch Electrocardiograms in Neonates and Children. *J. Pediatr.* **2022**, *253*, 40–45. [CrossRef] [PubMed]
56. Koshy, A.N.; Sajeev, J.K.; Nerlekar, N.; Brown, A.J.; Rajakariar, K.; Zureik, M.; Wong, M.; Roberts, L.; Street, M.; Cooke, J.; et al. Smart watches for heart rate assessment in atrial arrhythmias. *Int. J. Cardiol.* **2018**, *266*, 124–127. [CrossRef] [PubMed]
57. Abu-Alrub, S.; Strik, M.; Ramirez, F.; Moussaoui, N.; Racine, H.P.; Marchand, H.; Buliard, S.; Haïssaguerre, M.; Ploux, S.; Bordachar, P. Smartwatch Electrocardiograms for Automated and Manual Diagnosis of Atrial Fibrillation: A Comparative Analysis of Three Models. *Front. Cardiovasc. Med.* **2022**, *9*, 836375. [CrossRef] [PubMed]
58. Han, D.; Bashar, S.K.; Zieneddin, F.; Ding, E.; Whitcomb, C.; McManus, D.D.; Chon, K.H. Digital Image Processing Features of Smartwatch Photoplethysmography for Cardiac Arrhythmia Detection. *Annu. Int. Conf. IEEE Eng. Med. Biol. Soc.* **2020**, *2020*, 4071–4074.

59. Mannhart, D.; Lischer, M.; Knecht, S.; Lavallaz, J.D.F.; Strebel, I.; Serban, T.; Vögeli, D.; Schaer, B.; Osswald, S.; Mueller, C.; et al. Clinical Validation of 5 Direct-to-Consumer Wearable Smart Devices to Detect Atrial Fibrillation: BASEL Wearable Study. *JACC Clin. Electrophysiol.* **2023**, *9*, 232–242. [CrossRef] [PubMed]
60. Racine, H.-P.; Strik, M.; Van der Zande, J.; Abu-Alrub, S.; Caillol, T.; Haïssaguerre, M.; Ploux, S.; Bordachar, P. Role of Coexisting ECG Anomalies in the Accuracy of Smartwatch ECG Detection of Atrial Fibrillation. *Can. J. Cardiol.* **2022**, *38*, 1709–1712. [CrossRef] [PubMed]
61. Pengel, L.K.; Robbers-Visser, D.; Groenink, M.; Winter, M.M.; Schuuring, M.J.; Bouma, B.J.; Bokma, J.P. A comparison of ECG-based home monitoring devices in adults with CHD. *Cardiol. Young* **2023**, *33*, 1129–1135. [CrossRef]
62. Pepplinkhuizen, S.; Hoeksema, W.F.; Van Der Stuijt, W.; Wilde, A.A.M.; Smeding, L.; Van Steijn, N.J.; Winter, M.; Knops, R.E. Accuracy and clinical relevance of the single-lead Apple Watch electrocardiogram to identify atrial fibrillation. *Cardiovasc. Digit. Health J.* **2022**, *3*, s17–s22. [CrossRef]
63. Rajakariar, K.; Koshy, A.N.; Sajeev, J.K.; Nair, S.; Roberts, L.; Teh, A.W. Accuracy of a smartwatch based single-lead electrocardiogram device in detection of atrial fibrillation. *Heart* **2020**, *106*, 665–670. [CrossRef]
64. Wasserlauf, J.; Vogel, K.; Whisler, C.; Benjamin, E.; Helm, R.; Steinhaus, D.A.; Yousuf, O.; Passman, R.S. Accuracy of the Apple watch for detection of AF: A multicenter experience. *J. Cardiovasc. Electrophysiol.* **2023**, *34*, 1103–1107. [CrossRef] [PubMed]
65. Chang, P.-C.; Wen, M.-S.; Chou, C.-C.; Wang, C.-C.; Hung, K.-C. Atrial fibrillation detection using ambulatory smartwatch photoplethysmography and validation with simultaneous holter recording. *Am. Heart J.* **2022**, *247*, 55–62. [CrossRef] [PubMed]
66. Wyatt, K.D.; Poole, L.R.; Mullan, A.F.; Kopecky, S.L.; Heaton, H.A. Clinical evaluation and diagnostic yield following evaluation of abnormal pulse detected using Apple Watch. *J. Am. Med. Inform. Assoc.* **2020**, *27*, 1359–1363. [CrossRef] [PubMed]
67. Badertscher, P.; Lischer, M.; Mannhart, D.; Knecht, S.; Isenegger, C.; de Lavallaz, J.D.F.; Schaer, B.; Osswald, S.; Kühne, M.; Sticherling, C. Clinical validation of a novel smartwatch for automated detection of atrial fibrillation. *Heart Rhythm. $O_2$* **2022**, *3*, 208–210. [CrossRef] [PubMed]
68. Ford, C.; Xie, C.X.; Low, A.; Rajakariar, K.; Koshy, A.N.; Sajeev, J.K.; Roberts, L.; Pathik, B.; Teh, A.W. Comparison of 2 Smart Watch Algorithms for Detection of Atrial Fibrillation and the Benefit of Clinician Interpretation: SMART WARS Study. *JACC Clin. Electrophysiol.* **2022**, *8*, 782–791. [CrossRef] [PubMed]
69. Lee, C.; Lee, C.; Fernando, C.; Chow, C.-M. Comparison of Apple Watch vs. KardiaMobile: A Tale of Two Devices. *CJC* **2022**, *4*, 939–945. [CrossRef] [PubMed]
70. Roelle, L.; Ocasio, J.; Littell, L.; Fredman, E.; Miller, N.; Conner, T.; Van Hare, G.; Silvia, J.N.A. Expanding telehealth through technology: Use of digital health technologies during pediatric electrophysiology telehealth visits. *Cardiovasc. Digit. Health J.* **2022**, *3*, 256–261. [CrossRef] [PubMed]
71. Liao, M.-T.; Yu, C.-C.; Lin, L.-Y.; Pan, K.-H.; Tsai, T.-H.; Wu, Y.-C.; Liu, Y.-B. Impact of recording length and other arrhythmias on atrial fibrillation detection from wrist photoplethysmogram using smartwatches. *Sci. Rep.* **2022**, *12*, 5364. [CrossRef] [PubMed]
72. Dörr, M.; Nohturfft, V.; Brasier, N.; Bosshard, E.; Djurdjevic, A.; Gross, S.; Raichle, C.J.; Rhinisperger, M.; Stöckli, R.; Eckstein, J. The WATCH AF Trial: SmartWATCHes for Detection of Atrial Fibrillation. *JACC Clin. Electrophysiol.* **2019**, *5*, 199–208. [CrossRef]
73. Liu, X.; Fan, J.; Guo, Y.; Dai, H.; Xu, J.; Wang, L.; Hu, P.; Lin, X.; Li, C.; Zhou, D.; et al. Wearable Smartwatch Facilitated Remote Health Management for Patients Undergoing Transcatheter Aortic Valve Replacement. *J. Am. Heart Assoc.* **2022**, *11*, e023219. [CrossRef]
74. Feldman, K.; Duncan, R.G.; Nguyen, A.; Cook-Wiens, G.; Elad, Y.; Nuckols, T.; Pevnick, J.M. Will Apple devices' passive atrial fibrillation detection prevent strokes? Estimating the proportion of high-risk actionable patients with real-world user data. *J. Am. Med. Inform. Assoc.* **2022**, *29*, 1040–1049. [CrossRef] [PubMed]

healthcare

MDPI

*Systematic Review*

# Can Digital Technologies Be Useful for Weight Loss in Individuals with Overweight or Obesity? A Systematic Review

**Carmela Protano [1], Andrea De Giorgi [1], Federica Valeriani [2,*], Elisa Mazzeo [1], Stefano Zanni [1], Luigi Cofone [1], Gabriele D'Ancona [1], Anis Hasnaoui [3,4], Ivano Pindinello [1], Marise Sabato [1], Francesca Ubaldi [2], Veronica Volpini [2], Vincenzo Romano Spica [2], Matteo Vitali [1] and Francesca Gallè [5]**

1 Department of Public Health and Infectious Diseases, Sapienza University of Rome, 00185 Rome, Italy; carmela.protano@uniroma1.it (C.P.); andrea.degiorgi@uniroma1.it (A.D.G.); elisa.mazzeo@uniroma1.it (E.M.); stefano.zanni@uniroma1.it (S.Z.); luigi.cofone@uniroma1.it (L.C.); gabriele.dancona@uniroma1.it (G.D.); ivano.pindinello@uniroma1.it (I.P.); marise.sabato@uniroma1.it (M.S.); matteo.vitali@uniroma1.it (M.V.)

2 Department of Movement, Human, and Health Sciences, University of Rome Foro Italico, 00135 Rome, Italy; f.ubaldi@studenti.uniroma4.it (F.U.); v.volpini@studenti.uniroma4.it (V.V.); vincenzo.romanospica@uniroma4.it (V.R.S.)

3 Faculty of Medicine of Tunis, Tunis El Manar University, Rue Djebal Lakhdar, Tunis 1006, Tunisia; anis.hasnaoui@fmt.utm.tn

4 Signals and Smart Systems Lab L3S, National Engineering School of Tunis, Tunis El Manar University, Campus Universitaire Farhat Hached, Tunis 1068, Tunisia

5 Department of Medical, Movement and Wellbeing Sciences, University of Naples Parthenope, 80133 Naples, Italy; francesca.galle@uniparthenope.it

* Correspondence: federica.valeriani@uniroma4.it; Tel.: +39-(0)6-36733-257

**Abstract:** Digital technologies have greatly developed and impacted several aspects of life, including health and lifestyle. Activity tracking, mobile applications, and devices may also provide messages and goals to motivate adopting healthy behaviors, namely physical activity and dietary changes. This review aimed to assess the effectiveness of digital resources in supporting behavior changes, and thus influencing weight loss, in people with overweight or obesity. A systematic review was conducted according to the PRISMA guidelines. The protocol was registered in PROSPERO (CRD42023403364). Randomized Controlled Trials published from the database's inception to 8 November 2023 and focused on digital-based technologies aimed at increasing physical activity for the purpose of weight loss, with or without changes in diet, were considered eligible. In total, 1762 studies were retrieved and 31 met the inclusion criteria. Although they differed in the type of technology used and in their design, two-thirds of the studies reported significantly greater weight loss among electronic device users than controls. Many of these studies reported tailored or specialist-guided interventions. The use of digital technologies may be useful to support weight-loss interventions for people with overweight or obesity. Personalized feedback can increase the effectiveness of new technologies in motivating behavior changes.

**Keywords:** digital technologies; wearable devices; weight loss; overweight; obesity

## 1. Introduction

Obesity was classified as a disease as early as 1948, and due to the rising epidemic, the World Health Organization (WHO) has since defined obesity as "abnormal or excessive fat accumulation that may impair health", recognizing the need for action against this epidemic growth [1,2]. In the past two decades, the rates of obesity have rapidly increased across the developing world, and new statistics show that the prevalence of obesity is still growing [3]. It is also estimated that by 2030, obesity will affect over one billion people worldwide [4,5]. The continuous increase in the prevalence of overweight and obesity represents a major public health issue because scientific evidence has demonstrated that these conditions are a risk factor for several diseases, mainly chronic ones, such as diabetes, musculoskeletal disorders, cardiovascular diseases or even some cancers, such as gastroesophageal, breast, endometrial, ovarian, kidney and colon cancer [6–9]. Since the start of the International Obesity Task Force (IOTF) in 1995 [10], obesity has been calculated based on the body mass index (BMI) which is calculated based on the weight (in kg)/height (in $m^2$) ratio [11]. This measurement allows us to classify individuals into the "underweight", "normal weight", "overweight", or "obese" category. The WHO often classifies adult obesity in subclasses [Obese I, II, III] using BMI cutoffs [12]. This WHO classification is beneficial in distinguishing individuals who may have an increased risk of morbidity and mortality due to obesity [2]. Different determinants of health have been associated with obesity, such as individual, socio-economic, lifestyle and environmental factors [13]. It is widely acknowledged that there is a strong correlation between socio-economic status and malnutrition [14]. Some authors state that rapid urbanization can lead to "incorrect food choices" due to high consumption of ultra-processed food. The lack of time and education, in combination with the issue of poverty in this fast-paced world, can lead to poor food choices with a lack of nutritional value and quality and excessive sugar intake, along with a lack of physical activity (PA), which can lead to obesity [15,16]. Different methods for managing weight loss in individuals with overweight or obesity have been developed. These include different types of diets, pharmacotherapy and lifestyle interventions, alone or in combination. However, there is no one-size-fits-all approach, and new strategies are constantly being developed to keep up with changing population trends [17]. Furthermore, notwithstanding their effectiveness in determining weight loss, these methods may be ineffective in long-term body weight maintenance.

The introduction of new technologies has had a huge impact on lifestyle choices and health. In this modern era, in which connectivity and technological innovation are in, smartphones and wearables have rapidly gained popularity. Most of the population have their smartphones on or close to them throughout the day [18,19]. This increase in technology use has also contributed to the increasing adoption of sedentary lifestyle and to the consequent decrease in PA, which can be related to premature mortality and morbidity and an increased risk of major noncommunicable diseases [20]. On the other hand, many researchers have studied different ways to show how the use of digital eHealth or mHealth and new technology, such as wearable sensors, can actually enhance health promotion and prevention [21]. The term mHealth was first invented to describe emerging mobile communications and network technologies for healthcare [22], but later, the WHO defined mHealth as an integral part of eHealth, which refers to the cost-effective and secure use of information and communication technologies in support of health and health-related fields [23]. Good use of mobile phones and related apps can be effective in the delivery of information and improve the impact of treatment and healthcare delivery processes [24]. Likewise, wearable activity trackers such as fitness trackers, activity-tracking smartwatches and pedometers have shown to be very useful tools for overcoming physical inactivity and obesity. Many studies have shown that the use of these devices has been associated with increased PA, since they can support behavior-change techniques like self-monitoring and goal setting, as well as with improved BMI and lower risk of developing obesity [25–30]. In 2021, Berry et al. published a systematic review on the effectiveness of digital self-monitoring for weight loss in overweight and obesity, providing positive results in favor of new technologies [31]. In order to add further evidence to this field, the present review was performed to systematically analyze the available literature regarding behavioral weight loss interventions which aimed to increase participants' PA level by using digital technologies.

## 2. Materials and Methods

### 2.1. Selection Protocol and Search Strategy

This systematic review was conducted according to the Preferred Reporting Items for Systematic Review and Meta-Analysis (PRISMA) guidelines [32]. The protocol was then registered in PROSPERO with the number CRD42023403364. The research question of the present systematic review was: "Are digital technologies effective to support weight loss in behavioral interventions for individuals with overweight or obesity?". Thus, the review question was conceived using the "PICOS" Framework (P = Patient, problem or population; I = Intervention; C = Comparison, control or comparator; O = Outcome(s); S = Study type) according to the following eligibility criteria: (P) population: humans with overweight or obesity; (I) intervention: weight loss behavioral intervention based on electronic devices, mobile apps, artificial intelligence or smartphones/watches; (C) comparison: obese and overweight patients who did not undergo weight loss intervention based on electronic devices, mobile apps, artificial intelligence or smartphones/watches; (O) outcome: weight loss, BMI changes, anthropometric measures or body composition; (S) study: clinical trials. After a preliminary assessment of the literature, we decided to restrict the analysis to humans with obesity or overweight without any other comorbidities and to randomized clinical trials in order to obtain more consistent outcomes. Three electronic databases (PubMed, Scopus and Web of Science) were then scrutinized using the following search string: (obesity OR overweight) AND ("artificial intelligence" OR "machine learning" OR "mobile applications" OR "wearable electronic devices" OR smartphone OR smartwatch) AND ("dietary interventions" OR "nutritional status" OR "personalized nutrition" OR "weight control" OR "diet control" OR "weight loss"). Table S1 reports the search strategy for PubMed.

All databases were searched by title, abstract, and MeSH terms and keywords. The last search was performed from database inception to 8 November 2023.

### 2.2. Inclusion and Exclusion Criteria

This review was based on the use of electronic devices and new technologies to increase physical activity with the aim of achieving weight loss. In order to be eligible, studies were selected based on the following inclusion criteria: studies must be in English or Italian; weight loss must be associated with the use of electronic devices, mobile apps, artificial intelligence, or the use of a smartphone/smartwatch to manage/promote physical activity. Only randomized clinical trials were included. Furthermore, all studies which included underage individuals (<18 years) or patients who had other comorbidities or did not present with obesity or overweight were excluded from this systematic review. Reviews, meta-analysis, observational studies, case studies, proceedings, qualitative studies, editorials, commentary studies, pilot studies and any other type of article were also excluded. The references of reviews and meta-analyzes regarding the same issue were checked in order to identify further articles that did not come up on the baseline research results.

All results, from the beginning until to 8 November 2023, were then retrieved to reference software Zotero Systematic Review Manager v 6.0.26 for further screening and for the removal of duplicates. Ten authors (A.D.G., S.Z., E.M., F.U., V.V., L.C., M.S., G.D.A., I.P., A.H.) then proceeded with the selection of studies by Title and Abstracts according to the selection criteria listed above. All full texts were then read, independently, by the same authors and discussed further. Doubts and disagreements were settled by the other three authors (C.P., F.G., F.V.).

### 2.3. Data Extraction and Quality Assessment

Data were extracted from the selected studies by ten authors (A.D.G., S.Z., E.M., F.U., V.V., L.C., M.S., G.D.A., I.P., A.H.), according to specific characteristics which were previously approved by all authors. The data extraction table was constructed as follows: author, year, country, study design, study population, sample size, type of device, type of intervention, duration, frequency, comparison, main outcomes and secondary outcomes and results. These data were then arranged according to the type of study and the confounding factors.

Each included article was assessed using the Checklist to Evaluate a Report of a Nonpharmacological Trial (CLEAR NPT) [33]. This checklist has been specifically developed for measuring the quality of randomized clinical trials assessing nonpharmacological treatments. Indeed, the evaluation of nonpharmacological treatments such as technical devices, behavioral or psychological therapy involves some specific methodological considerations. For example, in nonpharmacological treatment trials, it is frequently impossible to carry out the blinding of care providers and participants, and the success of the treatment often depends on the experience and skill of the care providers. Besides, this kind of study is difficult to standardize [33]. Thus, according to several systematic reviews evaluating nonpharmacological treatment [34–37], the CLEAR NPT checklist was used [33]. This checklist contains 10 parameters, and for each item the choice was between "Yes", "No" or "Unclear". By adding up the answers, all authors could attribute a score. The score was between 10 and 8 for a low risk of bias, between 7 and 5 for a median risk of bias and lower than 5 for a high risk of bias.

The quality assessment was performed independently by ten authors (A.D.G., S.Z., E.M., F.U., V.V., L.C., M.S., G.D.A., I.P., A.H.) and the score was then verified by the other three authors (C.P., F.G., F.V.).

## 3. Results

A total of 1762 studies were retrieved from the following databases: PubMed, Web of Science, and Scopus. Of these, 796 duplicates were removed and 966 were screened by title and abstract. After the full-text assessment of the 133 articles that remained, 102 articles were excluded, 42 of them because they did not pertain to our question, 12 because the individuals were affected by other comorbidities, 16 because they were a different type of study from RCT, 7 because they considered a young age population (<18 years), 4 because did not have control groups, and 21 because they did not consider the assessment of changes in PA. Finally, we included 31 articles that met the inclusion criteria (Figure 1) [38–68].

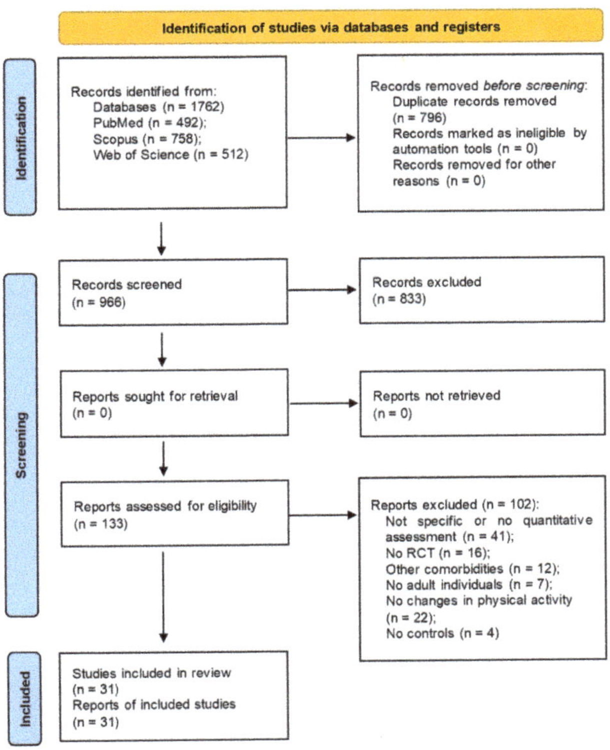


**Figure 1.** PRISMA flowchart for search strategy.

The main characteristics and findings of the interventions, as well as the primary and secondary weight-related outcomes assessed alongside weight loss, are shown in Table 1.

**Table 1.** Characteristics of the included studies.

| Author Year Country | Sample Size Study Population | Type of Device | Type of Intervention, Duration, Frequency | Comparison | Main and Secondary Outcomes | Results | Quality |
|---|---|---|---|---|---|---|---|
| Apinaniz et al., 2019 Spain [38] | 110, 54 intervention and 56 controls; 38.5 ± 5 years; 72% F and 28% M; BMI 32.7 ± 4.9 kg/m$^2$ | Smartphone app AKTIDIET | The AKTIDIET app on patients' smartphones provided reinforced health advice, including exercise programs, food intake tracking and instructional videos. Patients followed up at 1, 3 and 6 months. The program required daily self-reporting of diet and exercise, with personalized feedback and weekly assignments. The examination was repeated at 16 and 38 weeks | Usual care and motivational advice including recommendations on diet and physical exercise | Body weight after 6 months and adherence to dietary and exercise recommendations | There were no significant differences in weight change, nor in the adherence to dietary or physical exercise recommendations | 6 Yes, 3 No, 1 Unclear; Medium Bias Risk |
| Balk-Møller et al., 2017 Denmark [39] | 566, 355 intervention and 211 controls; 47 ± 10 years; 92.2% F and 7.8% M; BMI 73.8 ± 15.4 kg/m$^2$ | Web and smartphone app SoSu-life | Daily self-reporting of diet and exercise, personalized feedback about specific health issues related to the chosen pledge, with weekly assignments and challenges. The examination was repeated at 16 and 38 weeks | No activities | Change in body weight and anthropometric markers | The SoSu-life group had a larger decrease in body weight (−1.01 kg, $p = 0.03$), body fat percentage (−0.78%, $p = 0.03$), and WC (−1.79 cm, $p = 0.007$) after 38 weeks compared with the control group. The SoSu-life group had a larger decrease in body weight (−1.54 kg, $p < 0.001$) and a decrease in body fat percentage of −0.81% ($p = 0.003$) compared with the control group during the first 16 weeks | 9 Yes, 0 No, 1 Unclear: Low Bias Risk |

**Table 1.** *Cont.*

| Author Year Country | Sample Size Study Population | Type of Device | Type of Intervention, Duration, Frequency | Comparison | Main and Secondary Outcomes | Results | Quality |
|---|---|---|---|---|---|---|---|
| Beatty et al., 2020 USA [40] | 72, 37 intervention and 35 controls; 37.7 ± 15.3 years, 65.3% F and 34.7% M; BMI 31.3 ± 3.2 $kg/m^2$ | A wrist-worn ELMM device capable of tracking bites, displayed after each meal, as well as the number of steps taken by the user. | WD for 8 weeks. Workbook offered education regarding eating rate, energy intake and energy expenditure. | WO | Weight loss | No significant difference between WD and WO groups with respect to weight change [−0.46 (1.11) vs. 0.26 (0.82) kg, respectively, $p = 0.40$] | 4 Yes, 2 No, 4 Unclear; High Bias Risk |
| Block et al., 2015 USA [41] | 339, 163 intervention and 176 controls; 55 ± 8.9 years; 31.3% F and 68.7%; BMI 31.2 ± 4.4 $kg/m^2$ | Alive-PD program via Web, smartphone and automated phone calls | The program offered personalized dietary and PA goals, tracking tools, health information, quizzes, social support, feedback and reminders via web, email, IVR phone calls and mobile. The program lasted for a year, with regular goal setting and contact. Users received goals weekly for the first six months and bi-weekly thereafter, plus midweek reminders. | No contact from Alive-PD system except reminders to complete a 3-month and 6-month online follow-up questionnaire | Changes in body weight, BMI, WC | Reductions in weight, BMI and WC were all significantly greater in the intervention group than the control group ($p = 0.01$) | 9 Yes, 0 No, 1 Unclear; Low Bias Risk |

**Table 1.** *Cont.*

| Author Year Country | Sample Size Study Population | Type of Device | Type of Intervention, Duration, Frequency | Comparison | Main and Secondary Outcomes | Results | Quality |
|---|---|---|---|---|---|---|---|
| Burke et al., 2022 USA [42] | 502, 251 intervention and 251 controls; 45.0 ± 14.4 years; 79.5% F and 20.5% M; BMI 33.7 ± 4.0 kg/m$^2$ | Fitbit Charge 2, smartphone app | SM+FB of diet, PA and weight in a behavioral weight-loss intervention at 6 and 12 months. The calorie goal was determined based on the person's baseline body weight and real-time synced SM data to send messages that were responsive to the participants' SM entries; wrist-worn Fitbit Charge 2 was used to self-monitor PA with an aim of 150 min/week by 12 weeks. Participants weighed themselves daily. In-app messages were sent 3 times daily over the 12-month intervention | SM | Weight loss and changes in BMI from baseline to 6 months, percentage of body fat, WC | At 6 months, there was a significant percentage of weight change in both groups (SM+FB: −3.16%, 95% CI: −3.85% to −2.47%, $p < 0.0001$; SM: −3.20%, 95% CI: −3.86% to −2.54%, $p < 0.0001$) but no significant between-group mean difference (−0.04%, 95% CI: −0.99% to 0.91%, $p = 0.940$). | 9 Yes, 0 No, 1 Unclear; Low Bias Risk |
| Cho et al., 2020 Republic of Korea [43] | 129, 88 intervention and 41 controls; 49.2 ± 7.7 years; 51.2% F and 48.8% M; BMI 26.3 ± 3 kg/m$^2$ | Smartphone app | An app-based diet and exercise self-logging group (app only), or app-based self-logging and personalized coaching from professional dieticians and exercise coordinators group. The app delivered structured health-related curricula and personalized feedback based on reviews of the user's logs. Assessments were performed at baseline, week 6, week 12 and week 24 | Baseline education; no apps | Weight changes, body fat mass, WC between baseline and follow-up assessments | Those using the app with the personalized coaching group had greater body weight reductions (control −0.12 ± 0.30 kg; app only −0.35 ± 0.36 kg, $p = 0.67$; app with personalized coaching −0.96 ± 0.37 kg, $p = 0.08$), specifically by body fat mass reduction (control −0.13 ± 0.34 kg; app only −0.64 ± 0.38 kg, $p = 0.22$; app with personalized coaching −0.79 ± 0.38 kg, $p = 0.08$) | 9 Yes, 0 No, 1 Unclear; Low Bias Risk |

**Table 1.** *Cont.*

| Author Year Country | Sample Size Study Population | Type of Device | Type of Intervention, Duration, Frequency | Comparison | Main and Secondary Outcomes | Results | Quality |
|---|---|---|---|---|---|---|---|
| Duncan et al., 2020 Australia [44] | 116, 39 Enhanced, 41 Traditional and 36 Control; 44.5 ± 10.4 years; 70.7% F and 29.3% M; BMI 31.7 ± 3.9 kg/m$^2$ | Smartphone app Balanced, Fitbit, Accelerometer (Geneactiv) | In a 6-month intervention, Enhanced and Traditional group participants received personalized dietary recommendations, access to the 'Balanced' smartphone app, a calorie-counting platform, a face-to-face dietary consultation, a Fitbit activity tracker, body weight scales and a handbook. | The waitlist control group was asked to maintain current weight, PA and dietary intake | Weight change | At 6 months, weight was not significantly different between the pooled intervention groups and control group (difference = −0.92, 95% CI (−3.33, 1.48)) or 12 months (difference = 0.00, 95% CI (−2.62, 2.62)). | 8 Yes, 2 No, 0 Unclear; Low Bias Risk |
| Farage et al., 2021 USA [45] | 191, 103 intervention and 88 controls; 34.8 ± 7.6 years; 51.8% F and 48.2% M; BMI 46% 25–30 and 54% over 30 kg/m$^2$ | Smartphone app Lose it! | Electronic diet and exercise self-monitoring and weight loss interventions on 4- and 12-month weight loss; 28 phone calls over 12 months with counselors, regular feedback through email and weight monitoring using the BodyTrace e-scale. In addition, the participants received a personalized exercise plan based on their self-reported baseline PA. They were asked to gradually increase aerobic exercise from their baseline level until reaching 225–250 min weekly | Self-paced participants received assistance upon request | Weight change | At 4 months, the counselor-initiated treatment group lost an average of 3.7 kg (SD 3.6), and the self-paced treatment group lost 0.6 kg (SD 3.1). At 12 months, the counselor-initiated treatment lost 2.4 kg (SD 5.0) on average and the self-paced treatment group gained 0.2 kg (SD 5.1). | 7 Yes, 2 No, 1 Unclear; Medium Bias Risk |

**Table 1.** *Cont.*

| Author Year Country | Sample Size Study Population | Type of Device | Type of Intervention, Duration, Frequency | Comparison | Main and Secondary Outcomes | Results | Quality |
|---|---|---|---|---|---|---|---|
| Fukuoka et al., 2015 USA [46] | 61, 30 intervention and 31 controls; 55.2 ± 9.0 years; 77% F and 23% M; BMI 33.3 ± 6.0 kg/m$^2$ | Smartphone app and Omron pedometer | The intervention lasted 5 months and consisted of six in-person sessions and a home-based exercise program. A study-developed mobile phone app and pedometer augmented the intervention and providing self-monitoring tools (recording weight, activity and caloric intake). It was also used to deliver interactive intervention content through daily messages, video clips and quizzes | The control group used the pedometer, but the settings were changed to display the number of steps. No specific step goals were provided. Research staff removed the run-in mobile app from the participant's iPhone or collected the iPhone if one had been provided | Percentage change in weight and BMI from baseline to 5-month follow-up, hip circumference, objectively measured (via pedometer) PA | The intervention group (n = 30) lost an average of 6.2 (5.9) kg (−6.8% [5.7%]) between baseline and 5-month follow-up compared to the control group's (n = 31) gain of 0.3 (3.0) kg (0.3% [5.7%]) ($p < 0.001$). The intervention group had greater reductions in hip circumference ($p < 0.001$) | 6 yes, 2 no, 2 unclear; Medium Bias Risk |
| Hernández-Reyes et al., 2020 Spain [47] | 90, 45 intervention and 45 controls; 41.5 ± 11.3 years; 100% F; BMI 31.8 ± 5.3 kg/m$^2$ | Automatic push notifications | Objectives for diet and PA through exclusive access to specific functionalities of the app and automatic push notifications on specific days with personalized health-related and motivational messages | No access to functionalities related to the self-monitoring of weight at home, gamification or prescription of PA | Body fat loss, muscle mass and weight loss at 6 months | Receiving notifications during the intervention increased body fat loss (mean −12.9% [SD 6.7] in the intervention group vs. mean −7.0% [SD 5.7] in the control group; $p < 0.001$) and helped to maintain muscle mass (mean −0.8% [SD 4.5] in the intervention group vs. mean −3.2% [SD 2.8] in the control group; $p < 0.018$). These variations between groups led to a non-significant difference in weight loss (mean −7.9 kg [SD 3.9] in the intervention group vs. mean −7.1 kg [SD 3.4] in the control group; $p > 0.05$). | 4 Yes, 3 No, 3 Unclear; High Bias Risk |

**Table 1.** *Cont.*

| Author Year Country | Sample Size Study Population | Type of Device | Type of Intervention, Duration, Frequency | Comparison | Main and Secondary Outcomes | Results | Quality |
|---|---|---|---|---|---|---|---|
| Hong et al., 2022 Republic of Korea [48] | 29, 12 intervention and 17 controls; 80 ± 3.3 years; 100% F; Weight 58.63 ± 8.17 kg | Smartphone, 24-inch LCD display monitor and a smartphone mirroring device (Miracast MRC-01, Actto) | Smartphone mirroring-based telepresence exercise Program with exercise instructor who had a major in exercise physiology, in which participants exercised in their homes for 20–40 min three times a week for 12 weeks. Nutrition advice and fitness monitoring once a month. | Same exercise program at the senior citizen center | Weight loss, body composition and physical function | Weight ($p = 0.006$) significantly decreased in the control group, body fat percentage decreased significantly in the intervention ($p = 0.026$) and in the control ($p = 0.001$) groups, and skeletal muscle mass ($p = 0.44$) significantly increased in the control group. Two-way repeated-measures ANOVA revealed no significant interaction effects on all variables. | 8 Yes, 0 No, 2 Unclear; Low Bias Risk |
| Hurkmans et al., 2018 Belgium [49] | 102, 80 intervention and 22 controls; 45.5 ± 10.3 years; 70% F and 30% M; BMI 32 ± 2.0 kg/m$^2$ | Smartphone app | All intervention groups received the same advice from a registered dietician and a qualified PA coach during a 12-week period. The methods used included a conventional face-to-face weight loss program, a weight loss app program (app group) and a partial face-to-face and partial app program (combi group) | The control group did not receive any information during the same period | Weight reduction (5% decrease), BMI, metabolic risk factors, dietary pattern and PA | In the conventional group, app group, and combi group, BMI decreased significantly ($p = 0.004$, $p = 0.005$, and $p < 0.001$, respectively), no significant decrease was found in the control group. A significant time x group effect was found for BMI ($p = 0.006$), with the control group being significantly different compared with all other intervention groups.<br>No significant differences were found between the conventional group and the app group and between the conventional group and the combi group ($p = 0.41$). However, the combi group had significantly higher decrease in BMI compared with the app group ($p = 0.03$). | 8 Yes, 0 No, 2 Unclear; Low Bias Risk |

**Table 1.** *Cont.*

| Author Year Country | Sample Size Study Population | Type of Device | Type of Intervention, Duration, Frequency | Comparison | Main and Secondary Outcomes | Results | Quality |
|---|---|---|---|---|---|---|---|
| Hutchesson et al., 2018 Australia [50] | 57, 29 intervention and 28 controls; 27.1 ± 4.7 years; unspecified gender; BMI 29.4 ± 2.5 kg/m$^2$ | Advice via smartphone app, SMS, emails and website | Six-month weight loss program delivered using e-Health technologies only, comprising five delivery modes (website, app, email, text messages and social media) and using social cognitive theory and control theory theoretical frameworks. Participants received automated personalized email feedback from their accredited practicing dietitian. Individualized energy intake and energy expenditure goals were set for each participant based on their estimated energy expenditure and creating a 2500 kJ/day energy deficit to help facilitate a 0.5–1 kg weight loss/week, goals to be achieved by modifying eating and physical habits | No intervention for six months: they were instructed to continue their usual eating and PA habits | Weight change at six months | No significant between-group differences were observed for weight ($p > 0.05$); significant mean difference favoring the intervention group was observed for body fat (kg) (−3.10 (−5.69, 0.52), $p = 0.019$). | 8 Yes, 0 No, 2 Unclear; Low Bias Risk |

**Table 1.** *Cont.*

| Author Year Country | Sample Size Study Population | Type of Device | Type of Intervention, Duration, Frequency | Comparison | Main and Secondary Outcomes | Results | Quality |
|---|---|---|---|---|---|---|---|
| Jakicic et al., 2016 USA [51] | 471, 237 intervention and 234 controls; mean 30.9 years; 71% F and 29% M; mean BMI 31.2 $kg/m^2$ | Wearable device and web interface | Low-calorie diet, PA, and group counseling sessions. At 6 months, telephone counseling sessions and text message prompts were added to the interventions, with self-monitoring of diet and PA using a website (standard intervention) or a wearable device (enhanced intervention). Group-based sessions were scheduled weekly for the initial 6 months and monthly between months 7 and 24. | Same intervention but only with self-monitoring; no website or wearable devices | Weight change, body composition | At 24 months, weight loss was 2.4 kg (95% CI, 1.0 to 3.7) lower in the enhanced intervention group compared with the standard intervention group ($p = 0.002$). In post hoc analysis, the percent weight loss differed significantly between the standard intervention and enhanced intervention groups ($p < 0.001$). Both groups had significant improvements in body composition, with no significant difference between groups. | 9 Yes, 0 No, 1 Unclear; Low Bias Risk |

**Table 1.** *Cont.*

| Author Year Country | Sample Size Study Population | Type of Device | Type of Intervention, Duration, Frequency | Comparison | Main and Secondary Outcomes | Results | Quality |
|---|---|---|---|---|---|---|---|
| Jiang et al., 2021 China [52] | 272, 136 intervention and 136 controls; 31.8 ± 5 years; 41.2% F and 58.8% M; BMI 32.5 ± 3.5 kg/m$^2$ | Smartphone app and daily online instructions | Six-month intervention. Companion-Intensive Multi-aspect Weight Management (CIMWM) strategy focusing on a combination of online and offline medical interventions with daily lifestyle supervision and guidance of diet and exercise. Participants received an individualized calorie-restricted diet which was developed by registered dietitians. Individualized exercise plans were created by health managers for each participant based on their health status and exercise capacity. Participants in the CIMWM group were provided with two Fit Nutrition Bars daily as well as monthly face-to-face guidance and daily online instructions via the mobile application "Medical Weight Management", which allowed them to upload data regarding their daily weight, as well as food diaries, lifestyle supervision and guidance of diet and exercise. | Traditional multi-aspect weight management was required to complete daily self-monitoring instead of being offered as daily online instructions | Clinically significant weight loss (defined as weight loss ≥ 5%), anthropometric measures and determination of metabolic indexes | Significant changes in BMI, body fat and skeletal muscle mass-to-visceral fat area ratio from baseline to 6 months were observed between two groups ($p < 0.05$). | 5 Yes, 2 No, 3 Unclear; Medium Bias Risk |

**Table 1.** *Cont.*

| Author Year Country | Sample Size Study Population | Type of Device | Type of Intervention, Duration, Frequency | Comparison | Main and Secondary Outcomes | Results | Quality |
|---|---|---|---|---|---|---|---|
| Johnson et al., 2019 USA [53] | 30, 20 intervention and 10 controls; 43.2 ± 11 years; BMI 36.1 ± 6.8 kg/m$^2$ | Wireless watches and weight scales to sync with personal smartphones | Participants assigned to the VCIP group received individualized health coaching by a multidisciplinary team (registered dietitian, exercise physiologist, certified athletic trainer and medical doctor) based on data uploaded over the 12-week intervention period | m-health devices; no health coaching sessions, nor team member feedback on steps per day nor calories uploaded | Weight change | There was a significant ($p < 0.001$) difference for post-intervention weight loss between VC (8.23 kg) compared to IP (3.2 kg) and CG (2.9 kg) | 7 Yes, 1 No, 2 Unclear; Medium Bias Risk |
| Johnston et al., 2013 USA [54] | 292, 147 intervention and 145 controls; 46.5 ± 10.5 years; 90% F and 10% M; BMI 33 ± 3.6 kg/m$^2$ | WW smartphone application and WW online tools | WW program based on food and activity plan, group support and skills to change behavior, followed through weekly meetings. Weights and self-reported use of access modes were measured at baseline and at 3 and 6 months | Self-help group with publicly available printed materials explaining basic dietary and exercise guidelines for safe weight loss | Reductions in BMI and weight | WW subjects lost 4.6 kg and self-help subjects lost 0.6 kg at 6 months. Participants in the WW group significantly decreased their weight (F = 34.5, $p < 0.001$) and BMI at 6 months (F = 36.7, $p < 0.001$) compared with those in the self-help group | 6 Yes, 3 No, 1 Unclear; Medium Bias Risk |
| Laing et al., 2014 USA [55] | 212, 105 intervention and 107 controls; 43.1 ± 14.5 years; 73.1% F and 26.9% M; BMI 33.4 ± 7.09 kg/m$^2$ | Smartphone app | 6 months of usual care without (n = 107) or with (n = 105) MyFitnessPal; dietary intake, PA and weight self-monitoring, goal setting, and feedback | Control group patients were free to "choose any activities you'd like to lose weight," without specifying any particular interventions | Weight loss at 6 months, 3 self-reported behavioral mediators of weight loss (exercise, diet and self-efficacy in weight loss) at baseline and at 3 and 6 months | At 3 months, participants in the control group gained an average of 0.24 kg, whereas those in the intervention group lost 0.03 kg (between-group difference 0.27 kg [95% CI, 1.13 to 0.60 kg]; $p = 0.53$). At 6 months, participants in the control group gained an average of 0.27 kg and those in the intervention group lost 0.03 kg (between-group difference 0.30 kg [CI, 1.50 to 0.95 kg]; $p = 0.63$) | 7 Yes, 1 No, 2 Unclear; Medium Bias Risk |

**Table 1.** *Cont.*

| Author Year Country | Sample Size Study Population | Type of Device | Type of Intervention, Duration, Frequency | Comparison | Main and Secondary Outcomes | Results | Quality |
|---|---|---|---|---|---|---|---|
| Lugones-Sanchez et al., 2020 Spain [56] | 440, 231 intervention and 209 controls; 48.1 ± 10 years; 69.3% F and 30.7% M; BMI 32.8 ± 3.4 kg/m$^2$ | Smartphone app (EVIDENT 3 APP) and Smart band (Mi Band 2, Xiaomi) | 3-month intervention with counseling, smartphone app and smart band (Mi Band 2, Xiaomi). After 7 days, subjects were trained to use the device and the app to allow the dietary intake to be self-reported daily and PA data were collected automatically from the smart band. Once all of the daily information was collected, the app integrated the data to create personalized recommendations based on the subjects' characteristics and specific objectives and goals for weight loss. | Controls only had counseling | Weight loss and changes in some parameters of body composition at baseline and 3 months | The mHealth intervention produced a greater loss of body weight (−1.97 kg, 95% CI −2.39 to −1.54) relative to standard counseling at 3 months (−1.13 kg, 95% CI −1.56 to −0.69): $p < 0.01$. A significant between-group difference was noted only in BMI (−0.54 kg/m$^2$, 95% CI −0.84 to −0.24); $p < 0.01$. | 8 Yes, 1 No, 1 Unclear; Low Risk of Bias |
| Lugones-Sanchez et al., 2022 Spain [57] | 650, 318 intervention and 332 controls; 48.3 ± 9.6 years; 68.5% F and 31.5% M; BMI 33.04 ± 3.5 kg/m$^2$ | Smartphone app, wristband, brief counseling | The intervention group received training to use the app and the smart band for 3 months; self-monitoring, tailored feedback and a PA record. The app integrated the data to create personalized healthy food recommendations. The smart band was set to congratulate the user when reaching 10,000 steps/day, and the app displayed this step recommendation | Brief counseling | Weight loss, body composition | At 12 months, significant mean differences were found between groups for weight −0.26 (−1.21 to 0.70), BMI −0.06 (−0.41 to 0.28), waist circumference −0.48 (−1.62 to 0.66), hip circumference −0.69 (−1.62 to 0.25) and body adiposity index −0.33 (−0.77 to 0.11) | 8 Yes, 1 No,1 Unclear; Low Bias Risk |

**Table 1.** *Cont.*

| Author Year Country | Sample Size Study Population | Type of Device | Type of Intervention, Duration, Frequency | Comparison | Main and Secondary Outcomes | Results | Quality |
|---|---|---|---|---|---|---|---|
| Martin et al., 2015 USA [58] | 40, 20 intervention and 20 controls; 44.4 ± 11.8 years; 82.5% F and 17.5% M; BMI 29.8 ± 2.9 kg/m$^2$ | Smartphone app Smartloss and accelerometer | SmartLoss participants (n = 20) were prescribed a 1200 to 1400 kcal/d diet and were provided with a smartphone, body weight scale and accelerometer that wirelessly transmitted body weight and step data to a website. Participants received feedback and treatment recommendations once a week based on their weight graph, while counselors educated each participant that the weight graph was used to objectively quantify adherence to the calorie prescription and to guide counseling and treatment recommendations | Attention-matched health education with health tips on smartphone | Change in body weight and waist circumference | Weight loss was significantly larger in the SmartLoss (least squares mean ± SEM: −9.4 ± 0.5%) compared with the Health Education group (−0.6 ± 0.5%), $p < 0.001$; Mean ± SEM waist circumference change for the SmartLoss group was 21.6 ± 1.00, 25.3 ± 1.01, and 26.9 ± 1.00 cm while in the Health Education group was 1.3 ± 1.04, 1.7 ± 1.04, and 1.7 ± 1.00 cm at weeks 4, 8, and 12, respectively, $p < 0.05$. | 6 Yes, 1 No, 3 Unclear; Medium Bias Risk |
| Martínez-Rodríguez et al., 2022 Spain [59] | 80, 40 intervention and 40 controls; 45.7 ± 8.5 years; BMI 32.9 ± 5.1 kg/m$^2$ | Smartphone app | Dietary and activity recommendations provided with a wearable device (Fitbit Charge 2) and the dietary supplement Metabolaid®+ an activity bracelet for monitoring+ smartphone app | Dietary and activity recommendations provided with Fitbit Charge 2 and the dietary supplement + an activity bracelet for monitoring | Weight loss, body composition, anthropometric measurements | Both groups lost a significant amount of body weight ($p < 0.001$), while the group using the app also lowered their fat mass ($p < 0.005$). | 3 Yes, 4 No, 3 Unclear; High Bias Risk |

**Table 1.** *Cont.*

| Author Year Country | Sample Size Study Population | Type of Device | Type of Intervention, Duration, Frequency | Comparison | Main and Secondary Outcomes | Results | Quality |
|---|---|---|---|---|---|---|---|
| Nakata et al., 2022 Japan [60] | 141, 72 intervention and 69 controls; 43.2 ± 9.3 years; 26% F and 74% M; BMI 27.6 ± 3.5 kg/m$^2$ | Smartphone app Healthcare, CALO mama Plus | 3-month intervention. Smartphone healthcare application CALO mama Plus registered daily diet, exercise, calculated dietary intake and provided advice using artificial intelligence technology. The participants wore the device for at least 10 h/day for more than 3 days | No intervention; they continued their current lifestyle without any dietary apps | Body weight change over 3 months | The change in body weight was −2.4 ± 4.0 kg and −0.7 ± 3.3 kg in the intervention and control groups, respectively, with a significant between-group difference in body weight change (−1.60 kg; 95% confidence interval −2.83 to −0.38; $p = 0.011$). | 6 Yes, 3 No, 1 Unclear; Medium Bias Risk |
| Roth et al., 2023 Finland [61] | 150, 77 intervention and 73 controls; 43.4 ± 10.9 years; 91.3% F and 8.7% M; BMI 35.8 ± 3.2 kg/m$^2$ | Smartphone app | 12 months of healthy lifestyle that supported sustainable weight loss through physical therapy and proper nutrition | No app or electronic devices | Weight loss and changes from baseline to 12 months in body fat distribution | The intervention group lost, on average, 7.75% (95% CI: 9.66% to 5.84%) of their initial body weight after 12 months, whereas the weight of the controls did not change (mean = 0.00% [95% CI: 1.98% to 1.99%]); $p < 0.001$. | 6 Yes, 3 No, 1 Unclear; Medium Bias Risk |

**Table 1.** *Cont.*

| Author Year Country | Sample Size Study Population | Type of Device | Type of Intervention, Duration, Frequency | Comparison | Main and Secondary Outcomes | Results | Quality |
|---|---|---|---|---|---|---|---|
| Saldivar et al., 2021 USA [62] | 371, 185 intervention and 186 controls; 54.1 ± 10.5 years; 82.8% F and 17.2% M; BMI 43.1 ± 9.53 kg/m$^2$ | Smartphone app and text messages | 12-week and 20-week texting program—POWER Program with three text messages per week, which included appointment reminders, health and wellness tips and educational information related to care and disease management. The 12- and 20-week programs allowed patients to set goals around exercise or nutrition. The 20-week program also included motivational, mental health and stress management messages to help encourage healthy lifestyle changes | Only medical group visits without any text messages | Weight loss | Both POWER and POWER + 20-week texting groups had a significant reduction in weight at their final group visit compared to their baseline (POWER, 114 ± 27 kg vs. 112 ± 26 kg, $p < 0.001$; POWER + 20-week texting, 111 ± 28 kg vs. 109 ± 28 kg, $p < 0.01$), but not the 12-week texting group (114 ± 29 kg vs. 113 ± 29 kg, $p = 0.22$), with no differences between the groups. | 3 Yes, 2 No, 5 Unclear; High Bias Risk |
| Spring et al., 2017 USA [63] | 96, 32 Standard, 32 Technology supported, 32 Self-guided; 39.3 ± 11.7 years, 84.4% F and 15.6% M; BMI 34.6 ± 3.0 kg/m$^2$ | Smartphone app ENGAGED and wireless accelerometer | 6 month intervention. STND and TECH groups received eight 90 min in-person weekly group sessions. TECH used a smartphone application with social networking features and wireless accelerometer, and received 2 to 4 personalized messages per week by trained coaches with at least a bachelor's degree who reviewed the self-monitoring and goal attainment and helped participants solve problems. If fidelity fell below 90%, the coach was retrained by a doctoral-level staff member | Self-guided (SELF) and Standard (STND) used paper diaries to self-monitor diet, activity and weight | Primary weight loss and behavioral adherence | Weight loss was greater for TECH and STND than SELF at 6 months (25.7 kg [95% confidence interval: 27.2 to 24.1] vs. 22.7 kg [95% confidence interval: 25.1 to 20.3], $p < 0.05$) but not at 12 months.<br>TECH and STND did not differ except that more STND (59%) than TECH (34%) achieved 5% weight loss at 6 months ($p < 0.05$). | 9 Yes, 1 No, 0 Unclear; Low Bias Risk |

**Table 1.** *Cont.*

| Author Year Country | Sample Size Study Population | Type of Device | Type of Intervention, Duration, Frequency | Comparison | Main and Secondary Outcomes | Results | Quality |
|---|---|---|---|---|---|---|---|
| Stephens et al., 2017 USA [64] | 62, 31 intervention and 31 controls; median 20 years; 71% F and 29% M; BMI 28.5 kg/m$^2$ | Smartphone app | Smartphone application + health coach intervention and counseling sessions, providing health coach with the ability to monitor and track all participant progress on a real-time basis and text messages focused on current diet or PA status. Participants were encouraged to exercise at least 150 min/week at moderate intensity | Counseling session | Weight, BMI, WC, dietary habits, PA habits and self-efficacy for healthy eating and PA at 3 months | The control group gained a slight amount of weight (0.3 kg) from baseline to 3 months, while participants in the Smartphone + Health Coach group lost a significant amount (−1.8 kg, $p < 0.01$); the difference in weight change between groups was statistically significant ($p = 0.026$). The smartphone group also had a significant decrease in BMI ($p < 0.01$) and WC ($p < 0.01$) | 3 Yes, 2 No, 5 Unclear; High Bias Risk |
| Thomas et al., 2020 USA [65] | 146, 72 intervention and 74 controls; 58.3 ± 10.3 years; 78.1% F and 21.9% M; BMI 91.4 ± 15.6 kg/m$^2$ | Website and smartphone app | 6 months of no-cost access to the online web-based virtual reality program, accessible via website and mobile app. Half of the participants were randomized to also receive the ES) program, which consisted of four separate 'scenarios' focused on challenges at home, the workplace, the gym and social gatherings that were made available to participants at weeks 2, 4, 6 and 8, respectively, with daily points goals personalized according to sex, age, starting weight and activity level | Online weight management program alone (WW) | Body weight loss, satisfaction with the weight-loss program | Both groups achieved statistically significant weight loss across the trial, with no difference in mean ± standard error weight loss between WW and WW + ES at 3 months (2.7 ± 1.1 kg vs. 4.2 ± 1.1 kg, respectively; $p = 0.086$) but greater weight loss in WW + ES at 6 months (2.6 ± 1.3 kg vs. 4.9 ± 1.3 kg, respectively; $p = 0.042$) | 8 Yes, 0 No, 2 Unclear; Low Bias Risk |

**Table 1.** *Cont.*

| Author Year Country | Sample Size Study Population | Type of Device | Type of Intervention, Duration, Frequency | Comparison | Main and Secondary Outcomes | Results | Quality |
|---|---|---|---|---|---|---|---|
| Thorgeirsson et al., 2022 Iceland [66] | 146, 95 intervention and 51 controls; 46.8 ± 11.7 years; 92.5% F and 7.5%; BMI 36.3 ± 5.2 kg/m$^2$ | Smartphone app Sidekick | Standard treatment supplemented with a digital therapeutic mobile application designed to increase frequency of healthy behaviors through goal-setting, self-monitoring and completion of health-related tasks in nutrition, PA and stress management for 4 months | Standard weekly coaching sessions for 4 months | BMI at 4 months | The weight loss was 3.6% among those treated per-protocol (n = 70), and 1.5% among those not treated per-protocol (n = 76) ($p <$ 0.0001). BMI reductions of 1.4 kg/m$^2$ (treated per-protocol) and 0.5 kg/m$^2$ (not treated per-protocol) ($p < 0.0001$) were achieved. | 5 Yes, 3 No, 2 Unclear; Medium Bias Risk |
| Vaz et al., 2021 USA [67] | 28, 13 intervention and 15 controls; 43.25 ± 2.48 years; 86% F and 14% M; BMI 34.40 ± 0.96 kg/m$^2$ | A wrist-worn three-axis accelerometer (Fitbit Charge Heart Rate™), a smartscale (Fitbit Aria™) smartphone app Fitbit™ and commercially available messaging and photo-sharing apps | Participants were instructed to step on the smartscale every morning. The app was programmed to automatically send out a reminder to motivate participants to meet the target for PA for that day, based on continuous activity data obtained from the wearable activity tracker, with remote professional coaching by the physician. Participants were instructed to wear the activity tracker as close as possible to 24 h per day, 7 days per week, and any day with <500 recorded steps indicated a tracking problem. They received conventional outpatient weight-management visits every 3 months for 6 months of the duration of the intervention | Controls received only weight-management visits | Change in weight at 6 months, changes in waist circumference | At 6 months, the intervention group experienced a statistically significant weight change of 7.16 ± 1.78 kg (mean ± SE, 95% CI −11.05 to −3.26, $p < 0.01$), which differed from the weight change in controls (−3.00 ± 1.05 kg (95% CI −5.27 to −0.73, $p < 0.05$) by −4.16 ± 2.01 kg (95% CI −8.29 to −0.02, $p < 0.05$). Waist circumference significantly improved (intervention vs. control: $p <$ 0.01). | 6 yes, 2 no, 2 unclear; Medium Bias Risk |

**Table 1.** *Cont.*

| Author Year Country | Sample Size Study Population | Type of Device | Type of Intervention, Duration, Frequency | Comparison | Main and Secondary Outcomes | Results | Quality |
|---|---|---|---|---|---|---|---|
| Zhang et al., 2023 China [68] | 642, 440 intervention and 202 controls; 46.1% F and 53.9% M; 70.1 ± 5.3 years; BMI 27.67 ± 2.63 $kg/m^2$ | Smartphone app | The remote dietary and PA intervention group (group DPI), and the remote PA intervention group (group PI) used the app for health information collection, health assessment, guidance and feedback and follow-up. The treatment duration was 3 months. Nutritional professionals provided one-on-one personalized dietary guidance and feedback to the participants according to their age, gender, weight, food intake, chronic disease situation, choice of food type, and portion size, 3 to 5 times a week | Health education book on a reasonable diet | Weight at day 45 (time 2), and day 90 (time 3) | Compared with groups PI and controls, group DPI showed a significant decrease in weight (−1.56 vs. −0.86 kg and −1.56 vs. −0.66 kg, respectively; $p < 0.05$) and BMI (−0.61 vs. −0.33 $kg/m^2$ and −0.61 vs. −0.27 $kg/m^2$, respectively; $p < 0.05$) at time 2. Compared with groups PI and controls, group DPI showed a significant decrease in body weight (−4.11 vs. −1.01 kg and −4.11 vs. −0.83 kg, respectively; $p < 0.05$) and BMI (−1.61 vs. −0.40 $kg/m^2$ and −1.61 vs. −0.33 $kg/m^2$, respectively; $p < 0.05$) at time 3. | 9 Yes, 0 No, 1 Unclear; Low Bias Risk |

Eat Less, Move More (ELMM); workbook plus device (WD); workbook only (WO); self-monitoring (SM); feedback (FB); videoconferencing (VC); in-presence (IP); Weight Watchers (WW);
MyFitnessPal app (MyFitnessPal); preventing obesity with eating right (POWER); standard (STND); technology-supported (TECH); experience success (ES); Automated Interactive Voice
Response (IVR); body mass index (BMI); confidence interval (CI); physical activity (PA); standard deviation (SD); waist circumference (WC).

The included articles were published between 2013 [54] and 2023 [61,68], and 15 of them were performed in the USA [40–42,45,46,51,54,55,58,62–65,67], 9 in Europe [38,39,47,49,56,57,59,61,66], 5 in Asia [43,47,52,60,68] and 2 in Australia [44,50]. Both genders were represented in most studies, except in two studies that did not report this information [50,54], and two studies that included only women [47,48]. The overall sample size had a range from 28 [67] to 650 [57]. As for participants' age, individuals aged 18–80 years were included [48]. All of the studies assessed a BMI mean value with standard deviation, except for that of Hong et al. [48], which reported only the population mean weight.

In concern to quality assessment, 14 studies were considered with a "Low Bias Risk", 12 with a "Medium Bias Risk" and 5 with a "High Bias Risk".

Many of the evaluated studies used smartphone apps to carry out the intervention, matched with other procedures such as motivational phone calls [41] and text messages [50,62], and a good number of them also assessed the use of wearable devices such as smartwatches, smart bands or accelerometers [44,48,51,54,56–58,63,67].

The majority of the studies included a specific duration of each session and frequency of intervention, with a minimum of 8 weeks [40] and a maximum of 24 months [51] for the duration, and with frequency varying from three times daily [42] to monthly [51], except for a few where these characteristics were kept generic, specifying neither duration nor frequency [47,58,59,64].

All but one [48] of the studies were aimed at achieving weight loss through improvements in both diet and PA.

In six studies, no activity was assigned to the control group [39,47,49,50,59,61], and in two studies, the control group had the only task of self-monitoring [42,51].

As for the results, a weight reduction related to the technologies used was observed in the majority of the studies [39,41,43,45,46,49,52–54,56–61,64–68]. Additionally, six studies described a reduction in body fat among participants [39,41,57,58,64,67] and in nine papers, a decrease in BMI was also showed beyond weight loss [41,49,52,54–57,64,66,68]. Moreover, some authors reported waist or hip circumference reductions in the intervention groups [39,41,46,57,58,64,67]. Ten studies reported no significant differences in the outcomes between users and controls [38,40,42,44,47,48,50,55,62,63]. Hernandez et al. reported a decrease in body fat, despite no significant difference in weight loss [47], while the study by Jakicic et al. reported a significantly different weight loss in the favor of standard treatment [51].

## 4. Discussion

The findings of this review suggest that using digital technologies may be useful for supporting interventions aimed at reducing excess weight when employed to modify weight-related behaviors, namely PA and diet. In fact, the majority of the controlled trials analyzed reported significantly better outcomes related to weight loss among participants who used some kind of electronic devices or applications than among non-users [39,41,43,45,46,49,52–54,56–61,64–68].

The adoption of new technologies is rapidly spreading in several areas of our lives, such as in health promotion and control [69]. In this context, several devices and applications have been proposed as digital solutions to improve health-related behaviors, such as PA and diet, especially since the beginning of the COVID-19 pandemic [70]. As for PA, nowadays, the use of even more sophisticated wearable devices goes beyond the mere tracking of steps or other movements and may help users to reach their activity goals, increase their PA levels and reduce health risk related to inactivity [71]. The integration of gamification and/or social support elements can increase their effectiveness in movement promotion, both in adults and children [72–74].

With regard to diet monitoring and management, several digital technologies have been developed and evaluated in different subgroups, with inconsistent results [75,76]. Digital resources can reach many people at a low cost and have the potential to support lifestyle changes, enabling individuals to self-regulate their behaviors [77–79]. As for employing these technologies for weight loss, a systematic review and meta-analysis published by Berry et al. in 2021 analyzed the potential role of a digital diet and PA self-monitoring in supporting weight loss among adults with overweight or obesity [31]. Their results showed a statistically significant effect of digital self-monitoring in weight loss, moderate PA increase and calorie intake reduction. Furthermore, they reported that tailored interventions were significantly more effective than nontailored ones, highlighting the importance of tailored advice. In line with this, the review by Irvin et al., which was aimed at examining the status of digital exercise program delivery, found that apps may be useful for a low-intensity approach and can improve adherence to programs through self-monitoring [70]. However, the authors stated that tailored interventions can produce significant findings for weight loss and that individuals need specialist support to achieve their weight goals. Interestingly, this has also been proven for digital interventions used in studies aimed at dietary behavior change [80]. Although it was established that digital interventions have the potential to determine proper changes in the eating behavior of individuals, the efficiency of these interventions increases when coupled with tailored feedback and counseling. This should be considered in the perspective of the long-term maintenance of healthy habits after the conclusion of weight loss interventions.

Keeping this in mind, the evidence coming from our review underlines the usefulness of digital technologies in supporting weight loss, since two-thirds of the analyzed studies showed that their usage resulted in significantly greater weight loss. Furthermore, eighteen of the included studies reported tailored interventions, and only four of these did not find significant differences between participants and controls [42,47,50,63]. In addition, only three [48,50,63] out of the eleven interventions which involved specialists in their implementation reported non-significant differences. The study published by Jakicic et al. was the only reporting that the digital technologies employed for physical activity monitoring and feedback did not offer an advantage over standard behavioral approaches, since the weight reduction observed in its intervention group, although significant, was lower than that observed in controls [51]. Notably, this intervention was not tailored or specialist-driven.

Digital self-monitoring enables individuals to monitor their health behaviors, either through the input of their own data or through the automatic tracking of sensors or wearable technology. Such solutions can allow individuals to receive tailored, automated and real-time feedback. The integration of these systems into usual weight management services may also inform obesity treatment and address service provision, increasing their effectiveness in weight loss and long-term maintenance [31].

However, some considerations are needed in this regard. In general, internal (i.e., motivation and self-efficacy), social (i.e., supporters and saboteurs) and environmental (i.e., an obesogenic environment) factors have been shown to influence the outcomes of a weight loss program, as well as the acceptability of the intervention [81]. Considering the barriers to exercise and PA that people with overweight or obesity may encounter, digital solutions have the potential to provide convenient and equitable support in weight loss based on behavior change [70]. However, as evidence shows that individualized and interactive tools may improve adherence to intervention and facilitate behavior change, those factors which can drive or hinder the use of digital technologies should be also considered when designing a digital-based intervention. In 2022, Jakob et al. reported that user-friendly and technically stable app design, customizable push notifications, personalized app content, passive data tracking, integrated app tutorials, gratuitousness and personal support represent intervention-related characteristics, which can positively influence adherence to mHealth apps for preventing or managing noncommunicable diseases [82]. As for individual-related factors, lack of technical competence, low health literacy, low self-efficacy, a low education level, mental health burden, lack of experience with mHealth apps, privacy concerns, low expectations of the app, low trust in healthcare professionals conducting the intervention, lack of time, age, gender and pre-existing conditions were the user characteristics frequently associated with low mHealth app adherence [82].

In addition, due to the availability of different technological solutions, it should also be considered that some of them can be more effective in supporting certain categories than others in behavior change. In a review published in 2018, Cheatham et al. assessed the efficacy of wearable activity tracking technology in assisting behavior change and weight loss, showing that its use in short-term interventions may lead to better results in middle-aged and older adults, but not in younger adults [83]. Belegoli et al. showed that web-based digital health interventions can be more effective in short-term but not in long term weight loss and lifestyle habit changes interventions with respect to offline interventions for overweight and obese adults [84].

Therefore, further research in this field should focus on the individualization of digital-based interventions based on subjects' characteristics. This could imply the choice of the most adequate behavior change technique to motivate people, but also the implementation of educational interventions to increase their digital literacy, and subsequently their adherence to the weight loss program.

This review has some limitations. First of all, the heterogeneity of the studies examined was high due to the characteristics of the interventions and, in particular, due to the variety of technologies employed and the type of activity (or non-activity) assigned to controls. This did not allow us to compare the studies and to perform a meta-analysis of their results. Furthermore, it should be noted that, in a part of the studies, digital technologies were used to address participants' dietary behaviors together with PA, while in other interventions, diet was only self-reported or in some cases not controlled at all. This may limit the reliability of the findings related to the effectiveness of each technology in determining a specific behavior change and then weight loss, due to possible confounding bias. Moreover, it should be noted that participants in the studies showed differences in gender, age and health conditions. Although we selected only those studies which involved healthy subjects, it is possible that different categories of subjects, mainly those who perceived themselves as at risk for some disease, complied differently with the intervention and this may have influenced the outcomes. In order to obtain stronger evidence about the effectiveness of technology in weight loss, future research should be focused on specific population subgroups and type of device/application. However, it is also possible to highlight the strengths related to this review. In particular, the analysis was specifically focused on randomized controlled studies involving healthy subjects in order to obtain more reliable evidence. Furthermore, this review was intended to explore the possible employ of digital technology in the context of behavioral interventions aimed at reducing body weight, besides the exclusive use of monitoring devices such as activity trackers.

## 5. Conclusions

As the development of digital technologies advances, their use in healthcare settings increases. Electronic devices and mobile applications may be useful to support weight loss lifestyle-based interventions for people with overweight or obesity. However, evidence suggests that tailored automated feedback or specialists' advice can increase the effectiveness of these resources by enhancing individuals' motivation to change their behaviors.

**Supplementary Materials:** The following supporting information can be downloaded at: https://www.mdpi.com/article/10.3390/healthcare12060670/s1, Table S1 reports the search strategy used for PubMed.

**Author Contributions:** Conceptualization, C.P., F.V. and F.G.; methodology, A.D.G., E.M. and S.Z.; software, A.D.G., E.M. and S.Z.; validation, C.P., F.V., A.D.G., E.M., S.Z. and F.G.; formal analysis, A.D.G., E.M., S.Z., L.C., G.D., A.H., I.P., M.S., F.U. and V.V.; data curation, F.G., F.V. and C.P.; writing original draft preparation, C.P., A.D.G., F.V., E.M., S.Z. and F.G.; writing—review and editing, C.P., F.V., V.R.S., M.V. and F.G.; supervision, M.V. and V.R.S.; project administration, C.P., F.V. and F.G. All authors have read and agreed to the published version of the manuscript.

**Funding:** This research did not receive any specific grant from funding agencies in the public, commercial, or not-for-profit sectors.

**Institutional Review Board Statement:** Not applicable.

**Informed Consent Statement:** Not applicable.

**Data Availability Statement:** Raw data will be made available, if necessary, upon request to the corresponding author.

**Conflicts of Interest:** The authors declare no conflicts of interest.

## References


1. James, W. WHO recognition of the global obesity epidemic. *Int. J. Obes.* **2008**, *32*, 120–126. [CrossRef]
2. World Health Organization. Obesity and Overweight. In *Fact Sheets*; no 311 January 2015; Available online: https://www.who.int/news-room/fact-sheets/detail/obesity-and-overweight (accessed on 1 December 2023).
3. Nguyen, N.T.; Nguyen, X.T.; Lane, J.; Wang, P. Relationship between obesity and diabetes in a US adult population: Findings from the National Health and Nutrition Examination Survey, 1999–2006. *Obes. Surg.* **2011**, *21*, 351–355. [CrossRef]
4. World Obesity Atlas. World Obesity Federation. London. 2022. Available online: https://s3-eu-west-1.amazonaws.com/wof-files/World_Obesity_Atlas_2022.pdf (accessed on 1 December 2023).
5. Chong, B.; Jayabaskaran, J.; Kong, G.; Chan, Y.H.; Chin, Y.H.; Goh, R.; Kannan, S.; Ng, C.H.; Loong, S.; Kueh, M.T.W.; et al. Trends and predictions of malnutrition and obesity in 204 countries and territories: An analysis of the Global Burden of Disease Study 2019. *EClinicalMedicine* **2023**, *57*, 101850. [CrossRef]
6. Huang, C.Y.; Yang, M.C.; Huang, C.Y.; Chiu, P.S.; Liu, Z.S.; Chang, R.I. Design and implementation of a dynamic healthcare system for weight management and health promotion. In Proceedings of the IEEE International Conference on Industrial Engineering and Engineering Management (IEEM 2017), Singapore, 10–13 December 2017; pp. 2386–2390. [CrossRef]
7. Pi-Sunyer, X. The Medical Risks of Obesity. *Postgrad. Med.* **2009**, *121*, 21–23. [CrossRef]
8. Argyrakopoulou, G.; Dalamaga, M.; Spyrou, N.; Kokkinos, A. Gender Differences in Obesity-Related Cancers. *Curr. Obes. Rep.* **2021**, *10*, 100–115. [CrossRef] [PubMed]
9. National Cancer Institute. Obesity and Cancer Factsheet. Available online: https://www.cancer.gov/about-cancer/causes-prevention/risk/obesity/obesity-fact-sheet (accessed on 1 December 2023).
10. World Obesity Federation. World Obesity (Formerly IASO) History. Available online: https://www.worldobesity.org/about/about-us/history (accessed on 1 December 2023).
11. Cole, T.J.; Lobstein, T. Extended international (IOTF) body mass index cut-offs for thinness, overweight and obesity. *Pediatr. Obes.* **2012**, *7*, 284–294. [CrossRef] [PubMed]
12. Weir, C.B.; Jan, A. BMI Classification Percentile and Cut Off Points. In *StatPearls [Internet]*; StatPearls Publishing: Treasure Island, FL, USA, January 2023. Available online: https://nih.gov (accessed on 21 January 2024).
13. Yumuk, V.; Tsigos, C.; Fried, M.; Schindler, K.; Bussetto, L.; Misic, D.; Toplak, H. European Guidelines for Obesity Management in Adults. *Eur. Guidel. Obes. Manag. Adults* **2015**, *8*, 402–424. [CrossRef] [PubMed]
14. Marmot, M. The health gap: The challenge of an unequal world. *Lancet* **2015**, *386*, 2442–2444. [CrossRef] [PubMed]
15. Marceca, M.; Sabato, M.; Aloise, I.; Baiocchi, N.; Mancini, G. Public Health Approach to Outdoor Urban Health. In *Equity in Health and Health Promotion in Urban Areas. Green Energy and Technology*; Battisti, A., Marceca, M., Ricotta, G., Iorio, S., Eds.; Springer: Cham, Switzerland, 2023. [CrossRef]
16. Popkin, B.M.; Adair, L.S.; Ng, S.W. Global nutrition transition and the pandemic of obesity in developing countries. *Nutr. Rev.* **2012**, *70*, 3–21. [CrossRef]
17. Twells, L.K.; Harris Walsh, K.; Blackmore, A.; Adey, T.; Donnan, J.; Peddle, J.; Ryan, D.; Farrell, A.; Nguyen, H.; Gao, Z.; et al. Nonsurgical weight loss interventions: A systematic review of systematic reviews and meta-analyses. *Obes. Rev.* **2021**, *22*, e13320. [CrossRef]
18. Ellis, D.A. Are smartphones really that bad? Improving the psychological measurement of technology-related behaviors. *Comput. Hum. Behav.* **2019**, *97*, 60–66. [CrossRef]
19. Ratan, Z.A.; Parrish, A.M.; Zaman, S.B.; Alotaibi, M.S.; Hosseinzadeh, H. Smartphone Addiction and Associated Health Outcomes in Adult Populations: A Systematic Review. *Int. J. Environ. Res. Public Health* **2021**, *18*, 12257. [CrossRef] [PubMed]
20. Lee, I.M.; Shiroma, E.J.; Lobelo, F.; Puska, P.; Blair, S.N.; Katzmarzyk, P.T. Lancet Physical Activity Series Working Group. Effect of physical inactivity on major non-communicable diseases worldwide: An analysis of burden of disease and life expectancy. *Lancet* **2012**, *380*, 219–229. [CrossRef]
21. Martínez-Pérez, B.; de la Torre-Díez, I.; López-Coronado, M. Mobile Health Applications for the Most Prevalent Conditions by the World Health Organization: Review and Analysis. *J. Med. Internet Res.* **2013**, *15*, e120. [CrossRef] [PubMed]
22. Istepanian, R.; Laxminarayan, S.; Pattichis, C.S. (Eds.) *M-Health: Emerging Mobile Health Systems*; Springer Science & Business Media: Berlin, Germany, 2007. [CrossRef]
23. World Health Organisation. Global Observatory for eHealth. Available online: https://www.who.int/observatories/global-observatory-for-ehealth (accessed on 3 December 2023).

24. Free, C.; Phillips, G.; Watson, L.; Galli, L.; Felix, L.; Edwards, P.; Patel, V.; Haines, A. The effectiveness of mobile-health technologies to improve health care service delivery processes: A systematic review and meta-analysis. *PLoS Med.* **2013**, *10*, e1001363. [CrossRef] [PubMed]
25. Ang, G.; Edney, S.M.; Tan, C.S.; Lim, N.; Tan, J.; Müller-Riemenschneider, F.; Chen, C. Physical Activity Trends Among Adults in a National Mobile Health Program: A Population-Based Cohort Study of 411,528 Adults. *Am. J. Epidemiol.* **2023**, *192*, 397–407. [CrossRef]
26. Braakhuis, H.E.M.; Berger, M.A.M.; Bussmann, J.B.J. Effectiveness of healthcare interventions using objective feedback on physical activity: A systematic review and meta-analysis. *J. Rehabil. Med.* **2019**, *51*, 151–159. [CrossRef]
27. Bravata, D.M.; Smith-Spangler, C.; Sundaram, V.; Gienger, A.L.; Lin, N.; Lewis, R.; Stave, C.D.; Olkin, I.; Sirard, J.R. Using pedometers to increase physical activity and improve health: A systematic review. *JAMA* **2007**, *298*, 2296–2304. [CrossRef]
28. Brickwood, K.J.; Watson, G.; O'Brien, J.; Williams, A.D. Consumer-Based Wearable Activity Trackers Increase Physical Activity Participation: Systematic Review and Meta-Analysis. *JMIR Mhealth Uhealth* **2019**, *7*, e11819. [CrossRef]
29. Lyons, E.J.; Lewis, Z.H.; Mayrsohn, B.G.; Rowland, J.L. Behavior change techniques implemented in electronic lifestyle activity monitors: A systematic content analysis. *J. Med. Internet Res.* **2014**, *16*, e192. [CrossRef]
30. Duan, Y.; Shang, B.; Liang, W.; Du, G.; Yang, M.; Rhodes, R.E. Effects of eHealth-Based Multiple Health Behavior Change Interventions on Physical Activity, Healthy Diet, and Weight in People With Noncommunicable Diseases: Systematic Review and Meta-analysis. *J. Med. Internet Res.* **2021**, *23*, e23786. [CrossRef] [PubMed]
31. Berry, R.; Kassavou, A.; Sutton, S. Does self-monitoring diet and physical activity behaviors using digital technology support adults with obesity or overweight to lose weight? A systematic literature review with meta-analysis. *Obes. Rev.* **2021**, *22*, e13306. [CrossRef] [PubMed]
32. Page, M.J.; Moher, D.; Bossuyt, P.M.; Boutron, I.; Hoffmann, T.C.; Mulrow, C.D.; Shamseer, L.; Tetzlaff, J.M.; Akl, E.A.; Brennan, S.E.; et al. PRISMA 2020 explanation and elaboration: Updated guidance and examples for reporting systematic reviews. *BMJ* **2021**, *372*, n160. [CrossRef]
33. Boutron, I.; Moher, D.; Tugwell, P.; Giraudeau, B.; Poiraudeau, B.; Nizard, R.; Ravaud, P. A checklist to evaluate a report of a nonpharmacological trial (CLEAR NPT) was developed using consensus. *J. Clin. Epidemiol.* **2005**, *58*, 1233–1240. [CrossRef] [PubMed]
34. Alkaduhimi, H.; Saarig, A.; van der Linde, J.A.; Willigenburg, N.W.; van Deurzen, D.F.P.; van den Bekerom, M.P.J. An assessment of quality of randomized controlled trials in shoulder instability surgery using a modification of the clear CLEAR-NPT score. *Shoulder Elb.* **2018**, *10*, 238–249. [CrossRef] [PubMed]
35. Kamioka, H.; Tsutani, K.; Mutoh, Y.; Okuizum, H.; Ohta, M.; Handa, S.; Okada, S.; Kitayuguchi, J.; Kamada, M.; Shiozawa, N.; et al. A systematic review of nonrandomized controlled trials on the curative effects of aquatic exercise. *Int. J. Gen. Med.* **2011**, *4*, 239–260. [CrossRef] [PubMed]
36. Liu, F.; Cui, J.; Liu, X.; Chen, K.W.; Chen, X.; Li, R. The effect of tai chi and Qigong exercise on depression and anxiety of individuals with substance use disorders: A systematic review and meta-analysis. *BMC Complement. Med. Ther.* **2020**, *20*, 161. [CrossRef]
37. Protano, C.; Fontana, M.; De Giorgi, A.; Marotta, D.; Cocomello, N.; Crucianelli, S.; Del Cimmuto, A.; Vitali, M. Balneotherapy for osteoarthritis: A systematic review. *Rheumatol. Int.* **2023**, *43*, 1597–1610. [CrossRef]
38. Apiñaniz, A.; Cobos-Campos, R.; Sáez de Lafuente-Moríñigo, A.; Parraza, N.; Aizpuru, F.; Pérez, I.; Goicoechea, E.; Trápaga, N.; García, L. Effectiveness of randomized controlled trial of a mobile app to promote healthy lifestyle in obese and overweight patients. *Fam. Pract.* **2019**, *36*, 699–705. [CrossRef]
39. Balk-Møller, N.C.; Poulsen, S.K.; Larsen, T.M. Effect of a Nine-Month Web- and App-Based Workplace Intervention to Promote Healthy Lifestyle and Weight Loss for Employees in the Social Welfare and Health Care Sector: A Randomized Controlled Trial. *J. Med. Internet Res.* **2017**, *19*, e108. [CrossRef]
40. Beatty, J.A.; Greene, G.W.; Blissmer, B.J.; Delmonico, M.J.; Melanson, K.J. Effects of a novel bites, steps and eating rate-focused weight loss randomised controlled trial intervention on body weight and eating behaviours. *J. Hum. Nutr. Diet.* **2020**, *33*, 330–341. [CrossRef]
41. Block, G.; Azar, K.M.; Romanelli, R.J.; Block, T.J.; Hopkins, D.; Carpenter, H.A.; Dolginsky, M.S.; Hudes, M.L.; Palaniappan, L.P.; Block, C.H. Diabetes Prevention and Weight Loss with a Fully Automated Behavioral Intervention by Email, Web, and Mobile Phone: A Randomized Controlled Trial Among Persons with Prediabetes. *J. Med. Internet Res.* **2015**, *17*, e240. [CrossRef] [PubMed]
42. Burke, L.E.; Sereika, S.M.; Bizhanova, Z.; Parmanto, B.; Kariuki, J.; Cheng, J.; Beatrice, B.; Cedillo, M.; Pulantara, I.W.; Wang, Y.; et al. Effect of tailored, daily feedback with lifestyle self-monitoring on weight loss: The SMARTER randomized clinical trial. *Obesity* **2022**, *30*, 75–84. [CrossRef] [PubMed]
43. Cho, S.M.J.; Lee, J.H.; Shim, J.S.; Yeom, H.; Lee, S.J.; Jeon, Y.W.; Kim, H.C. Effect of Smartphone-Based Lifestyle Coaching App on Community-Dwelling Population With Moderate Metabolic Abnormalities: Randomized Controlled Trial. *J. Med. Internet Res.* **2020**, *22*, e17435. [CrossRef] [PubMed]
44. Duncan, M.J.; Fenton, S.; Brown, W.J.; Collins, C.E.; Glozier, N.; Kolt, G.S.; Holliday, E.G.; Morgan, P.J.; Murawski, B.; Plotnikoff, R.C.; et al. Efficacy of a Multi-component m-Health Weight-loss Intervention in Overweight and Obese Adults: A Randomised Controlled Trial. International. *Int. J. Environ. Res. Public Health* **2020**, *17*, 6200. [CrossRef]

45. Farage, G.; Simmons, C.; Kocak, M.; Klesges, R.C.; Talcott, G.W.; Richey, P.; Hare, M.; Johnson, K.C.; Sen, S.; Krukowski, R. Assessing the Contribution of Self-Monitoring through a Commercial Weight Loss App: Mediation and Predictive Modeling Study. *JMIR Mhealth Uhealth* **2021**, *9*, e18741. [CrossRef]
46. Fukuoka, Y.; Gay, C.L.; Joiner, K.L.; Vittinghoff, E. A Novel Diabetes Prevention Intervention Using a Mobile App: A Randomized Controlled Trial With Overweight Adults at Risk. *Am. J. Prev. Med.* **2015**, *49*, 223–237. [CrossRef]
47. Hernández-Reyes, A.; Cámara-Martos, F.; Molina Recio, G.; Molina-Luque, R.; Romero-Saldaña, M.; Moreno Rojas, R. Push Notifications From a Mobile App to Improve the Body Composition of Overweight or Obese Women: Randomized Controlled Trial. *JMIR Mhealth Uhealth* **2020**, *8*, e13747. [CrossRef]
48. Hong, J.; Kim, S.W.; Joo, H.; Kong, H.J. Effects of smartphone mirroring-based telepresence exercise on body composition and physical function in obese older women. *Aging Clin. Exp. Res.* **2021**, *34*, 1113–1121. [CrossRef]
49. Hurkmans, E.; Matthys, C.; Bogaerts, A.; Scheys, L.; Devloo, K.; Seghers, J. Face-to-Face Versus Mobile Versus Blended Weight Loss Program: Randomized Clinical Trial. *JMIR Mhealth Uhealth* **2018**, *6*, e14. [CrossRef]
50. Hutchesson, M.J.; Callister, R.; Morgan, P.J.; Pranata, I.; Clarke, E.D.; Skinner, G.; Ashton, L.M.; Whatnall, M.C.; Jones, M.; Oldmeadow, C.; et al. A Targeted and Tailored eHealth Weight Loss Program for Young Women: The Be Positive Be Healthe Randomized Controlled Trial. *Healthcare* **2018**, *6*, 39. [CrossRef]
51. Jakicic, J.M.; Davis, K.K.; Rogers, R.J.; King, W.C.; Marcus, M.D.; Helsel, D.; Rickman, A.D.; Wahed, A.S.; Belle, S.H. Effect of Wearable Technology Combined With a Lifestyle Intervention on Long-term Weight Loss: The IDEA Randomized Clinical Trial. *JAMA* **2016**, *316*, 1161–1171. [CrossRef]
52. Jiang, W.; Huang, S.; Ma, S.; Gong, Y.; Fu, Z.; Zhou, L.; Hu, W.; Mao, G.; Ma, Z.; Yang, L.; et al. Effectiveness of companion-intensive multi-aspect weight management in Chinese adults with obesity: A 6-month multicenter randomized clinical trial. *Nutr. Metab.* **2021**, *18*, 17. [CrossRef]
53. Johnson, K.E.; Alencar, M.K.; Coakley, K.E.; Swift, D.L.; Cole, N.H.; Mermier, C.M.; Kravitz, L.; Amorim, F.T.; Gibson, A.L. Telemedicine-Based Health Coaching Is Effective for Inducing Weight Loss and Improving Metabolic Markers. *Telemed. J. E-Health* **2019**, *25*, 85–92. [CrossRef]
54. Johnston, C.A.; Rost, S.; Miller-Kovach, K.; Moreno, J.P.; Foreyt, J. A randomized controlled trial of a community-based behavioral counseling program. *Am. J. Med.* **2013**, *126*, 1143.e19–1143.e24. [CrossRef] [PubMed]
55. Laing, B.Y.; Mangione, C.M.; Tseng, C.H.; Leng, M.; Vaisberg, E.; Mahida, M.; Bholat, M.; Glazier, E.; Morisky, D.E.; Bell, D.S. Effectiveness of a smartphone application for weight loss compared with usual care in overweight primary care patients: A randomized, controlled trial. *Ann. Intern. Med.* **2014**, *61*, S5–S12. [CrossRef]
56. Lugones-Sanchez, C.; Sanchez-Calavera, M.A.; Repiso-Gento, I.; Adalia, E.G.; Ramirez-Manent, J.I.; Agudo-Conde, C.; Rodriguez-Sanchez, E.; Gomez-Marcos, M.A.; Recio-Rodriguez, J.I.; Garcia-Ortiz, L. EVIDENT 3 Investigators. Investigators. Effectiveness of an mHealth Intervention Combining a Smartphone App and Smart Band on Body Composition in an Overweight and Obese Population: Randomized Controlled Trial (EVIDENT 3 Study). *JMIR mHealth uHealth* **2020**, *8*, e21771. [CrossRef]
57. Lugones-Sanchez, C.; Recio-Rodriguez, J.I.; Agudo-Conde, C.; Repiso-Gento, I.; GAdalia, E.; Ramirez-Manent, J.I.; Sanchez-Calavera, M.A.; Rodriguez-Sanchez, E.; Gomez-Marcos, M.A.; Garcia-Ortiz, L. EVIDENT 3 Investigators. EVIDENT 3 Investigators. Long-term Effectiveness of a Smartphone App Combined with a Smart Band on Weight Loss, Physical Activity, and Caloric Intake in a Population with Overweight and Obesity (Evident 3 Study): Randomized Controlled Trial. *J. Med. Internet Res.* **2022**, *24*, e30416. [CrossRef]
58. Martin, C.K.; Miller, A.C.; Thomas, D.M.; Champagne, C.M.; Han, H.; Church, T. Efficacy of SmartLoss, a smartphone-based weight loss intervention: Results from a randomized controlled trial. *Obesity* **2015**, *23*, 935–942. [CrossRef] [PubMed]
59. Martínez-Rodríguez, A.; Martínez-Olcina, M.; Mora, J.; Navarro, P.; Caturla, N.; Jones, J. New App-Based Dietary and Lifestyle Intervention on Weight Loss and Cardiovascular Health. *Sensors* **2022**, *22*, 768. [CrossRef] [PubMed]
60. Nakata, Y.; Sasai, H.; Gosho, M.; Kobayashi, H.; Shi, Y.; Ohigashi, T.; Mizuno, S.; Murayama, C.; Kobayashi, S.; Sasaki, Y. A Smartphone Healthcare Application. CALO mama Plus, to Promote Weight Loss: A Randomized Controlled Trial. *Nutrients* **2022**, *14*, 4608. [CrossRef]
61. Roth, L.; Ordnung, M.; Forkmann, K.; Mehl, N.; Horstmann, A. A randomized-controlled trial to evaluate the app-based multimodal weight loss program zanadio for patients with obesity. *Obesity* **2023**, *31*, 1300–1310. [CrossRef] [PubMed]
62. Saldivar, P.; Mira, V.; Duran, P.; Moldovan, C.; Ang, G.; Parikh, N.; Lee, M.L.; Friedman, T.C. Implementing texting programs in the P.O.W.E.R. (preventing obesity with eating right) medical group visit for weight loss. *Obes. Sci. Pract.* **2021**, *7*, 583–590. [CrossRef] [PubMed]
63. Spring, B.; Pellegrini, C.A.; Pfammatter, A.; Duncan, J.M.; Pictor, A.; McFadden, H.G.; Siddique, J.; Hedeker, D. Effects of an abbreviated obesity intervention supported by mobile technology: The ENGAGED randomized clinical trial. *Obesity* **2017**, *25*, 1191–1198. [CrossRef] [PubMed]
64. Stephens, J.D.; Yager, A.M.; Allen, J. Smartphone Technology and Text Messaging for Weight Loss in Young Adults: A Randomized Controlled Trial. *J. Cardiovasc. Nurs.* **2017**, *32*, 39–46. [CrossRef] [PubMed]
65. Thomas, J.G.; Goldstein, C.M.; Bond, D.S.; Hadley, W.; Tuerk, P.W. Web-based virtual reality to enhance behavioural skills training and weight loss in a commercial online weight management programme: The Experience Success randomized trial. *Obes. Sci. Pract.* **2020**, *6*, 587–595. [CrossRef] [PubMed]

66. Thorgeirsson, T.; Torfadottir, J.E.; Egilsson, E.; Oddsson, S.; Gunnarsdottir, T.; Aspelund, T.; Olafsdottir, A.S.; Valdimarsdottir, U.A.; Kawachi, I.; Adami, H.O.; et al. Randomized Trial for Weight Loss Using a Digital Therapeutic Application. *J. Diabetes Sci. Technol.* **2022**, *16*, 1150–1158. [CrossRef]
67. Vaz, C.L.; Carnes, N.; Pousti, B.; Zhao, H.; Williams, K.J. A randomized controlled trial of an innovative, user-friendly, interactive smartphone app-based lifestyle intervention for weight loss. *Obes. Sci. Pract.* **2021**, *7*, 555–568. [CrossRef]
68. Zhang, N.; Zhou, M.; Li, M.; Ma, G. Effects of Smartphone-Based Remote Interventions on Dietary Intake, Physical Activity, Weight Control, and Related Health Benefits Among the Older Population with Overweight and Obesity in China: Randomized Controlled Trial. *J. Med. Internet Res.* **2023**, *25*, e41926. [CrossRef]
69. Yeung, A.W.K.; Torkamani, A.; Butte, A.J.; Glicksberg, B.S.; Schuller, B.; Rodriguez, B.; Ting, D.S.W.; Bates, D.; Schaden, E.; Peng, H.; et al. The promise of digital healthcare technologies. *Front. Public Health* **2023**, *11*, 1196596. [CrossRef]
70. Irvin, L.; Madden, L.A.; Marshall, P.; Vince, R.V. Digital Health Solutions for Weight Loss and Obesity: A Narrative Review. *Nutrients* **2023**, *15*, 1858. [CrossRef] [PubMed]
71. Bassett, D.R.; Toth, L.P.; LaMunion, S.R.; Crouter, S.E. Step Counting: A Review of Measurement Considerations and Health-Related Applications. *Sport. Med.* **2017**, *47*, 1303–1315. [CrossRef]
72. Mamede, A.; Noordzij, G.; Jongerling, J.; Snijders, M.; Schop-Etman, A.; Denktas, S. Combining Web-Based Gamification and Physical Nudges with an App (MoveMore) to Promote Walking Breaks and Reduce Sedentary Behavior of Office Workers: Field Study. *J. Med. Internet Res.* **2021**, *23*, e19875. [CrossRef]
73. Valeriani, F.; Protano, C.; Marotta, D.; Liguori, G.; Romano Spica, V.; Valerio, G.; Vitali, M.; Gallè, F. Exergames in Childhood Obesity Treatment: A Systematic Review. *Int. J. Environ. Res. Public Health* **2021**, *18*, 4938. [CrossRef] [PubMed]
74. Memon, A.R.; Masood, T.; Awan, W.A.; Waqas, A. The effectiveness of an incentivized physical activity programme (Active Student) among female medical students in Pakistan: A Randomized Controlled Trial. *J. Pak. Med. Assoc.* **2018**, *68*, 1438–1445.
75. Scarry, A.; Rice, J.; O'Connor, E.M.; Tierney, A.C. Usage of Mobile Applications or Mobile Health Technology to Improve Diet Quality in Adults. *Nutrients* **2022**, *14*, 2437. [CrossRef] [PubMed]
76. Barnett, A.; Wright, C.; Stone, C.; Ho, N.Y.; Adhyaru, P.; Kostjasyn, S.; Hickman, I.J.; Campbell, K.L.; Mayr, H.L.; Kelly, J.T. Effectiveness of dietary interventions delivered by digital health to adults with chronic conditions: Systematic review and meta-analysis. *J. Hum. Nutr. Diet.* **2023**, *36*, 632–656. [CrossRef]
77. Teixeira, P.J.; Marques, M.M. Health behavior change for obesity management. *Obes. Facts* **2018**, *10*, 666–673. [CrossRef]
78. Chaudhry, U.A.R.; Wahlich, C.; Fortescue, R.; Cook, D.G.; Knightly, R.; Harris, T. The effects of step-count monitoring interventions on physical activity: Systematic review and meta-analysis of community-based randomised controlled trials in adults. *Int. J. Behav. Nutr. Phys. Act.* **2020**, *17*, 129. [CrossRef]
79. Brindal, E.; Hendrie, G.; Freyne, J.; Coombe, M.; Berkovsky, S.; Noakes, M. Design and Pilot Results of a Mobile Phone Weight-Loss Application for Women Starting a Meal Replacement Programme. *J. Telemed. Telecare* **2013**, *19*, 166–174. [CrossRef]
80. Chen, Y.; Perez-Cueto, F.J.A.; Giboreau, A.; Mavridis, I.; Hartwell, H. The Promotion of Eating Behaviour Change through Digital Interventions. *Int. J. Environ. Res. Public Health* **2020**, *17*, 7488. [CrossRef]
81. Tay, A.; Hoeksema, H.; Murphy, R. Uncovering Barriers and Facilitators of Weight Loss and Weight Loss Maintenance: Insights from Qualitative Research. *Nutrients* **2023**, *15*, 1297. [CrossRef]
82. Jakob, R.; Harperink, S.; Rudolf, A.M.; Fleisch, E.; Haug, S.; Mair, J.L.; Salamanca-Sanabria, A.; Kowatsch, T. Factors Influencing Adherence to mHealth Apps for Prevention or Management of Noncommunicable Diseases: Systematic Review. *J. Med. Internet Res.* **2022**, *24*, e35371. [CrossRef]
83. Cheatham, S.W.; Stull, K.R.; Fantigrassi, M.; Motel, I. The efficacy of wearable activity tracking technology as part of a weight loss program: A systematic review. *J. Sports Med. Phys. Fit.* **2018**, *58*, 534–548. [CrossRef]
84. Beleigoli, A.M.; Andrade, A.Q.; Cançado, A.G.; Paulo, M.N.; Diniz, M.F.H.; Ribeiro, A.L. Web-Based Digital Health Interventions for Weight Loss and Lifestyle Habit Changes in Overweight and Obese Adults: Systematic Review and Meta-Analysis. *J. Med. Internet Res.* **2019**, *21*, e298. [CrossRef]

MDPI AG
Grosspeteranlage 5
4052 Basel
Switzerland
Tel.: +41 61 683 77 34

*Healthcare* Editorial Office
E-mail: healthcare@mdpi.com
www.mdpi.com/journal/healthcare

www.ingramcontent.com/pod-product-compliance
Lightning Source LLC
Chambersburg PA
CBHW040825250926
51850CB00007BA/1266
*9783725850792*